Old people's homes and the production of welfare

Library of Social Work

General Editor:
Noel Timms
Professor of Social Work Studies
University of Newcastle upon Tyne

Old people's homes and the production of welfare

Bleddyn Davies
Professor of Social Policy
University of Kent

Martin Knapp
Lecturer in economics
and research fellow in the
Personal Social Services Research Unit
University of Kent

Routledge & Kegan Paul
London, Boston and Henley

First published in 1981
by Routledge & Kegan Paul Ltd
39 Store Street, London WC1E 7DD,
9 Park Street, Boston, Mass 02108, USA and
Broadway House, Newtown Road,
Henley-on-Thames, Oxon RG9 1EN
Set in Press Roman 10pt by Columns, Reading
and printed in Great Britain by
Biddles Ltd, Guildford

British Library Cataloguing in Publication Data

Davies, Bleddyn

Old people's homes and the production of
welfare. − (Library of social work
ISSN 0305-4381).
1. Old age homes − Economic aspects −
Great Britain
I. Title   II. Knapp, Martin   III. Series
338.4'736261'0941   HV1481.G5   80-41185

ISBN 0 7100 0700 0

Contents

Preface   vii

Part one   Introduction   1

1   The production of welfare   3
   1.1   Inputs and outputs   5
   1.2   Output and the social welfare paradigm   9
   1.3   The production relations approach   12
   1.4   The state of the literature   15

Part two   Outputs   21

2   The psychological well-being of residents   25
   2.1   Engaged activity   26
   2.2   Psychological well-being   29

3   Other outputs   54
   3.1   Benefits to residents not contributing
          directly to psychological well-being   55
   3.2   Outputs enjoyed principally by residents'
          significant others   61

Part three   Inputs and the production process   65

4   Resource inputs: labour and capital   69
   4.1   The manpower input   69
   4.2   The capital input   88
   4.3   Conclusion   106

Contents

5   **Social environment**   108
    5.1   The general environment of the home   108
    5.2   Theoretical perspectives on social
          environment   110
    5.3   Some important dimensions of social
          environment   132
    5.4   Conclusion   146

6. **Personal characteristics and experiences**   147
    6.1   Resident personality   147
    6.2   Experiences prior to admission to the
          home   149
    6.3   Individual characteristics at the point
          of entry   152
    6.4   The stages of admission, adjustment and
          institutionalisation   155

Part four   Conclusion   163

7   **Concluding discussion**   165
    7.1   Applying the production relations
          approach   165
    7.2   The production relations approach and
          understanding the causes of welfare   185
    7.3   The production relations approach and
          policy   188

Appendix A   **The Life Satisfaction Rating Scale of Neugarten,
                 Havighurst and Tobin**   201

Appendix B   **The use of Bradburn's Affect Balance Scale with
                 the elderly in residential care**
                 Sheila Peace, John Hall and Graham Hamblin   204

Notes   210

Bibliography   218

Index   243

Preface

The Personal Social Services Research Unit was set up to investigate resource problems of social care. Three streams of work were established at its foundation: analyses of variation between areas in local provision in relation to needs; the evaluation of innovations in the domiciliary care of the elderly; and the exploration of the dependence of welfare outcomes on resources and other factors. Despite some differences in emphasis and analysis, the three streams have much in common. In particular, central to all of them, is the study of the relations between resources, other factors and outcomes.

This book is an output of the third of these streams: what we call the cost and production relations programme. In the past the literature has lacked a study applying this approach to residential care of the aged, or indeed to any other form of social care for any of the main client groups of social services departments. It also lacks a study using this intellectual framework — or indeed any other framework of its breadth — which emphasises argument about what determines the welfare outcomes produced in such facilities. So, although the Unit's philosophy puts great emphasis on handling empirical evidence in the development of theory and policy argument, it seemed in this case necessary to lay the foundations for future empirical work by producing a theoretical review of such arguments, drawing as widely as possible on the international literature. This book is the outcome of that attempt. We hope that residential care was the ideal focus for such work since both capital and recurrent resources were of importance, since the big and sophisticated international literature on the subject is hardly known in this country, and since the effects of resource and other factors are principally felt by a clearly definable group of recipients.

An attempt to pull together other people's arguments may be a necessary condition for the advancement of knowledge. However, the ideas described in this book are drawn from research on institutions which do not exactly parallel our old people's homes and from cultures which are in other ways dramatically different from our own. Our labours therefore will bear fruit if we are able to build an empirical study on this theoretical work. Currently there are no data sets which would allow us to describe and quantify production relations in residential homes, nor could there have been unless an attempt had been made to show what kinds of phenomena must be measured and what parameters estimated for such a study. However, we have been able to obtain data sets which allow us to explore some questions; where relevant, these explorations are cited in the text.

We owe our thanks to many people. The work has been funded by the DHSS. Constitutional conventions prevent us from naming individual officials. Their help has always been dedicated and often inspired. So important are the similarities between the types of the work conducted in the three sections of the Unit that this work has gained greatly from work on other programmes. No academics working on similar areas could fail to gain from the scholarly, industrious and talented work of persons like Andrew Bebbington and David Challis. Our thanks must also be expended to publishers for their co-operation and permission to reprint material. This work first saw the light of day in December 1975 as a fifteen-page discussion paper with just a handful of references. It has grown through many stages to its present size and has been typed and retyped with infinite patience and good humour by Carole Phillips. To all of these people we are very grateful for their assistance and naturally we absolve them from all responsibility.

This has been a happy collaboration. It has not been of the kind where we can easily describe who did what: like many happy marriages it would be difficult to remember who peeled the potatoes a week last Tuesday far less a year last Tuesday. In all parts of the book we have each privately seen passages whose inanities and infelicities could only have been our own and not those of our collaborator. However BD knows that far more of MK's time has been devoted to it than his own. What praise is due for the book's merits should be enjoyed more by him and what blame should be incurred for its weakness should be borne by the other author.

Part one

Introduction

Chapter 1

The production
of welfare

During the mid-1970s, residential care of the elderly has increasingly been the subject of analytic writing. One theme of the literature has been criticism of the vagueness with which providers specify ends, means, and their interconnection. Great interest has been shown in those homes whose management is most self-conscious in its commitment to an articulated set of principles. The new literature, though most is still theoretically vague and analytically partial, acknowledges the complexity of means, ends and their interconnection more than the literature of the 1960s.

A second theme has been the implications for policy of the systemic interdependence of residential with other provision: it is recognised that services can be combined in packages or be alternatives to one another to some degree for many clients. Crude argument around this theme has been deployed for thirty years or more. What is newer is the strength of interest amongst policy-makers in increasing the variety of residential and other provision, and the range of prototype schemes now running, though without formal evaluation. There is now much greater variety of resource inputs and assumptions than in the past. Examples are the 'do-it-yourself' co-operative home in Finsbury with substantial care input from relatives and others not on the pay-roll; homes which segregate the ill (particularly the dying) by placing them in 'extra care' units or sick bays; homes that segregate the confused to differing degrees; homes whose managers reflect to an exceptional degree the beliefs of the 'therapeutic community' movement in the psychological import of the mundane; nursing homes provided by health authorities; the home in Hillingdon created by adapting council houses and providing intensive domiciliary support; the special housing in Hammersmith occupied by persons similar in their needs to entrants to homes and provided with intensive domiciliary support; homes providing day care which can ease the transition to residential care as well as provide immediate support; homes which operate with different proportions of residents in short-stay, and different proportions of the physicially dependent and confused; the Derbyshire 'home-by-home' scheme — features of sheltered housing with a small residential unit; homes which have substituted part-time staff for full-time staff working split shifts; homes that are the centre of a complex providing a range of services, 'the core from which community-based developments of all kinds can issue' (Allen, 1977). This increased variety first raises questions about the relative cost-effectiveness of alternatives, and second has increased the degree of substitution possible between services of which at least the prototypes exist and can be evaluated, and so made that much more complex the answers to the central questions of how cost-effective are alternatives for clients of different characteristics.

In the innovations we see not just the greater articulation of premises and the self-conscious subordination of *modus operandi* to explicit argument about causality and role, but also the progressive erosion of boundaries. In some schemes it is the boundary between the home and the rest of society that has been removed. In others, it is the traditional administrative boundaries of action and responsibilities between sections of the social services department, between the social services department and health and housing authorities, even to some extent between public authorities and informal community support systems; erosion that has enabled local authorities to exploit a wider range of real and financial resources and opportunities as well as increase the variety of forms of care. The voluntary sector has begun to rethink its role in residential care in the light of at least some of these changes (Age Concern and National Corporation for the Care of Old People, 1977). With such innovation and variety it is not surprising that the Personal Social Services Council has called for the formulation of a 'philosophy of residential care' (PSSC, 1977). Research is an essential prerequisite for developing such a philosophy and for contributing to our perception of the aims of residential care and how they can be most cost-effectively achieved. It is our aim in this book to contribute to these.

This book is therefore a critical review of theory about old people's homes and particularly about what determines the quality of life of residents in old people's homes. It discusses the objectives of homes and describes causal arguments contained in the literature about what influences the quality of living of residents; and in doing so, it attempts to make explicit a number of important differences in the theoretical stances of writers. Inevitably, much of the literature that has contributed to our argument is not specifically about homes, and some of it is not about the aged: our criterion of relevance has been that the literature contributes to theory about what determines quality of life in old people's homes.

A reading of the British literature and our acquaintance with practice in social work education in this country have left us with the impression that the education of social workers in this body of scholarship is more rudimentary than their education in similar fields.[1] That this is so cannot be healthy. The elderly comprise well over half the clients of social services departments, and account for approximately one half of social service department resources (Department of Health and Social Security, 1977; Plank, 1978). Decisions about these clients are often greatly influenced, if not effectively made, by professional social workers, and many leaders of the profession argue that qualified workers should bear a greater responsibility for the elderly than is current practice in many authorities.

The book has two themes: the exposition, criticism and development of causal argument; and the collection and handling of evidence to test, develop and make practically useful the theory thus explicated. In practice, this amounts to a discussion of the indicators of the theoretical concepts and their validity, and the light that the use of the indicators has thrown on the validity of the theories. The quantification of theory is just as important as the statement and assessment of the causal argument. Indeed, the former is indispensible to the latter, since the evidence we use to assess the validity of the causal argument is mainly quantitative, and since the usefulness to policy of causal arguments depends greatly on their quantitative importance. In this introductory chapter we introduce the concepts and nomenclature of the *Production of Welfare* perspective on old people's homes, focusing in particular on inputs, outputs and production relations.

1.1 Inputs and outputs

Following the conventions of the analysis of production relations, let us call 'quality of life' in all its dimensions, and other benefits derived from the provision of residential care, the *outputs*, and their determinants, the *inputs*. This essay is about the relationship between inputs and outputs in old people's homes.

Outputs

Outputs include all those consequences that so directly reflect aspects of welfare that they are valued in their own right.[2] Since the old people's home is in practice often almost a self-contained community, nearly all aspects of the quality of life could well be influenced by inputs. Therefore, a theory that seeks to explain the relationship between inputs and the quality of life must attempt to explain a formidable range of phenomena. Moreover, there is no reason why all aspects of quality of life should be so highly correlated that they can be treated as a single outcome. Residents who perceive the quality of food to be high, need not necessarily perceive affective relationships with other residents to be satisfying, since these two aspects of the quality of life are likely to be affected by quite different resource inputs, expectations, and personal characteristics. The theory must therefore explain variations in different aspects of the quality of life. Yet perceptions of the quality of the food and satisfaction with the nature of the relationships with other residents may have causes in common. Indeed, the satisfaction with the latter may affect the perception of the former. One of the major tasks of a theoretical discussion is to consider what aspects of the quality of life tend to be found together, and what tend not to be; and how the achievement of some will influence the achievement of others. Such a theory of outputs is a necessary prerequisite for a coherent policy for residential care. Such policy could have only a weak basis in knowledge without the quantitative description of the variations in the present combinations of outputs, because only with knowledge of the present mix can judgments be made about the value to be placed on the different combinations possible.

An intelligent being from outer space, foreign to the practices and performance of social services departments but committed to both the application of reason and to the values on which our social policies are based, would treat as welfare consequences valuable in their own right few other than those for the residents themselves and their significant others. He would see as only *indirectly* important most of the consequences for the welfare of others, like the staff of homes. Most such consequences he would consider important only because of their effect on the quality of life of the residents and the perceptions of significant others. However, there are perhaps two types of consequence that are major exceptions. First, Richard Titmuss argued that social services were not 'merely utilitarian instruments of welfare' but were also 'agents of altruistic opportunity' (Titmuss, 1972). This he argued both because altruistic behaviour promotes social integration and because it is a satisfaction in its own right. A change in social arrangements that increases altruistic behaviour makes altruistic behaviour by others more likely; and, probably still more, makes likely (among other quasi-altruistic behaviour) behaviour whose content is the same but whose motivations more reflect a calculus of self-interest. In this way, it sets into operation a process that leads to the enhancement of social integration that Gouldner calls the 'reciprocity multiplier' (Gouldner, 1963). If possible, one must count among the outputs the effects of social integration both of the altruistic behaviour that is the stimulus for the multiplier process, and of the altruistic and quasi-altruistic behaviour that is thus generated. The argument has been given a new cogency by Hirsch's lucid argument about the way some powerful social trends are increasingly making less likely altruistic and quasi-altruistic behaviour (Hirsch, 1977, especially chapter 3), and by the way collective welfare interventions can themselves reduce such behaviour (Abrams, 1977). Second, if salary payments were lower because of the joys of altruistic service, it would be legitimate to include the extent of this satisfaction as a separate output, probably doing so in practice by including a quantitative estimate of the extent to which these salary levels were depressed. But our rational man from outer space would find that the most important consequences that he would count as *outputs* would be those enjoyed by clients and their significant others.

Indeed, it is not just that it is the satisfaction of clients and significant others that is mainly important. It is that the quality of life of *individuals* must be *separately* counted. One reason is that individuals enjoy different immediate experiences as residents of homes. The characteristics of other residents with whom they share a room count greatly for the quality of their life; and the contacts of residents of the same home with individual care staff can vary greatly, and care staff may contribute very differently to the welfare of residents. Another reason why the quality of life of individuals must be separately counted is that their needs differ, as is acknowledged by the emphasis on personal treatment plans. People respond differently to similar environments. There is a sense in which the individual is a part of the process which produces his own welfare.[3] This is one reason why outputs must be measured as late in the process of the production of welfare as is feasible. Therefore an important aspect of the task is to measure the consequences valued for their own sake as far along the process of the production of welfare as is compatible with the development of reliable and valid indicators.

Inputs

The causal arguments presented in this book are about the relationship between inputs and outputs. Inputs include both non-resource and resource factors — and so encompass all influences upon output. In this book we distinguish three kinds of input: resource inputs, non-resource inputs, and quasi-inputs. *Resource inputs* are the conventional inputs or factors of production distinguished in economics and in the present context include the staff, physical capital, provisions and other consumables. *Non-resource inputs* and *quasi-inputs* are those determinants of final and intermediate output which are basically intangible: staff attitudes, characteristics of the social environment, resident experiences prior to admission, and so on. The distinction between these two is that the non-resource inputs lie inside, and the quasi-inputs outside, the domain of control of the producing unit or producer. Thus, for example, many aspects of the social milieu will reflect the attitudes and perceptions of the head of the home, whereas the personalities of elderly people entering care are rather more exogenous influences upon the outcome of the care intervention. The distinction between the non-resource inputs and the quasi-inputs is an important one for policy. The question of endogeneity — that is, the question of what factors are influenced by others whose causation is itself the subject of argument, and which are therefore intermediate in causal priority in the argument — is largely empirical and our discussion in chapters 4, 5 and 6 will cast some light upon it.[4] Maintaining the distinction between the three input concepts allows us to state the basic premise of the *Production of Welfare* perspective: outputs are determined by the levels and modes of combination of the resource and non-resource inputs (which are mainly under the control of the administrator or policy-maker, albeit sometimes only after the elapse of a considerable period of time), given the exogenously determined values of the quasi-inputs.

Perhaps it is because there is an assumption that non-resource and quasi-inputs are more important than resource inputs that the latter are neglected in most of the literature. It may well be that variations in the attitudes, assumptions and role perceptions of staff have a greater effect on outputs than the nature of buildings or money spent on current resources, but it will become clear to the reader of this book that resource, non-resource and quasi-inputs are related in ways that make it vital to consider them in conjunction with one another. One reason is that they are likely to be correlated. Quite apart from the impact of labour resources on the time that staff give to individuals, it might well be that staff are more concerned with individuals in homes whose resource inputs are most generous. If the various inputs are correlated, one could not make an unbiased estimate of the effects of variations in resource inputs merely by observing variations in outputs, without taking into account the simultaneous variations in non-resource and quasi-inputs. However, the interrelationships between inputs are likely to be more complex. For example, a minimum level of resource inputs may be a prerequisite for variations in some other inputs to have a really strong effect. To describe production relations accurately, it is therefore necessary not just to allow for variations in both resource and other inputs, but also to interrogate the argument and evidence contained in the literature about the precise ways in which they operate to produce outputs in conjunction with one another.

The neglect by researchers of the influence of resource inputs severely limits the practical usefulness of the literature. Resource inputs are more controllable by high level decision-makers than most other inputs. If our desire is to develop a theory that contributes directly to the betterment of the quality of the lives of the most deprived residents in homes, it is important that the effects of such controllable factors should be carefully assessed. It is not just that the theory must predict the effects of overall resource inputs. Since the objective is theory which will contribute to management practice, the level of aggregation of resource inputs about whose effects we must seek to generalise should correspond to the choices made by management. For instance, a theory that does not distinguish between types of manpower is less practically useful than one that distinguishes between types of care and other staff; and distinguishes those categories of staff that have relevance to management decisions about task specification and training. Therefore, if we cannot present and test precise theoretical argument about the effect of using different types of manpower, we can undertake only speculative discussion — discussion which can at best only suggest items for an agenda of empirical research.

1.2 Output and the social welfare paradigm

The concept 'output' remains ill-defined in all the social services and particularly in residential care. Most attempts to define and study outputs have not been based directly on the theoretical foundations of social welfare interventions. Generally, most have relied instead on the declared aims of the professionals and other actors in decision processes, or what could be inferred about them from their behaviour. Though a useful approach in many circumstances, and certainly an easier one than attempting to work out objectives from higher order principles, the dangers of following it are great when the actors themselves are uncertain about objectives in other than the most general terms. This is particularly so for residential care of the elderly, as was made explicit in a recent study by the DHSS (1976a) and in a report of a working party set up by the PSSC (1975). The study of 478 residential establishments by the Social Work Service of the DHSS (1976a, p.4) observed that:

> An unspoken understanding between management and heads of homes about the purposes of residential care in general or in a particular home undoubtedly existed, but at the time there appeared to have been little conscious examination of this. Consequently it would have been surprising if individual heads of homes had been clear about the aims and objectives they saw except in a rather limited way.

The PSSC working party lamented the absence of 'a philosophy' of residential care: 'The present lack of such philosophy largely explains why there is no understanding, either by the public or by those in the field, of what should be the essential objectives of this form of care' (PSSC, 1975, p.15) — a specification of objectives to which the report and one of the working papers made useful and practical contributions. 'The purpose and objectives of residential care should be agreed and

9

stated within a clear philosophy upon which all such provisions can be based' (ibid., p.15). 'Our major concern has been to define the objectives of care in order to ask why residential care becomes necessary for some individuals, and to assess its contribution within the range of social service provision' (ibid., p.16).

The PSSC Report was not alone in stressing the separate identity but interdependence of social care and other aspects of service processes. Kushlick long ago made the distinction between 'administrative' and 'client-orientated' criteria of efficient service (Kushlick, 1967). Partly because of work such as his, there is now a general acceptance of the argument, if no great agreement about what exactly the outputs are and how they should be measured. The definition we put forward in section 1.1, consequences of interventions valued for themselves, is compatible with that provided by the Institute of Municipal Treasurers and Accountants (1972): that the 'measurement of final output is the measurement of ultimate effectiveness or the extent to which the organisation is successful in achieving its policy objectives' (p.iv). 'Final outputs for those receiving assistance must be measured in terms of the improvement in their welfare ... compared to the condition ... in the absence of Personal Social Services (p.3). No doubt we might equally accept Billis's (1975) conception of outputs as 'positive change or deterioration in social functioning' (with presumably other aspects of care like accommodation and feeding and improvements or deterioration in psychological well-being), but that would not prevent us from finding reasons for disagreeing about what constituted these objectives, and what formed valid evidence about the degree of their attainment. As Billis himself has written (of the specification of the objectives of residential care by another author): 'most of the literature is immensely respectable but dumbfoundingly vague'.

Residential homes are to a greater or lesser extent surrogate communities. Do old people's homes therefore conform to what is perhaps the main characteristic of the total institution — a high degree of insulation from the outside world — to such an extent that it requires deliberate management to prevent them from acquiring the other characteristics of the total institution? Such management requires not just the proper accountability for care (as well as administrative efficiency) to the social services department, but a deliberate treatment programme; a programme that sets out to achieve personal growth through the creation of a prosthetic and therapeutic environment. Thus it is much more like the hospital (particularly the psychiatric hospital) than it might at first appear. We shall return to the implications of this.

Second, it follows from their relative insulation, and so from the characteristic of being surrogate communities, that one must include among their outputs all the most important dimensions of psychological well-being and quality of life. Moreover, the input of resources could potentially affect the degree to which many if not all of the dimensions of quality of life and psychological well-being are achieved. Therefore the outputs of residential homes are almost as multifarious and broad as those of concern to the so-called Social Indicators Movement; and the intellectual problems of specifying and measuring them have much in common. Again, the basic argument of the subjective social indicators school (that man does not live by bread alone, so that his welfare is not measured adequately just by indicators of his material condition)[5] is equally valid for residential homes.

However, there are differences which make other sources of intellectual inspiration more appropriate. First the Social Indicators Movement has a concern with all, not just the elderly. Far more important, the definition of the goals of a residential home is based on an explicit policy paradigm legitimated by being the outcome of focused political decision and a developed executive apparatus. It cannot be claimed that the definition of dimensions of life satisfaction and quality of life in the Social Indicators Movement has such a basis. The policy paradigm of social welfare provides the criteria for judging the validity of output measurement in a way that is impossible for the Social Indicators Movement since it reflects a coherent assumptive world which provides the rationale of policy interventions. In particular, the social welfare paradigm has an explicit intellectual basis, causal theories, supporting value assumptions and normative arguments.

Since the welfare paradigm is international, it allows the research worker to draw on a larger international literature yielding theoretical argument about what consequences are likely to be important, accounts of their causation, and instruments for collecting data to operationalise the theoretical concepts. Indeed the existence of a social welfare paradigm allows more. Not only does it permit the exploitation of literature which embodies its values, beliefs and assumptions, but also its own broader intellectual basis is clear enough to allow the research worker to make use of the broader intellectual base of the paradigm. For instance, since they embody similar values and assumptions to those embodied in the British social welfare paradigm, not only can use be made of the British and American social work literature and the American gerontological literature, but use can also be made of the work of the personality theorists on whose work so much social work writing is explicitly based. This is far less reasonable in the study of quality of life in society as a whole, a main concern of the Social Indicators Movement. One reason for this is that although policy paradigms have a broad internal consistency, different policy paradigms are often quite inconsistent (Davies, 1975 and 1976). For instance, because the social welfare paradigm has political legitimacy and is in part based on the propositions of the fulfilment theorists of personality, it is more valid to draw on (say) a Maslovian framework for the analysis of psycholo-

11

gical well-being in a study of production relations in homes for the aged, than in a study of psychological well-being of general populations, like that by Allardt (1973).

It is also true that the existence of bodies of literature which make explicit the causes and consequences of social welfare intervention make more easy the identification of errors of commission or omission in empirical work. The more explicit is the basis for the argument about what dimensions of consequences are important, the less credible it is to constrain our measurement of output to some such easily measured dimensions as changes in physical capacity for self care only.[6] And equally the more explicit the intellectual basis, the more clearly it forces a choice between theoretical positions that are equally drawn on by practitioners of the paradigm that make incompatible predictions about issues salient to studies of production relations. Ultimately, progress will depend on making clear where the implications of causal arguments for the studies differ, even if it is not always possible to choose between the alternatives on the basis of evidence. Failure to make these implications clear can only result in the production of yet another vague approach to a field whose lack of theoretical precision makes it bewildering to those from other disciplines approaching it for the first time, and unsatisfying to those who seek to draw conclusions from it for other types of inquiry.

1.3 The production relations approach

The production relations approach contributes in three main ways. First, we have found in the literature many perspectives but no one paradigm which contains them, or indeed could contain them. The development of satisfactory theory can often be assisted by a meta-theoretical paradigm which specifies what it is that theory for a specific context should explain. Such meta-theory clarifies what are the important questions. The production relations approach does this. It suggests what relationships should be investigated and quantitatively estimated. For instance, one relationship that it suggests to be important is that between the scale of homes and the possibilities of transforming inputs into outputs. Several British studies have demonstrated the existence of scale effects in residential homes for the elderly. (See for instance, Wager, 1972; Davies and Knapp, 1978; and Knapp, 1978b.) The reasons for the effects of scale are manifold. Over the range of home sizes which are most common in the UK, staff and facilities can be more effectively used in larger homes. Indeed, it would be surprising if scale were not also to affect what would be the best combination of resources for producing outputs. The second example of a relationship of importance is the responsiveness of the quality of life to increases in total resource inputs. A third example is the degree to which one input can replace another to produce the same output. The deleterious consequences on some aspects of the quality of life of badly designed accommodation can be compensated for, in part at least, by additional labour (Knapp, 1979), and similarly a scarcity of care staff can be compensated for to some degree by more staff of other kinds.

Second, the production relations approach provides a convenient technical vocabulary for focusing upon and describing relationships. For example, the term 'elasticity of output with respect to total inputs' describes how the ratio of outputs to inputs varies with the size of the home. Other coefficients indicate how the most productive mix of inputs varies with the size of the establishment. Again the production relations approach provides methods for describing the technical substitutability of inputs in the production of outputs. These apply equally to resource and non-resource inputs.

Third, the approach provides a repertoire of statistical techniques for handling the logical problems that commonly arise in studies of the relationships between inputs and outputs, techniques for the handling of evidence that follow exactly the contours of the intellectual problem. This strikes the econometrician as the most obvious of the contributions of the approach, but it is a contribution whose importance is frequently underestimated even by statisticians of other sorts. Important though this is to the conduct of a production relations study, the literature on which this essay is based is not such that the repertoire of statistical techniques is further discussed below. But what must be asserted is that there is nothing about the production relations approach that encourages the researcher to perceive complex human relationships as simple and mechanistic. Indeed, the opposite is the case. The approach provides a repertoire that more nearly matches the complexity of reality that any of the alternatives so far developed. It suggests some of the complex alternative forms that relationships may take, and so encourages us to be precise about issues which might otherwise be fudged. It forces a more comprehensive account to be taken of the factors at work. It provides tests for the existence and stability of relationships which are too easily assumed to exist by those casually examining partial evidence in the light of preconceived ideas. No one can imagine that production relations in old people's homes are like those in the generation of electricity, or can forget how heterogeneous and self-determining are most of the human inputs into the production process. As long as we remember that we are arguing by analogy, that we are discussing a 'quasi-technology' based substantially on perceptions and assumptions of actors, and not a true technology based on machines, nothing but good can come from the fresh insights that the perspective can give.

However, there is no denying the striking similarity between the arguments of recent contributions to the application of the production relations approach to the social services to those of persons advocating a systems approach. (Perhaps the main difference is that most systems writing in social work is vague about actual relationships; as Martin Davies (1977, p.83) has argued, much of it is 'excessively abstruse'.) First, both the production relations and the systems approach have a preoccupation with goals and their specification. They are thus preoccupied because the approaches focus on courses of action, and on clarifying objectives in contexts where they are often extremely vague. Both the systems approach and the production relations approach accept that this reality is too complex to postulate a unique objective. Both acknowledge the existence of latent as well as manifest goals. Both also acknowledge that objectives need not be immutable.

Second, the arguments about the relationship of the client to his environment in an open systems approach to social work are strikingly similar to the types of argument developed in this essay's application of the production relations approach. The systems analyst's concept of 'environment' is equivalent to what would in the production relations approach be called 'exogenous' inputs and quasi-inputs: factors that influence the achievement of objectives but which are outside the system's control. Both acknowledge that clients and workers have different although overlapping environments − a form of argument whose importance is reflected in the emphasis given to congruence of resident and home in the chapters that follow. Equivalent to the endogenous variables in the production relations approach − namely, factors that are subject to the influence of the system − are what the systems analyst calls 'resources'. Both in systems theory and in the production relations approach, we argue that residents do not react passively but bring to bear attitudes, expectations, values, indeed whole personalities from their past experience. Again, both approaches avoid naive assumptions about causal relations presumed to exist independently of changes in the environment. Not only do both argue that causation between factors A and B can run both ways, but also that the causal relationship is dependent upon many other characteristics. Both approaches can equally well take account of a world of changing circumstances and of uncertainty. Both recognise the importance of simultaneously handling many aspects of social reality in theorising, and so neither predisposes the analyst to overemphasise the importance of single factors. Both focus on the problems of relationships, structure, and interdependence. Martin Davis's study provides a good example of all these features.

However, judging from the applications of the systems approach to social services of one kind and another, the production relations approach has more to offer to those collecting large-scale (and so statistical) evidence. First, it more systematically specifies the important questions, both theoretical and practical: it is a higher 'meta-theory', that is, a more highly developed body of general arguments which define the questions for more context-specific theoretical argument.[7] Second it offers a more highly developed repertoire of modelling techniques which are purpose-built to test arguments about relationships with statistical evidence and to answer those important questions. This wider range of circumstances for which modelling techniques have been developed allows the analyst to stretch his understanding more successfully in the process of interrogating the evidence. Third, it seems to us that attempts to apply the production relations approach in the analysis of actual large-scale evidence in social services like health and education have been the more successful. But it is not that the production relations approach is at odds with the systems approach; since at the level of abstract argument about what it is that characterises a good perspective they so obviously argue the same. It is that, when faced with the nitty-gritty task of collecting and analysing evidence, the researcher who knows his theoretical and applied production relations literature has more to help him than the researcher with a knowledge of systems approaches. It seems to us significant that the systems approach has been most applauded by two groups: social work academics who are unskilled in the handling of quantitative evidence in models that simulate the real world; and mathematicians who have least contact with the institutional context and who again are not directly concerned with the handling of evidence.

However, it is not our purpose to start an argument about the merits of approaches that have so much in common when such arguments are unlikely to be resolved by appeal to evidence. *Chacun à son goût.* We are at least confident that the argument of this book will be at least as intelligible to the devotees of systems analysis as their arguments are to us. We hope that they find ours as interesting.

1.4 The state of the literature

Analyses of production relations are of two general types: cost function studies and production function studies. The former, which estimate relations between costs and outputs, reflect the causal structures explicitly described by the latter; the equations describing the relationship between costs and outputs being derived from those that describe the production function.[8] The cost function yields much of the information provided by the production function, but its main purpose is the estimation of the costs of producing different combinations of output. (See, for instance, Davies and Knapp, 1978, and Knapp, 1978a or 1978b, for cost function studies of residential homes for the elderly.) The production function, which describes the relationship between outputs and inputs is more complex than the cost function.[9]

15

Introduction

It is the theory of the production function that provides the principal source of meta-theory for this essay.

A review of cost and production function studies of residential homes for the aged would be brief indeed if it restricted itself only to those which fell squarely within the genre. We have already alluded to one of the principal ways in which most of the literature fails to meet the specification of a production relations study. Whereas the essence of the production relations approach is that it quantifies the contribution of physical resources to outputs allowing for the effects of other inputs, almost none of the studies that use measures of output that are content-valid by the criteria of the social welfare paradigm systematically assesses the importance of resource inputs while controlling for other important inputs. Indeed, those strands of the American literature which have got nearest to measuring the dimensions of output most central to the social welfare paradigm have completely ignored the consequences of different structures of inputs. In the rare cases in which physical inputs, costs, and aspects of standards are examined, they are merely correlated.

Some of the studies that come closest to adopting the production relations approach illustrate these generalisations. For instance, Greenwald and Linn (1971) simply present intercorrelations of costs, staffing patterns, physical facilities, patients' satisfaction, cleanliness, size and services for a small sample of twenty-six homes. Only vague inferences about causality can be made from these intercorrelations. Other studies are even more limited. Curry and Ratliff (1973) look only at the effects of home size on scores on the Life Satisfaction Index (discussed in chapter 3 below) and an indicator of isolation. Probably the closest that the gerontological literature has come to a production function conceptualisation of social service provision is in the work of Lawton, Nahemow and Teaff (1975). The authors investigate the relationship between selected physical characteristics of planned housing environments (sponsorship, community size, building size, and building height) on the one hand and resident well-being on the other, controlling for a variety of personal variables. Nevertheless, this study is still insufficiently comprehensive in its collection of resources data and too constrained in its exploitation of regression analysis to be called a production function study. McCaffree and Harkins (1976) have set out what amounts to a production relations type of study for American nursing homes, examining the relationship between the outcomes of care and the structure and environment of the home.

Other studies, that equally fall short of the full production function mode, have used indicators of 'intermediate', not final, output; indicators of consequences not valued in their own right, but for their contribution to consequences that are so valued.[10] In particular, they use indicators of the 'quality of care'. Whilst none of these researchers would hold to the view in principle, in practice many of them implicitly equate quality of care with quality of resident life, an identification which is both invalid and dangerous. Townsend (1962) was one of the first to attempt to measure quality of care and since then a number of attempts have been made to measure such intermediate outputs (which are often no more than composites of inputs) and relate them to such factors as ownership, size of facility, social integration of residents and of 'professionalism' of staff. (For recent surveys of this literature see Lawton, 1970a; Levey *et al.*, 1973; Kart and Manard, 1976.)

Finally, in this introductory chapter, mention should perhaps be made of the few previous suggestions for an *explicit* economic model of residential care services for the elderly. Binstock (1966) set out a number of serious deficiencies in gerontological research in relation to its usefulness for the establishment of social welfare programmes. His comments, though now a decade old, have gone largely unheeded. He argued, for example, that the production function model was probably the most useful approach to adopt. Lawton (1970a) discussed the five major components of organisations originally set out by Katz and Kahn (1966), laying particular stress on the need for research of the production component, and Wiseman and Silverman (1974) proposed a similar emphasis. Berliner (1972, chapter 10) couched his discussion of the generation of individual welfare in economic terms and in so doing highlighted both the applicability of the 'economic' model and its concomitant problems in this gerontological setting.

With regard to British services for the elderly, support for an economic conceptualisation of the problem comes from many quarters. The York research into the measurement of quality of life of the elderly and of the outputs of care services is being conducted by a team which includes a number of economists, and although there are few explicit references to a production relations model, the overall approach and nomenclature of the York research is very much in accordance with the approach described in this book. (See Williams, 1977; Williams and Anderson, 1975; Wright, 1974.) The 'Balance of Care' model underlying the research of Fanshel (1975) and Mooney (1978) is particularly interesting. Fanshel's systems analytic approach to the study of the welfare of the elderly has, as noted above, a number of elements in common with the production relations approach. Fanshel suggests operationalising the concept of service benefits by measuring the change in dependency state of the elderly. At a second stage this would then be related to service inputs in order to estimate the input-output, production, or transfer function. In seeking to develop a broad comprehensive macro-model of the welfare of the elderly in all sectors of the community, however, he sacrifices the insight given by a discussion that shows a deep understanding of context. He also fails to exploit the repertoire of both economic and gerontological theories, and his conceptualisation of benefit or output is limited, paying little regard to the emerging consensus of opinion among social welfare theorists and practitioners as to the objectives of care services for the elderly. Mooney's recent study of the balance of care services for the elderly in Aberdeen 'fails to measure output, effectiveness and benefit [and therefore] has severe limitations' (Mooney, 1978, p.150), but nevertheless breathes a breath of fresh economic air upon an important policy question. He is concerned with the optimal balance of care between community services, residential homes and hospitals, and to this end sets out an interesting theoretical approach to establish the optimum. In its basic line of approach and nomenclature Mooney's methodology is generally consistent with the perspective discussed in this book. However, the simplicity of his methodology may harbour considerable difficulties when one introduces *multiple* outputs or benefits. As with Fanshel's systems analysis model, the robustness and usefulness of Mooney's suggested approach will be more thoroughly tested with a more content-valid data set, and particularly one which focuses upon the output variables suggested by the social welfare paradigm.

The focus of this study is therefore the feasibility of specifying what are the outputs of residential homes and the feasibility of measuring them; and also what are the non-resource and quasi-inputs which operate in conjunction with resources to produce the outputs.

Part two of this book, which consists of chapters 2 and 3, deals with outputs and their measurement. The theoretical concept of output discussed in this book, especially earlier in this chapter, is general to all social welfare contexts. The arguments of chapter 2 are specific to the elderly and those of chapter 3 specific to residential homes. Part three, consisting of chapters 4, 5 and 6, tackles the questions of definition and measurement of the inputs into the production process. The resource inputs, principally labour and capital, are discussed in chapter 4. These are the factors of most interest to economists, the factors probably most frequently mentioned in policy documents and also the factors most commonly neglected in the social welfare and gerontological literatures. Chapters 5 and 6 address the non-resource and quasi-inputs, particularly the social environment or caring milieu of the home, staff attitudes, salient resident characteristics, and resident experiences before, during and after admission to the home. These chapters may be read in isolation, but of course the resource, non-resource and quasi-inputs are all closely inter-related and cannot be taken in isolation in the production process.

Finally, chapter 7 summarises the arguments of the book, discussing the nature and logic of the production of welfare process as a consistent whole, and alluding to some of the main differences between approaches. Second, it mentions a number of latent and manifest policy issues in the light of the theory and evidence about the nature of production relations, and examines one of them — the policy framework for the independent sector — in more detail. It seems likely that the rate of expansion will be higher in the private than in the local authority or voluntary sectors. This final section is only a bare sketch of a policy essay but it helps to illustrate the way in which production relations knowledge could contribute to quite radical policy development.

Part two

Outputs

Movements from a general definition of 'output' in a personal social services context to a measure or set of measures operational in a study of a particular mode of care requires that we move through a number of theoretical and practical stages. In the previous chapter we presented a conceptualisation of output in terms of the consequences of intervention valued in their own right. In chapters 2 and 3 we are concerned with the problems of operationalising the chosen consequences.

The output concept is closely related to a concept more familiar to students of the personal social services — that of 'need'. Output, like need, is a 'shortfall' concept: indeed, output can be conceptualised in terms of the extent to which need is reduced, leading immediately to a practical research design which makes comparisons between individuals and over time. Also like need, outputs are flows through time, and so must be discounted to their present value; that is, applying to future benefits a rate of time preference in such a way that the lower value that we place on a benefit in the distant rather than the near future is duly taken into account in our evaluation. These two arguments raise a host of logical complications. We shall not explore them further. They are dealt with more than adequately in accessible literature.

In this book we do not discuss in any great detail those outcomes enjoyed principally by residents that are not central to their overall psychological well-being. Of the vast number of effects distinguished in the literature, only mortality and morbidity will be discussed at any length. There are a number of reasons for our emphasis on psychological well-being. First, there are already very many studies of these other outcomes spread widely throughout the literature. Second, any study of indicators and interrelationships would anyway warrant a monograph in its own right. Third, as we shall again argue in chapter 7, many of the outcomes distinguished by previous writers are important only because they exert an influence upon resident psychological

Outputs

well-being. As a result, these are often more reliably counted as inputs rather than outputs.

Chapter 2

The psychological
well-being of residents

The arguments of the previous chapter lead inexorably to a careful consideration of the psychological well-being of residents. This chapter therefore contains the core of our discussion of the measurement of the outputs of old people's homes: an analysis of the manner in which the literature has dealt with the psychological well-being, life satisfaction, morale, affect, or 'social adjustment', of residents.

In the first section we take a look at some recent literature on engagement and the measurement of engaged activity. Engaged activity, it has been argued, can be used as an indicator of the quality of life of elderly residents of care institutions. We shall find that this approach does not have universal value in the measurement of output. Engaged activity is not therefore the principal focus of the 'Production of Welfare' approach nor of this chapter. We move on in the second section of the chapter to an examination of psychological well-being — its theoretical underpinnings and its potential for practical research. We argue that the personalities of potential residents vary greatly and that as a result the social environments best suited to them will also vary to a considerable degree. This has not always been fully appreciated in much of the post-war literature which has tended, particularly in Britain, to focus more on the quality of *care* to the neglect of the quality of *life*. This variance in 'optimal' environments makes it essential to develop a framework for examining the fit between the needs of a resident and the social milieu surrounding him. In discussing the contribution of the literature to this end, the arguments of personality theorists are an essential background. Accordingly, some of the more salient points of the most important arguments of the personality theorists are outlined in section 2.2.2. Sections 2.2.3 to 2.2.7 evaluate approaches to the assessment of resident psychological well-being from this and other relevant perspectives. The degree to which the approaches involve the collection of data in a manner that is economical, and the degree to which they satisfy purely psychometric criteria for their judgment — like their reliability and construct validity — is considered in these sections. The Appendix to this chapter, prepared by Sheila Peace, John Hall and Graham Hamblin, describes the use of one particular scale — the Affect Balance Scale — in the recent North London Polytechnic study of residential homes for the elderly.

2.1 Engaged activity

A resident of an old people's home, or any elderly person in his or her environment, is said to be 'engaged' if he or she is 'interacting with materials or with people in a manner which is likely to maintain or develop . . . skills and abilities. A highly engaged person is constantly doing things . . . can be *seen* to be interacting with materials or people . . . ' (Blunden and Kushlick, 1974, p.5). Albert Kushlick, the most distinguished proponent of the engagement approach in the UK, argues that seeking to increase the level of engaged activity in old people's homes is consistent with other commonly expressed aims, such as 'meeting the needs of individuals, building self-confidence, or increasing self-control, independence, self esteem, or dignity' (ibid., p.6) and in addition has the advantage of being easily monitored. The American literature on which Dr Kushlick's work is based, notably that by Cataldo, Risley and others of the so-called 'Living Environments Group' of Kansas University Department of Human Development, argues that the higher the level of 'wholesome' client activity the higher the quality of life (see Kushlick, 1974, p.16). Similarly, some of Kushlick's Winchester colleagues assert that the 'effectiveness of a residential environment could be assessed by measuring the degree to which residents were still performing the various normal activities on which they spent their time previously' (Jenkins, Felce, Lunt and Powell, 1976). The approach has been applied to the very aged in geriatric facilities in the USA by McClannahan (1973a, 1973b, 1974), and has been applied by Dr Kushlick's team in Wessex in a number of studies of elderly residents of caring institutions (Kushlick and Blunden, 1974; Lunt *et al.*, 1977; Powell *et al.*, 1977).

The use of indicators of engaged activity offers a number of practical advantages. First it is claimed that it is a 'clear, simple, and reliable method' which should require a very short period of observer training before scores can be safely obtained. However, such data are not necessarily inexpensive. Observation of the whole waking day is necessarily time-consuming. There appear not to have been the comparative studies of a large number of individuals in different environments which could establish whether the concentration of time sampling on one or two periods of a single day could yield reliable indicators of engaged activity in general. That the time distribution of activity over the waking day varies substantially between persons suggests that the time sampling would need to be stratified for the effects of situational contexts to be found. Perhaps, therefore, the techniques as they are now used with a detailed study of a few units would be expensive to apply to the study of a large number of persons.

The second practical advantage claimed for indicators of engaged activity is that the techniques of measurement are salient to almost all residents, including substantial minorities of residents who are physically infirm, or mentally impaired. But not all engaged activity is equally engaging, so that activity scores should be weighted. Indeed, it follows from the argument of Maddi (1961, 1966) (and is implicit in the discussion by others of such concepts as approach and avoidance motives) that the degree of psychological activation from stimuli is not merely different in degree between people but different in kind; stimuli which tend to induce an approach motive for some can induce an avoidance motive (fear) for others. Therefore the ratings for the stimuli must vary between individuals. They must also take into account variations in the intensity of the activity (if not also of its meaningfulness and variety) since persons also vary in their preference for these. Thus to obtain indicators of the activation consequences of activity requires a much more complicated basis for recording engaged activity as well as a technique for assessing what weights should be attached for each individual to activity on each dimension. Much of the simplicity which helps make engaged activity attractive as the basis for measurement might be lost if it were to be developed thus. But the number of dimensions demanded by the Maddi theory exceeds the number so far used in observing engaged activity. Moreover, without such individualised rating systems, it is difficult to argue that scoring takes into account individual needs. Engaged activity depends on both personality characteristics internal to the person and stimuli provided by the environment. It must not be thought to be an indicator of the latter only. That it is both is implicit in the following quotation from Doke and Risley (1972): 'A measure of engagement in activities ... is a direct measure of the stimulation that the environment provides to the resident and the strength of beneficial consequences to the residents for admitting engaged behaviour' because it reflects both environmental and behavioural characteristics. Motivated activity is a function not only of the incentives provided by the environment but also of the personality of the subject. All the most likely forms which encapsulate the ways in which the strength of personal motivation and of environmentally determined incentives influence the amount of engaged activity would suggest that, for instance, the level of engaged activity will be very different for two persons facing similar congruent environments, but differing in that one is of a low activation personality type whereas the other is of a high activation type.

27

Conversely, the engaged activity of two such people could be the same in environments differing with respect to congruence. Equal amounts of engaged activity by the criteria of a uniform weighting system would not imply that their interests were equally catered for by the environment.

Of course, Kushlick and other proponents of the utility of measuring engaged activity do not argue otherwise. Their argument asserts far less, although a quick reading might cause some misunderstanding of their position, which is that 'active engagement implies that these individual "interests", etc., are being catered for. Similarly their disengagement or non-engagement implies that they are not being met' (Kushlick and Blunden, 1974, p.9). Here there is merely an assertion about the categories engagement, non-engagement, and disengagement, with no assertion as to differences in degree. We can certainly accept that a form of the function yielding such an outcome is highly plausible. Indeed Atkinson (1957), an associate of McClelland (whose work we draw upon in section 2.2.2) made a set of propositions which seem to imply a multiplicative form for the relationship between engaged activity, personal motivation and environmentally determined incentives. In such a form the complete absence of environmentally-generated incentives would cause zero activity, whilst minimal incentive would result in some engaged activity and meet the interests of the individual to some degree. But it is differences in degree that are of real interest. For this, the picture is more complicated.

There is some specific evidence for British old people's homes that the relationships between activity and well-being are complex. No doubt, it is generally true that where the degree of engaged activity is very low in relation to some 'typical' level of activation it could be argued that increased engagement would almost certainly improve the psychological well-being of all residents. At least an increase in engaged activity in such a context could safely be taken to imply an increased psychological well-being. However, it is not obvious that the degree of engaged activity would increase the psychological well-being of almost all residents. Certainly John Townsend and Ann Kimbell (1974, 1975) argued on the basis of some evidence for homes in Cheshire that attempts to increase the amount of engaged activity actually *diminished* some aspects of the psychological well-being of the residents. Similarly, the studies of community-residing elderly Britons by Crawford (1971) and Knapp (1977b) produced qualitative and quantitative evidence, respectively, to support a *disengagement* perspective of ageing. As we have argued above, the efficacy of engaged activity cannot be judged outside the environmental and personal context in which it occurs, a fact which is not often recognised by practitioners, researchers, or the general public. As one North American gerontologist so succinctly put it: 'although idleness and meditation may be acceptable for St Thomas and for the gurus of teenagers today, American activity-oriented middle-agers become distraught when grandpa sits on the porch in his rocking chair for undue lengths of time' (Rosencranz, 1974, p. 66).

However, this is not to argue that the measurement of engaged activity can play no part in a study of production relations in residential environments for the elderly. In particular, it might be a very useful outcome measure for those residents who are mentally or physically handicapped, but it would be necessary to base the measurement on a more complex recording of activities and individualised weighting systems than have so far been used, and to view it strictly within its particular environmental and personal context.

Having seen this approach to have been of definite though not universal value, we must find a different basis. The bases of the American literature have in common that they measure welfare in one way or another. Some of them are related explicitly to psychology and personality theory. We therefore first draw out some important strands of personality theory in order to subsequently examine the content validity of measures of well-being.

2.2 Psychological well-being

2.2.1 Output, social environment and individual fit

The general social environment of a home is not an output but a quasi-input, and one which need not have a powerful impact if the individual resident is able to find what one writer called a 'social niche' that compensates for inadequacies in the environment in general. In the absence of such social niches the impact of the social environment on individuals will probably differ greatly. It is clear throughout the entire literature on production relations in human and social services that the assumption that inputs have similar consequences for all recipients has very limited support. Therefore, what is important is the relationship between personal characteristics and environment. This subsection elaborates this proposition.

Aged persons are likely to differ more than the young. Neugarten (1964) argues that differences are likely to become greater with age, despite the experience of similar social roles in variants of a common culture, since educational, vocational and social events (their incidence influenced by continuities in personality) accumulate to enhance variation. However, Neugarten also asserts that the evidence about this is ambiguous, and most of it relates to the general population living in the community. But perhaps residents in homes are drawn more from some variants of the culture than others, and to a disproportionate degree possess some personality characteristics that affect social roles and perceptions. Whatever the force of that argument, there are clear enough indications of heterogeneity for us to expect far more powerful relationships in models which have as a central feature differences between individuals. For evidence we again turn to the American literature. First, the balance of evidence of the literature seems to support Kahana's position (1974, p.201):

> When considering programs for the elderly, their individual needs along the dimensions of activity-disengagement must be considered along with other factors, [for] apparently helpful environmental characteristics may be harmful to some elderly people while apparently undesirable features may benefit others.

Likewise Wolk and Telleen (1976, p.96) write about the relationship between activity and the accomplishment of the developmental tasks discussed by theorists of personality who postulate core tendencies towards fulfilment:

> To allow that simple activity level should strongly predict developmental task accomplishment is an oversimplification. Rather an individual must perceive the possibility for personal initiative and experimentation with new behaviours, since each set of developmental tasks characterizing an age span poses qualitatively new challenges.

The literature testing and elaborating theory about patterns of ageing has evolved from a bipolar, activity versus disengagement position of the early 1960s to one that stresses the diversity of individual strategies of ageing. The activity or 'lay' theory of ageing essentially asserts a positive relationship between the aged individual's level of participation in social activity and his subsequent life satisfaction or psychological well-being. This assertion stems from an assumption that the individual's role requirements or demands upon self and society remain fairly stable as he passes from middle to old age. It has often been claimed that the activity perspective on ageing is contradistinctive to the disengagement hypothesis of Cumming and Henry (1961). This non-developmental theory suggests that withdrawal or disengagement from social participation is actually functionally advantageous to both individual and society, and one would therefore expect to observe a negative association between social participation and well-being. Adherence to the bipolar viewpoint that one or other perspective, but not both, was appropriate, and the resultant efforts to test one against the other, only served to obscure the variety of ageing patterns (Knapp, 1977b). Later studies of alternative patterns of ageing yielded more realistic typologies, and the activity and disengagement theories have lost much of their practical relevance. It now seems that 'neither theory is sufficient by itself to explain all of the myriad patterns of ageing, many of which require further information of a sociological or social psychological nature to elaborate meaningfully' (Dowd, 1975, p.585). One of the most important pieces of further information is individual personality, which Havighurst (1968) has described as the 'pivotal dimension' in the explanation of observed associations between levels of activity and engagement, on the one hand, and psychological well-being on the other. Savage *et al.* (1977) confirm this finding in their study of the elderly in Newcastle-upon-Tyne.

Typologies of patterns of ageing based on differences in the personalities of elderly people have been developed. Reichard and her colleagues derived five patterns: mature, rocking-chair, armoured, angry, and self-haters. The longitudinal study of Neugarten and her colleagues yielded eight patterns of ageing, the elderly in each group being described as either reorganisers, focused, successfully disengaged, holders-on, constricted succourance-seeking, apathetic, or disorganised (Reichard *et al.*, 1962; Neugarten *et al.*, 1964; Neugarten, 1968; and see Havighurst, 1968). Savage *et al.* (1977) identified four patterns: the silent majority, introverted, perturbed, and mature tempered. These patterns of ageing can clearly be related to the theoretical arguments of Rogers and Maslow (who might be called 'core fulfilment' theorists) and Erikson (who is neither unambiguously a 'conflict' nor a 'fulfilment' theorist), and who postulate self-actualisation and ego-integration, and a sense of betrayal and despair. These theoretical arguments clearly suggest predictions about what constitutes a developmental task and what factors predispose towards its successful performance. The classifications of Reichard and Neugarten are not the same as those implicit in any particular typology of personality presented by the main personality theorists themselves but these empirical studies are of direct relevance in that they relate to the sub-population of the elderly that interests us here. For instance, the literature on the relocation of the elderly demonstrates associations between personal (and personality) characteristics and adjustments to relocation (Turner, 1969; Turner, Tobin and Lieberman, 1972; Yawney and Slover 1973; Tobin and Lieberman, 1976).

Important though they undoubtedly are, personality traits by themselves do not determine life satisfaction. Indeed, some evidence suggests that intra-psychic characteristics are not as stable or rigid as might be inferred from Freudian theory. Longitudinal studies of adulthood and adolescence show much evidence of changes in personality. For instance, Neugarten (1964, p.205) concluded a review of the literature:

As is true in childhood and adolescence, changes in personality occur throughout the long period of life we call adulthood. Although the evidence is inadequate, there are data to support the position that changes occur in intra-psychic processes as well as in more readily observable behaviour; such changes are orderly and developmental in nature. . . .

Commenting on the longitudinal studies (ibid., p.188), she wrote:

Whether the studies are test-retest or antecedent-consequent in design . . . the general picture with regard to consistency of adult personality can be summarised by saying that measures taken at long time intervals tend to produce statistically reliable, but relatively low, correlations . . . . The indication is that while there is continuity of personality measurable by present techniques, the larger proportion of the variance in the measures used at times two remains unaccounted for. Making allowances for the fallibility of measures with regard to reliability, the implication is that there is at least as much change as there is stability.

The precise degree of correlation between personality characteristics at two points of time among the elderly, and that among those most likely to enter old people's homes in particular, is important. Low correlations would undermine the argument that the personality needs of the elderly vary in ways which demand different environments. High correlations would have profound implications for the probability of achieving self-actualisation in a setting not perfectly congruent with those personality needs. The evidence from the longitudinal studies (which alone can distinguish cohort from ageing effects) seems to be slight, and the salient population is untypical of the elderly in general. Nevertheless, it is not surprising that what are stable personality characteristics — and so in a sense not a response to some external stimuli at that time, however caused — by themselves explain a relatively small part of variance in behaviour. Moos (1975) writes about a prediction 'sound barrier', an upper limit in the prediction of behaviour from variables describing individual differences found in such diverse fields as studies of military organisation, the prediction of violent behaviour, and absconding from correctional institutions. Indeed, it could be argued that the effects of interaction between person and setting are generally more important in a wide range of contexts than the separate effects of personal and environmental characteristics. Moos goes as far as to assert that there is little relationship between a person's behaviour inside a psychiatric or correctional institution and his behaviour outside. For instance, he asserts that there was little correlation between behaviour before entering hospital and (three weeks later) in hospital; and, quoting Ian Sinclair's conclusion, that the type of probation hostel has less impact on subse-

quent community behaviour than the environment to which the proba-
tioner returns (Sinclair, 1971).

Perhaps these more extreme assertions were stronger than is compatible even with Moos's own evidence. It would be perverse to ignore the
importance both of personality itself, and of personality-environment
interactions. The latter may be more influential than the former. One
of the central features of the explanation of outputs of residential
homes must therefore be the idea of fit between the person and his
environment. The quality of life and sense of psychological well-
being is substantially the outcome of two sets of causes: on the one
hand micro-environmental characteristics which change relatively
slowly, to which individual residents are not matched systematically
in relation to their psychological needs, and which they cannot substantially control; and on the other, personal characteristics of the
individual that both make him vary in the degree to which 'adjustment' — or, to use a more neutral term, psychological and behavioural adaptation — will be necessary, and will make that adaptation
more or less difficult. What is important is to develop the concept of
fit. Some, like Battista and Almond (1973), who distinguish fit with
respect to values, goals, needs and roles, have started to make it more
specific. It is a process we shall continue in chapter 5. Meanwhile,
having acknowledged the centrality of personality theory, we must
develop an argument about its implications for the measurement
of output.

2.2.2 Personality theory: core tendencies and inter-individual variation

The measurement of resident-benefiting outputs involves two key
issues: (a) the selection of dimensions among which must be sought
the environmental fit; and (b) the choice or development of instruments with which to measure these dimensions. In this regard the
social work paradigm, that is, the common assumptions, beliefs and
values shared by social work professionals, clearly accepts the psychologists' perception that personality and the congruence between personality and environment are the main causes of variation in psychological well-being between individuals. Our handling of these key
issues must therefore be guided by theories of personality, particularly those theories which have influenced social work assumptions,
and those which appear to make predictions compatible with available evidence.

Two features of personality theories are important. The first is
their assumption about the *core tendencies* of man — features inherent in him which do not vary greatly over the life-span and which
have a general and pervasive influence over the whole of his behaviour.
The second is their treatment of the *peripheral characteristics* of

33

personality, characteristics closer to behaviour which tend to change and develop over the life-span.

The social welfare paradigm clearly draws greatly from the writings of those humanist psychologists, like Erich Fromm, Carl Rogers or Abraham Maslow, who postulate a core tendency to seek self-fulfilment or self-actualisation (Fromm, 1947; Rogers, 1959, 1961; Maslow, 1959, 1970). There are differences between these writers. In Rogers's theory the core tendency is an attempt to actualise potentialities by seeking the 'positive regard' of others (that is the approval of persons significant to one's life) and 'positive self-regard' (that is the approval of, or satisfaction with oneself). How this actualising tendency would be expressed will depend partly upon a person's inherent potentialities and partly on the lessons he has learned from his environment about how to achieve a positive regard that is compatible with a positive self-regard. Like Rogers, Maslow makes the seeking for the actualisation of his inherent potentialities man's core tendency. However, the self-actualisation concept is less a focus of Maslovian writing, and Maslow postulates a tendency to seek physical and psychological survival — succourance not just in addition to, but prepotent over, fulfilment. Maslow discusses categories of need. In diminishing order of relevance to survival, and ascending order of relevance to fulfilment, they are: physiological, safety, belongingness and love, and esteem needs. Fromm's core tendency is not dissimilar to that of Maslow (or Allport) — a drive towards self-realisation. Fromm postulates needs for relatedness, and rootedness, the identity and transcendence to become a productive individual with a stable and consistent frame of reference with which to view the world. Thus Rogers, Maslow, Fromm and to a lesser degree Erikson, postulate fulfilment as the essential tendency. Other theorists put congruence with the environment at the centre. For instance McClelland's theory has as its core tendency the minimisation of large discrepancies between expectations and occurrence and the maximisation of small discrepancies, and so the avoidance of either intolerable uncertainty or unrelieved boredom (McClelland *et al.*, 1953). Fiske and Maddi (1961) postulate that a person will attempt to maintain the level of actuation to which he is accustomed (see also Maddi, 1961, 1966). These 'consistency' theories may not have had as great an impact on the social welfare paradigm as the fulfilment theories; but they gain some empirical support, and have considerable salience to the assessment of well-being in a context in which persons have undergone a sudden and dramatic change in their environment.

The second important feature is the extent to which personality theories differ with respect to peripheral characteristics. These peripheral attributes of personality are closer to behaviour, are variable between persons, are substantially learned, and have more circumscribed influence; for instance, they influence behaviour in some circumstances only. Erikson's (1963) 'eight stages of man' have been well integrated into the social welfare paradigm. The environment during each of Erikson's stages leaves marks on personality which are of direct salience to psychological well-being. Erikson's second stage is crucial to the development of autonomy, the ability of a person to make choices for himself; an unsatisfactory outcome of the second stage predisposes the person to an adult personality marked by doubt about his ability to function competently. A successful outcome of the third stage leads to capacity to take initiative and responsibility, and to avoid later feelings of unworthiness and irresponsibility and tendency to acquiescence. At the fourth stage a successful outcome leads to traits expressing industry rather than a sense of inferiority in the way the person operates in relation to the outside world. The successful outcome of the fifth stage is a very secure sense of identity rather than a scattered, fragmentary, diffuse and drifting sense of who the person is; that of the sixth stage is the achievement of personal intimacy rather than the slipping into isolation and consequent self-absorption; that of the seventh stage is the feeling and accomplishment of general activity rather than personal stagnation; and that of the eighth stage is ego-integrity rather than despair.

The ego-integrated person has, in Erikson's words: 'adapted himself to the triumphs and disappointments inherent to being by necessity the originator of others and the generator of things and ideas.' The state of mind reflects an assurance of its proclivity for order and meaning of life

> as an experience which conveys some world order and spiritual sense, . . . the acceptance of one's one and only life cycle as something that had to be and that, by necessity, permitted of no substitutions . . . a comradeship with the ordering ways of distant times and different pursuits . . . [a readiness] to defend the dignity of his own life style against all physical and economic threats.

If the individual is not successful at the eighth stage in securing ego-integration, the result is despair. Erikson (1963) explains how

> the lack or loss of this accrued ego-integration is signified by fear of death: the one and only life style is not accepted as the ultimate of life. Despair expresses the feeling that time is now short, so short for the attempt to start another life and to try out alternative roads to integrity. Disgust hides despair.

Thus Erikson's stages of life provide clear statements about what personality characteristics predict variations in psychological well-being. Not surprisingly, therefore, attempts have been made to use it as a basis for predicting variations in well-being (see for instance Sherwood and Nadelson, 1972). Environmental congruence in this case would thus entail an environment which encouraged persons to exercise the strength acquired from successful outcomes of early developmental stages, and which gave support in coping with the consequences of the relative lack of success in these stages. In particular it would provide support in achieving and maintaining ego-integrity. Satisfaction in the later years of life comes from ego-integrity, but an integrity which cannot be achieved solely from the internal adjustment of the individual. As Brearley has argued: 'Satisfaction and happiness . . . depend on the congruence of the inner mental state with external circumstances' (Brearley, 1977, p.34).

The first seven stages of the psychic development schema postulated by Erikson are concentrated in the earlier years of an individual's life, and the assumption of a single stage for middle and old age is clearly unrealistic. In its stead, Peck (1955) substituted seven steps, the last three representing crises of old age: ego differentiation versus work-role preoccupation (a reorientation from what one *does* to what one *is*); body transcendence versus body preoccupation (the dominance of social and mental sources of satisfaction over physical discomfort and decline); and ego transcendence versus ego preoccupation (acceptance of the inevitability of death and a positive reappraisal of one's worldly contribution). These steps will be characterised much less by chronological age than by sets of developmental tasks, each set requiring environmental support and the degree of success at each step determining in part the felt satisfaction of the elderly individual.

Rogers's theory yields only two personality types. One type, the fully functioning person, is open to experience rather than being defensive; lives fully in each and every moment (because his 'experiences are available to awareness') rather than acting upon some preconceived life-plan; trusts and reacts to experiences and changes his self-structure accordingly to maintain congruence; experiences unconditional self-regard; meets each new situation with unique and creative behaviour; and will live with others in 'maximum possible harmony, because of the rewarding character of reciprocal positive regard' (Rogers, 1959, pp.234-5). It is more difficult to specify precise behavioural characteristics conforming to these descriptions than it is to do so for the Erikson or Peck stages, because it is a matter of judgment what behaviour is compatible with each characteristic description in any context. Fromm's theory likewise did not propose a typology of personality which would predict variations of psychological well-being, though he did discuss the common traits of fully mature people in a way that was not unlike Rogers's description of the fully functioning person. However, it might be predicted from his theory that personality types orientated towards his different needs would achieve different overall levels of psychological well-being.

From McClelland's theory one would predict that psychological well-being would be greatest in a context in which there was the greatest congruence between environmental characteristics and the motives, traits and schemata learned by the individual. In McClelland's theory, motives are states of mind aroused by some stimulus situation that serves as a signal that a change in situation is imminent, a change that will either be pleasant or unpleasant. Motives are of two kinds: approach motives and avoidance motives. Environmental congruence demands that the environment provides the stimuli to approach motives but not to avoidance motives. The most important motives of both kinds relate to needs for achievement, affiliation, and power. Environment should also be compatible with personality traits which, according to McClelland, consist of a collection of habits without the goal-directedness of motives. McClelland's schemata are cultural characteristics like ideas, values and social roles, and symbolise past experience. Subcultural variations are of clear salience to environmental congruence in old people's homes (McClelland *et al.*, 1951, 1953).

The Maddi theory argues that people vary in the *pattern* of activation during the day, as well as in the *average degree* of activation. The latter is the more important. High activation people will spend the major part of their time and effort pursuing stimuli in order to keep up their activation levels; low activation people will tend to do the opposite. Both high activation and low activation people vary in their preference for intensity, meaningfulness, and variety; and also their degree of passivity. The passive person anticipates his activity requirement badly, being neither self-reliant nor an initiator, and so tends to fail to achieve differentiation and integration. Fiske and Maddi (1961) also draw a distinction between regulating impact by looking to sources of stimulation inside and outside the person.

These arguments from personality theories provide criteria for judging the content validity of instruments for measuring psychological well-being — criteria by which to judge whether the instruments adequately cover the range of relevant dimensions. They also suggest factors that should be taken into account because they have an effect on psychological well-being either independent of, or in conjunction with, variations in resource inputs. The arguments thus provide a basis for discussing the merits of alternative instruments, including merits not often mentioned in the literature on these instruments themselves. This literature has tended to focus not on the content but on the concurrent validity of the instruments in relation to professional judgment, and the construct validity — the degree to which instrument scores are correlated with other variables in a way which is compatible with predictions of well-established theory.

We shall now discuss the content, concurrent, and construct validity of some of the more established methods that have been evolved for measuring psychological well-being.

2.2.3 Morale, life satisfaction, and psychological well-being

The development of measures of morale, life satisfaction, affect, or psychological well-being is perhaps the most salient approach to the measurement of outputs pursued by social gerontologists. In fact, relatively few writers have given explicit accounts of the centrality of psychological well-being in outcome or output assessment (exceptions include Binstock, 1966; Kosberg, 1974; Sherwood, 1972; and Wylie, 1970), although implicit or covert support is considerable. Recognition of the dominance of psychological well-being was voiced by Paul Brearley in his essay on residential work with the elderly: '[The] fundamental rights to choice, respect, dignity, independence, individuality and privacy are relevant only in so far as they provide for satisfaction in old age.... Personal satisfaction seems to be a fundamental need' (Brearley, 1977, pp.33-4). The conceptual domination of satisfaction assessment follows most clearly from the focus of humanist psychologists and others upon an internal frame of reference, as we have noted in the previous section. In this and subsequent sections, therefore, we present and discuss some of the indicators or instruments that have been developed, validated and applied in gerontological settings for the measurement of psychological well-being.

Lawton (1976) and Larson (1978) have recently reviewed the large number of instruments (and vast accompanying literature) which have attempted to measure the internal or subjective state of well-being of elderly people, whether resident in the community or in some care facility. Larson's review covered only American literature, excluded studies 'which had insufficient sample sizes or inadequate sampling procedures to allow generalisation', and focused predominantly on the quantitative characteristics of measures of subjective well-being and their correlates. We shall have cause to refer to Larson's review in later sections and chapters of this book, but for the purposes of the present section it is Lawton's clarifying summary of concepts and dimensions that is most useful. Lawton's summary builds upon his own vast experience in the measurement of morale and general well-being, including the design, validation and operationalisation of the popular Philadelphia Geriatric Center morale scale (see section 2.2.7 below). The large number of alternative scales, indices and ratings are summarised under twelve heads:

(a) Life satisfaction. (Primarily the Life Satisfaction Rating of Neugarten, Havighurst and Tobin, 1961, the Life Satisfaction Index, and some of its derivatives.) (See sections 2.2.4 and 2.2.5 below.) Lawton suggests that 'life satisfaction' is the most useful general term under which to subsume aspects of morale not included in those to follow, or item sets with very mixed content (see also Lohmann, 1978).

(b) Happiness. A concept with 'a long history of attempted measurement' (Bradburn, 1969; Wilson, 1967) which is considered to be 'an ideology because of the cognitive element that enters into its estimation and averaging over time, in contrast to the more time-limited affects or moods'.

(c) Mood. A time limited state of happiness in which emotion and psychophysiology play an important role (Cameron, 1975; Bradburn and Caplovitz, 1965).

(d) Age-related morale. An ideology whose 'referent for the balance of positive and negative experiences relates to the period of old age, with either an explicit or implied comparison to earlier periods of life' (Lawton, 1972a, 1975a; Pierce and Clark, 1973).

(e) Continuity of self. 'The perception that one's essential Self has endured through chronological and event-related time' (Erikson, 1963; Peck, 1955; Rosow, 1963).

(f) Positive self-concept of self-esteem. An acceptable image of oneself as oneself (Coleman, 1976; Breytspraak and George, 1977).

(g) Intra-psychic symptoms. Such as anxiety, depression, fears, worry, delusions, and hallucinations (Hathaway and McKinley, 1951).

(h) Psychophysiological symptoms. (Langner, 1962; Morris, Wolf & Klerman, 1975).

(i) Satisfaction with the status quo. (Cumming and Henry, 1961).

(j) Self-rated health. (Pierce and Clark, 1973).

(k) Attitudes. Ideologies about objects or events outside the self, including anomie and other special attitudes (Srole, 1956; Schooler, 1970a).

(l) Loneliness. A concept directly related to the individual's external world (Burgess, Cavan and Havighurst, 1947).

The sad fact about this voluminous body of research, Lawton notes, is that many of the above named domains are related to one another more strongly than they are to their validity criterion. He then sets out a procedure whereby the dissatisfied researcher can develop his own scale of psychological well-being: starting with a large pool of seemingly salient items, the judicious use of cluster or factor analyses with successive deletion and addition of items will allow one to converge on a set with high homogeneity of content and a tendency to be highly correlated. Other, non-conceptual, problems in measuring morale — such as wording, psychometric characteristics, time-referents, and validity —

must also be taken into account in deriving and applying a subjective well-being scale. The set of dimensions produced by Lawton and such comparative work as that recently undertaken by Lohmann (1977, 1978) suggests that the available alternative scales overlap to a considerable extent. We now turn, therefore, to a more detailed consideration of four of the most reliable and most frequently used instruments: the Life Satisfaction Rating, the Life Satisfaction Index, the Affect Balance Scale, and the Philadelphia Geriatric Center Morale Scale.[1]

2.2.4 Life satisfaction ratings

In this subsection we discuss life satisfaction ratings; that is, life satisfaction assessments made by judges subsequent to interviews with the elderly person. The ratings are not based on the elderly person's own reported feelings of psychological well-being. The most popular and thorough rating is that of Neugarten, Havighurst and Tobin (1961).

Although Neugarten and her colleagues based the development of their rating scale on an analysis of previous scales and indices, its face validity must be judged in relation to the arguments of personality theory. Earlier work on psychological well-being had focused on overt behaviour in relation to social criteria of success and competence, and had thus assumed (implicitly or explicitly) that greater social participation meant greater well-being. The Life Satisfaction Rating (LSR) approach instead focused on an internal frame of reference — the individual's own evaluation of his present and past life satisfaction and happiness. In this way, Neugarten and her associates intended to reduce the arbitrariness of value judgments in some of the earlier scales and to escape from an implicit acceptance of the 'activity perspective' on ageing (compare Cavan *et al.*, 1949; Havighurst and Albrecht, 1953.) Previous attempts at a quantitative assessment of individual life satisfaction suffered from other weaknesses too. The Cumming and Henry (1961) morale index was biased against high activity — high scores were obtained by those aged individuals content with the status quo, a value based upon the disengagement model of the ageing process. The Kutner morale scale managed to avoid relying upon overt behaviour to indicate well-being, but instead stumbled in other respects. In common with virtually all early attempts to measure psychological well-being, the Kutner scale was vulnerable to the psychological defenses of subjects, had not been validated in relation to external criteria, was unidimensional and based on few items, and was 'well-behaved' only in the population originally studied. In attempting to overcome these and other weaknesses, the developmental work of Neugarten, Havighurst and Tobin produced a well-validated (but rarely used) LSR scale and two slightly less valid but very popular Life Satisfaction Indices LSI).

Psychological well-being was analysed into five constituent components:

(a) Zest (as against apathy). Enthusiasm in, and pleasure from, the activities of everyday life.
(b) Resolution and fortitude. The extent to which life is meaningful and the acceptance of all that has gone before.
(c) Congruence between desired and achieved goals. Feelings of success in achieving major objectives, taking opportunities.
(d) Self-concept. The (positive) image of self — physical as well as psychological and social attributes.
(e) Mood tone. Maintaining 'happy, optimistic attitudes and moods', pleasure from life, spontaneous positive affect.

(For full details, see Appendix A to this chapter). The ratings along each component, on a five-point scale, were made by two independent judges, using four rounds of interviews with each elderly individual. Application of the LSR to a general elderly population in Kansas City over a 2½ year period revealed a high degree of agreement between the judges (Pearson correlation coefficient of 0.78 for the 177 interviewees). All the judges were drawn from a 'student-faculty research seminar'. The ratings were further validated by the high degree of correlation found between the judges' ratings and those made by a clinical psychologist who interviewed the elderly respondents eighteen months later. Despite this passage of time, and despite other potentially harmful factors (see Neugarten *et al.*, 1961, p. 140) a satisfactorily high correlation of 0.64 was obtained for the eighty respondents interviewed by the psychologist. Thus the ratings had a concurrent validity[2] that made them potentially valuable in the measurement of life satisfaction.

The content validity can best be assessed by examining the criteria for rating in relation to the type of characteristics that developmental psychology would suggest to be important. By this criterion also, the scale appears satisfactory. The ideas of the fulfilment theorists clearly underlie much of the thinking behind the LSR. In particular, the rating is directly relevant to Erikson's ego-integrity (and thus to Peck's concept of ego transcendence); for instance, the resolution and fortitude component is explicitly based on Eriksons's concept. Again the component indicating congruence between desired and achieved goals is clearly related to the actualisation potentialities discussed by Rogers and Maslow, and the self-concept component is clearly related to Rogers's positive regard and positive self-regard. For example, the scale awards a high rating to a respondent 'who thinks of himself as wise, mellow (and thus comfortable in giving advice to others); who feels proud of his accomplishments; who feels he deserves whatever good breaks he has had; who feels he is important to someone else' (Neugarten *et al.*, 1961, p.138). A low rating, on the other hand, will

41

be given to someone who thinks of himself as a burden to others and who speaks disparagingly of himself. The first component (zest) catches Rogers's concept of the fully functioning person open to experience, living fully in each and every moment, rather than being defensive and living according to preconceived plans. The component is intended to catch 'enthusiasm of response and degree of ego-involvement', low scores being given 'for meaningless (and unenjoyed) hyper-activity'. A feeling of not being manipulated but being free to choose alternative courses of action and being creative is caught by the third component, measuring congruence between desired and achieved goals. This component also catches the passivity which Maddi associated with low psychological well-being.

As far as it goes, this is clearly a satisfactory basis for output measurement. Within its limits it has a considerable content validity as well as face validity,[3] although the method of collecting the data required consisted of 'lengthy and repeated interviews covering all aspects of the respondents life pattern, his attitudes and values'. By assumption, the LSR was developed for use with a general sample of the elderly population, and thus the data collected included information on the daily round and the usual weekend round of activities. It related to interaction with other household members, relatives, friends and neighbours, income and work, religion, voluntary organisations; included estimates of the amount of social interaction as compared to the amount at age 45; recorded attitudes towards old age, illness, death and immortality; and contained questions about loneliness, boredom and anger, and questions regarding the respondent's role models and his self-image.

One can best consider its usefulness by considering its application to a production relations study of British old people's homes. In such an application, it would be necessary to face three problems. First, the variance of life satisfaction might in fact be smaller than in the general population because of the constriction of activities imposed by infirmity and the social environment. Applied to a population with less variance in life satisfaction, ratings of the quality achieved by Neugarten *et al.* (1961) would result in lower validity and reliability. Second, the assessment of a sufficient number of persons for the production relations modelling would be expensive. Third, the interviews would have to be conducted by a professional if they were to have credibility and, given the greater probability of low validity, independently validated for a subsample of residents by an independent judge. (The LSR scale is described in detail in Appendix A at the end of this book.)

2.2.5 Life satisfaction Indices A and B

At least one long interview is needed in order to collect sufficient data to make a life satisfaction rating, the interviewer probably needing to be a professionally trained social worker, psychiatrist or psychologist. With this in mind, Neugarten and her associates (1961) set out to design two Life Satisfaction Indices based on short self-report questionnaires — one (Index A) using 'agree/disagree' responses, the other (Index B) having open-ended questions and check-list items scored on a three point scale. Their aim was to design indices which correlated highly with scores on the LSR but which did not require the skills of highly trained interviewers.

The precoded index A, hereinafter referred to as LSI-A, consists of the following twenty items, where the respondent is given a score of 1 if he agrees with questions with an (A) after them or disagrees with a question with a (D) attached, and a score of zero otherwise:

1. As I grow older, things seem better than I thought they would be. (A)
2. I have had more of the breaks in life than most of the people I know. (A)
3. This is the dreariest time of my life. (D)
4. I am just as happy as when I was younger. (A)
5. My life could be happier than it is now. (D)
6. These are the best years of my life. (A)
7. Most of the things I do are boring or monotonous. (D)
8. I expect some interesting and pleasant things to happen to me in the future. (A)
9. The things I do are as interesting to me as they ever were. (A)
10. I feel old and somewhat tired. (D)
11. I feel my age, but it does not bother me. (A)
12. As I look back on my life, I am fairly well satisfied. (A)
13. I would not change my past life even if I could. (A)
14. Compared to other people my age, I've made a lot of foolish decisions in my life. (D)
15. Compared to other people my age, I make a good appearance. (A)
16. I have made plans for things I'll be doing a month or a year from now. (A)
17. When I think back over my life, I didn't get most of the important things I wanted. (D)
18. Compared to other people, I get down in the dumps too often. (D)
19. I've had pretty much what I expected out of life. (A)
20. In spite of what people say, the lot of the average man is getting worse, not better. (D)

The open-ended questionnaire, upon which is based the other index (LSI-B), has twelve questions, responses to which are given scores of 0, 1 or 2 by the interviewer. A scoring key is attached to the list of questions. This second index has rarely been used in gerontological studies (exceptions include Mangold, 1977, and the ten-year study of elderly persons in Newcastle-upon-Tyne reported in Savage *et al.*, 1977), and we do not list its open-ended questions or check-lists here. The interested reader is referred to Neugarten *et al.* (1961, pp. 141-2.)

The validity of the two indices can be examined from a number of standpoints. First, scores on the indices can be compared with scores on the LSR scale and with each other.[4] Second, we can compare the index scores with the ratings of the clinical psychologist previously referred to in section 2.2.4.[5] Both comparisons suggest that the indices attain at least reasonable validity, the LSI-B recording slightly higher correlations. However, an examination of the constituent items reveals that LSI-A has greater *face* validity.[6]

Subsequent research which has either applied or examined the life satisfaction measures of Neugarten, Havighurst and Tobin has concentrated almost entirely upon LSI-A. This is not the place to review the large number of applications of the index (partial reviews are provided by Adams, 1971; and Larson, 1978) but it is important that we take a brief look at some of the subsequent refinements of the instrument. The validity of all three of Neugarten's life satisfaction measures was examined in the previously mentioned 'rural' study of Wood *et al.* (1969). As well as confirming the validity of the instruments, Wood and her colleagues suggested a reduction of the number of items in the LSI-A and modification of the scoring system.[7] A further refinement came from Adams (1969) as a result of factor analysis of the responses from just over 500 non-institutionalised, 'small town' persons aged 65 and over. In their original construction of the LSI-A, Neugarten *et al.* had taken the same five conceptual dimensions of psychological well-being as had been used in the derivation of the LSR scale (see section 2.2.4 above). Adams's intention was to marry up these five conceptual dimensions with the empirically determined dimensions obtained from his own multivariate analyses. In fact, only three usable factors were extracted and identified (mood tone, zest for life and congruence between desired and achieved goals) and a fourth extracted and tentatively identified (resolution and fortitude).[8] Despite the conceptual and empirical validity of this dimensionality for psychological well-being, researchers have been loath to use anything other than a total, unidimensional score. Knapp (1976), however, examined Adams's four dimensions *independently* in relation to a number of biographical, activity, and 'retirement experience' determinants, finding very different patterns of association between dimensions.[9] Finally, Bigot (1974) applied the LSI-A to a British sample of 150 manual and professional workers, before and after retirement, and produced two main factors.[10] He recommended that these factors be used as separate indicators of different facets of psychological well-being, a recommendation taken up by himself and by Knapp (1977b). Surprisingly, Bigot's exciting research has had very little impact on subsequent British gerontological research.

Thus the Neugarten scale has been fairly extensively re-examined, has been compared with other indicators of well-being (broadly defined), has been applied in a large number and a wide variety of gerontological settings, and has been used in conjunction with other indexing methods.[11] (As well as the references above, see Edwards and Klemmack, 1973; Havighurst et al., 1969; Wolk and Telleen, 1976.) However, its inherent multidimensionality has not been exploited sufficiently nor has it been extensively used for institutional populations. (Exceptions are the studies of Curry and Ratcliff, 1973, and Bultena, 1974.) How useful would it be in a study of production relations in residential homes? The multidimensionality problem is relatively easy to overcome. Nevertheless, the application of the LSI-A to an institutionalised population may be difficult for at least a couple of reasons. First, the environments of residents in old people's homes must be more similar than the environments of persons living outside; and second, substantial proportions of residents in homes are confused to a degree that would make invalid their responses to the questions (compare Schmidt, 1975). We must therefore take a look at some of the other psychological well-being measurement instruments that have been suggested.

2.2.6 The Affect Balance Scale

The voluminous literature concerned with the validation and application of the LSIs of Neugarten et al. (1961) is only slightly larger than that inspired by Norman Bradburn's research of the 1960s. Bradburn, basing his work loosely on almost hedonist reasoning, developed the ten-item Affect Balance Scale (ABS) on the basis of validation in studies of an intensity previously unknown (Bradburn and Caplovitz, 1965; Bradburn, 1969). Whilst being a latter-day enunciation of hedonism, the ABS does not imply the Benthamite assumption that all 'pleasures' are qualitatively alike and differ only in quantity, but instead postulates the existence of two distinct dimensions — positive and negative affect. The differential statistical behaviour of these two affect dimensions against external variables further suggests that this duodimensionality is not statistically artifactual.

The ABS has ten items, the first five representing positive affect, and the others negative affect. Each respondent is asked: 'During the past few weeks have you felt . . . ':

1 Pleased about having accomplished something?

2 That things were going your way?
3 Proud that someone complimented you on something you had done?
4 Particularly excited or interested in something?
5 On top of the world?
6 Bored?
7 Depressed or very unhappy?
8 Very lonely or remote from other people?
9 Upset because someone criticised you?
10 So restless that you couldn't sit long in a chair?

Of the positive affect items, two (items 1 and 3) are directly related to Rogers's concept of positive self-regard and a third (item 4) relates to activation. However, the complete absence of anything that might reflect the developmental tasks of the later stages in life is an unfortunate gap as far as the evaluation of services for the aged is concerned; for instance, there is no sign of a question related to Erikson's ego-integrity. The gap is not surprising, since the scale was developed from the self-reports of a population of middle-aged men (Bradburn, 1969, p.57). The negative affect items likewise reflect the developmental tasks of the later stages in life in only a very general way.

Bradburn's distinction between positive and negative affect forms the basis of his indicator of psychological well-being. The pilot study (Bradburn and Caplovitz) had found that the discrepancy between the scores on the positive and negative indices was the important element in determining the relationship between the affect indices and self reports of happiness. The predominance of positive over negative feelings indicates psychological well-being, and a reverse predominance, psychological ill-being. The choice of this indicator appears to have been as much a response to the pattern of correlations in the pilot study as to the theoretical adherence to hedonist philosophy. Quite different factors predicted positive affect than predicted negative affect — the latter reflecting interpersonal tensions, worries, anxieties and other variables associated with mental illness, whilst the former was correlated with, for example, involvement with the environment. Bradburn argued that it was quite plausible to find that quite different things caused positive and negative feelings and quoted precedents from the literature in doing so.

Subsequent work has established various relationships between the ABS and related variables which, together with the relationships reported by Bradburn (1969) contribute to the scale's apparent construct validity (for instance, see Thurnher, 1974). Moriwaki (1974) showed that the global ABS and its two subscales were able to discriminate between normal elderly and elderly psychotics attending an outpatients clinic. The ABS was also significantly related to the degree of role loss, role loss being of particular significance in relation to the developmental tasks of the elderly and the theories of Erikson and others, although Moriwaki did not establish whether the scales discriminated between those who accomplished the developmental task imposed by the role loss successfully. Furthermore, Moriwaki showed the ABS to be correlated (0.61) with the Rosow morale scale and the nine item mental health scale developed by Srole and others (Rosow, 1963; Srole, 1956). However, Moriwaki's conclusion that the ABS is the best role predictor of psychological well-being seems to go beyond his evidence. Graney's work also suggested construct validity (Graney, 1973 and 1975), whilst Bild and Havighurst (1976) recently showed the ABS to be correlated 0.66 with Neugarten's LSI-A scale. Such findings are clearly interesting from the point of view of both validation and simplification. Studies of the quality of life of the elderly in residential care may not need to apply more than one reliable morale measure.

Apart from a minor contribution by Graney, the most considerable development of the ABS was made by Beiser (1974) who added further items, and after factor analysis, added a third dimension which he christened long-term satisfaction. He argued that Bradburn's item about feeling 'on top of the world' (item 5) was meaningless, finding it to have no significant pattern of co-variation with the other four variables defining positive affect. The three items added by Beiser were:

11　Considering the way your life is going at the moment, would you:
　　(a) like it to continue in much the same sort of way?
　　(b) like to change some parts of it?
　　(c) like to change many parts of it?
12　How successful have you been at planning your life, in your work, and with your family? Would you say:
　　(a) very;　(b) somewhat;　(c) undecided?
　　(d) a little unsuccessful?
　　(e) very unsuccessful?
13　Do you feel you have accomplished most of the things you would have liked to, up to this point in your life?
　　Answer yes or no.

These items have far greater face validity as indicating success in developmental task adjustment by the criteria of Erikson and Rogers than the items composed by Bradburn. Beiser showed that each of the three subscales, (positive affect — which he retitled 'pleasurable involvement', negative affect, and long-term satisfaction) were useful as predictors in a regression analysis of answers to the global question: 'Would you say you are very happy, pretty happy, not too happy?' Each dimension contributed to the prediction. Beiser's paper therefore confirms

Outputs

Bradburn's finding that the absence of factors promoting negative affect does not automatically ensure the emergence of positive affect and vice versa, and added to it the argument that items constituting the long-term satisfaction scale demand the long-term time referent and the pleasurable involvement responses. Beiser argued that his respondents clearly made this distinction, and the accumulated case material suggested the dependence of the level of long-term satisfaction upon the availability of, as well as the ability to respond to, emotional ties and the satisfaction that emanates from a long-term relationship. As we shall see below, in this and other respects, there are similarities between the ABS items and those of the Philadelphia Geriatric Center (PGC) morale scale. Appendix B to this chapter (at the end of the book) written by Sheila Peace, John Hall and Graham Hamblin, reports an application of the ABS in a sample of residents in old people's homes in Britain.

2.2.7 The Philadelphia Geriatric Center morale scale

One of the most useful scales to have emerged from that strand of the literature developing indicators of psychological well-being is Lawton's morale scale (Lawton, 1972a, 1975a). The Philadelphia Geriatric Center (PGC) scale was developed in order to meet the needs for 'a multi-dimensional definition of morale, . . . a scale appropriate for the very old; and . . . a scale of such length as to afford reasonable reliability, while at the same time not causing undue fatigue or inattention' (Lawton, 1972a, p.146). There is much evidence that the capacity to take up information declines with age and also that there is a tendency towards more cautious response (Drevenstedt, 1975). Earlier scales for the elderly had been applied mainly to groups who were in their sixties and were less than ideal for application to those of extreme age. Lawton's morale scale was intended to sacrifice the precision hopefully obtained from a large number of sophisticated questions in order to achieve a reliable questionnaire designed to make the task of the aged respondent simpler. The initial development was based upon a pool of fifty items taken from existing scales chosen to represent those components and content areas thought to be related to morale.

In this process of choosing items Lawton selected some aspects as being essential components of the concept. In particular his discussion focused on

(i) 'a basic sense of satisfaction with oneself . . . a feeling of having attained something in life, of being useful' at present, and thinking of oneself as adequate;
(ii) 'a feeling . . . that the people and things in one's life offer some satisfaction to the individual'; doing things with zest

48

in a way that shows a response to the environment; and a struggle for mastery which shows that the life lived is worth struggling with;

(iii) 'a certain acceptance of what cannot be changed', an appreciation of both the positive and negative aspects of old age.

The original pool of fifty items was reduced in three stages to a scale of twenty-two items, following three item analyses and a factor analysis applied to data obtained from 300 residents of an apartment dwelling, and a home for the elderly. These final twenty-two items (with the correct response indicated in parentheses) were:

1 Things keep getting worse as I get older. (No)
2 I have as much pep as I did last year. (Yes)
3 How much do you feel lonely? (Not much)
4 Little things bother me more this year. (No)
5 I see enough of my friends and relatives. (Yes)
6 As you get older you are less useful. (No)
7 If you could live where you wanted, where would you live? (Here)
8 I sometimes worry so much that I can't sleep. (No)
9 As I get older, things are (better, worse, same) than/as I thought they would be. (Better)
10 I sometimes feel that life isn't worth living. (No)
11 I am as happy now as I was when I was younger. (Yes)
12 Most days I have plenty to do. (Yes)
13 I have a lot to be sad about. (No)
14 People had it better in the old days. (No)
15 I am afraid of a lot of things. (No)
16 My health is good/not so good. (Good)
17 I get mad more than I used to. (No)
18 Life is hard for me most of the time. (No)
19 How satisfied are you with your life today? (Satisfied)
20 I take things hard. (No)
21 A person has to live for today and not worry about tomorrow. (Yes)
22 I get upset easily. (No)

Items operationalising the desired characteristics (i) — (iii) above would have considerable face validity in the context of personality theory; seeing the positive and negative sides of the ageing process is clearly related to ego-integrity, the basic sense of satisfaction is much the same as what Rogers called positive self-regard, and zest is a characteristic of a fully functioning person, just as the struggle for mastery is equivalent to a drive for self-actualisation. However, in the event, the individual items do not appear to cover the main characteristics dis-

Outputs

tinguished by personality theory with as much precision as LSI-A. Item 6 is clearly related to positive (or rather negative) self-regard, item 12 relates to the level of activation, and item 10 is related to lack of zest. A number of the items reflect what might be a failure to achieve ego-integrity and certainly capture the vulnerability, apprehension and anxiety that follow the losses which precipitate entry into a home. Like the ABS, the items altogether lack the time perspective needed to assess developmental task adjustment. But the items have far more face validity if one's point of reference is psychiatric symptomatology among the aged than if one's reference is normal human growth and development in later life. The presence of negative affect items associated with psychiatric disorder is not necessarily a weakness in measuring psychological well-being of residents in homes for the aged. It is clear that the prevalence of such symptoms in noninstitutionalised aged populations receiving social services is considerable. (Hence the emphasis on some of the symptoms in Goldberg *et al.*, 1970, and their coverage in, for instance, Wright, 1974 and 1978.) Lawton himself suggested that the full coverage of morale should include more items on positive affect so that one could indeed test whether positive and negative affect were independently determined (Lawton, 1975a, p.88). He also suggested 'better representation of items relating to self-perceived discontinuity of personality and . . . a more subtly phrased group of items evaluating the environment' (Lawton, 1972a, p.162), though these would be more valuable as an indicator of quasi-input than as one of the outputs in the context of our approach.

However, one must not judge an instrument simply by the face validity of its items; the PGC morale scale showed considerable internal consistency and test-retest correlations of 0.75 and 0.91, though admittedly on small samples. (Further reliability tests have been carried out by other users of the scale, notably Morris and Sherwood, 1975; and McCaffree and Harkins, 1976.) The initial investigation did not, however, provide an adequate test of concurrent validity, Lawton himself admitting that the validity criterion was based on 'casual observations gained from people whose primary activity in relation to subjects was other than that of rating their morale' (Lawton, 1972a, p.159).[12] An attempt was thus made to apply Neugarten's life satisfaction ratings on the basis of an interview lasting between thirty minutes and one hour (Neugarten *et al.* had based their ratings for most subjects on a number of interviews). Correlation with the life satisfaction ratings was 0.57, which was not very different from the correlation (of 0.55) derived by Neugarten *et al.* (1961) for LSI-A (and markedly better if one accepts Lawton's arguments for revision of the Neugarten validity test). However, it is not clear from the paper whether or not the *same* psychologist undertook both the LSR rating and the informal rating —

presumably not, since some contamination of the LSR rating would otherwise have been likely. Moreover, Lawton looked at the correlation with LSR only in those cases in which a psychologist and an administrator were in agreement in their judgment. These could well have been the most clear-cut cases, but conversely Lawton's validity test would apply to an older and more institutionalised sample. One would expect the application of a rating or a scale to such a sample to yield scores a higher proportion of whose variance would be due to error. This would be expected because there would be less environmental variation to cause variation in well-being itself, and since a high proportion of the older and more institutionalised sample would have difficulty in coping with the items. Thus it is not obvious that the apparently worse face validity of the PGC items necessarily resulted in a less useful scale.[13]

Almost as important as the face validity of the items is the stability and meaning of the factor structure yielded by them. Lawton initially found a six-dimensional factor structure (surgency; attitude toward own ageing; acceptance of status quo; agitation; easy-going optimism; and lonely dissatisfaction) which he subsequently abandoned in the light of analyses undertaken by Morris and Sherwood (1975) in a large study of institutionalised populations. These authors found only three factors in common with those of Lawton — tranquillity (a factor that corresponds to Lawton's agitation), satisfaction with life progression (corresponding to Lawton's attitude towards ageing), and lonely dissatisfaction. Lawton's (1975a) analysis of further data confirmed the stability of these dimensions.[14] The agitation dimension is closely related to the ABS negative affect concept (compare items in section 2.2.6), and is itself a manifest anxiety scale.

The three dimensions distinguished by Lawton are not very different from morale concepts found in other work, such as that of Pierce and Clark (1973) and Schooler (1970b). Schooler's study added to twenty-one of the original PGC items a further twenty morale items and four items from the Srole Anomie scale. His results were interesting not only because they reproduced the three factors from Morris and Sherwood and showed item consistency, but also because the factor analysis reproduced as a fourth dimension the Srole Anomie Scale. The anomie among residents of homes is clearly regarded as important by British writers like Meacher (1972), on the confused elderly, and Tunstall (1966) on old people living in the community. It may be that together the three factors (a) — (c) and an anomie dimension reflect stable entities of real importance for populations which include many who recently have undergone a major crisis to which they have not yet adjusted.[15]

In this chapter we have looked at a number of conceptual and empirical attempts to assess the psychological well-being of elderly individuals, and particularly those persons living in old people's homes. The later sections focused on three important and substantial bodies of gerontological literature — those relating to, and inspired by, the life satisfaction perspective of Neugarten et al. (1961), the affect balance model of Bradburn (1969), and the morale scaling procedure of Lawton (1972a). Each perspective has been examined from both theoretical and practical standpoints and each has been found to have relative advantages and disadvantages when compared with the developmental models of some psychologists and personality theorists and when subjected to comprehensive batteries of reliability and validity checks.

Of course, this is not to suggest that there have been no other psychological well-being measures. The gerontological literature itself harbours a very large number of morale and life satisfaction measurement instruments, and the so-called subjective social indicators movement has produced a similar number. Unfortunately, far too many of the suggested 'scales' and 'indices' of well-being, happiness, morale, or life satisfaction to be found in the gerontological literature are little more than random collections of arbitrarily scored items. Even the most rudimentary piloting procedures are ignored.[16] In stark contrast to these unreliable 'measures' stand the impressive, and generally impeccably prepared, subjective well-being scales of the social indicators movement.

Some of these subjective social indicators conceptualise global psychological well-being as the sum of satisfactions in different domains of living, which are in turn conceptualised as the sums of scores of items at a subdomain level (Campbell and Converse, 1970; OECD, 1974). Hall (1976) and his former colleagues of the SSRC Survey Unit have applied this approach in the UK. However, the approach, because of its simplicity and theoretical agnosticism, applied to a situation in which defences are likely to be aroused by questions about satisfaction with the environment, might well result in indicators with rather more substantial bias than those approaches discussed above. The 'domains of living' model has nevertheless been used in some gerontological settings. For example, Cavan, Burgess, Havighurst and Goldhamer (1949) used a seventy-item Attitude Inventory which included questions on the elderly person's satisfaction in relation to family, friends, work, recreation, religion, social organisation, health, and economic status. Two decades later a cross-national study also administered from Chicago looked at satisfaction in some of the domains of living (Havighurst et al., 1969), and there are other similar examples (e.g., Jackson, et al., 1977).

Another strand of the social indicators movement has adopted the approach pioneered by Cantril (1965) and in particular his so-called life satisfaction 'ladder'. The respondent is shown a ten-rung ladder (marked zero to nine), with the top rung representing the 'best possible life' and the bottom rung the 'worst possible life', and asked to indicate his own current life position. The Cantril ladder has been used in a longitudinal study of ageing by Palmore and his colleagues at the Duke Center for the Study of Aging and Human Development, North Carolina (Palmore, 1974; Palmore and Luikart, 1972). Recently, Palmore and Kivett (1977) examined *changes* in life satisfaction over a four-year period among a sample of nearly 400 community residents, aged between 46 and 70, using the same ladder. Whilst such longitudinal evidence is extremely interesting (and virtually unique), the face validity of the ladder remains rather doubtful in the light of some of the theoretical considerations reviewed above if it purports to measure anything other than very global affect or happiness.

The wealth of previous research, both theoretical and empirical, has thus produced a number of reliable and reasonably valid instruments eminently suitable for the measurement of psychological well-being in residential populations of elderly people. British applications of these various instruments have, in the past, been relatively few and far between. We would hope, therefore, that the encouraging recent surge of interest in the morale, life satisfaction and psychological well-being of the residents of British old people's homes pays due care and attention to the experiences of North American research in this area. In such a way it should be possible to avoid many of the pitfalls there encountered, and to move very much closer towards an output concept valid by the criteria of the social welfare paradigm.

Chapter 3

Other outputs

In this chapter we continue our discussion of the outputs of residential care of the elderly. The previous chapter was concerned with probably the most important general dimension of output — the psychological well-being of residents. We now therefore turn to a consideration of two other general dimensions of residential home output:

    (a) outputs other than those that contribute directly to resident psychological well-being but which are received principally by residents; and

    (b) outputs enjoyed principally by residents' 'significant others', generally their kith and kin.

Our treatment of these two general dimensions of residential home output, and particularly of the former, 'resident', dimensions, will be seen to diverge a little from previous studies of the outputs or outcomes of social care of the elderly. The key to this divergence is the production of welfare model outlined in the opening chapter of this essay (see also chapter 7). Outputs are defined as those consequences of care that so directly reflect aspects of welfare that they are valued in their own right. Thus, it is immediately obvious that some outcomes or effects of residential care are, in the nomenclature of our model, not final outputs at all, but rather intermediate outputs or inputs. We therefore postpone our detailed discussion of these factors until Part three. Of course, some of these 'resident intermediate outputs' will themselves be extremely important in the determination and definition of outputs enjoyed principally by the relatives and friends of residents. The psychological well-being of relatives, for example, may well be enhanced more by perceptions of an adequate quality of *care* than by the resident's own perceptions of quality of *life*. These points we shall take up again in the sections that follow.

3.1 Benefits to residents not contributing directly to psychological well-being

Resident psychological well-being, life satisfaction, or morale is seen to play a central part in both the theoretical and empirical studies of residential care of the elderly. As Morris (1974, p.61) states: 'Morale records a person's overall level of satisfaction with his life and the events upon which it has been, and is now being, built'. Among the advantages inherent in the use of self-report morale as an 'impact criterion' (Wylie, 1970) or output indicator are that it obviates the need for:

(a) establishing an external set of standards for performance;
(b) deciding on the applicability of external sets of standards for an elderly sample who, in many ways, are independent of tight societal expectations and controls (Bennett, 1963);
(c) deciding on what behaviour to observe, and for how long; and
(d) deciding how to integrate contradictory behaviour (Morris, 1974)

However, this is not to suggest that psychological well-being and its constituent dimensions, should be the sole focus of attention. There are a number of other dimensions of individual resident well-being whose importance has long been recognised from a variety of standpoints. It is to these that we briefly turn in this section.

3.1.1 Mortality

There are a great many aspects of mortality that are salient to our 'production model' of residential care services for the elderly. The question of predicting survival in a residential context has been addressed by many generations of gerontologists, geriatricians and social administrators. Equally important, however, are the problems of bereavement and grief, of coping with death and dying, of 'social death', and of the social role of the dying person. Feelings of bereavement, loss and grief on the part of relatives and friends of the deceased resident will generally be mixed with feelings of relief and acceptance of the inevitability of death, just as the ageing resident will himself approach death with an ambivalence of emotions. Some of the American literature makes 'death with dignity' one of the half dozen most significant objectives of long-term care (Callahan, 1979).

The question of bereavement is therefore taken up again in section 3.2.[1] Death is not only a physiological state or process, but also a social phenomenon (Atchley, 1977, p.180):

People are socially dead when we no longer treat them as people but as unthinking, unfeeling objects. Social death has occurred when people talk *about* the dying person rather than to the dying person even when the dying person is capable of hearing and understanding what is being said. Thus, social death sometimes occurs *before* physical death.

Thus it is possible to observe residents of old people's homes who have been 'assigned the social role of dying person', often signifying the total dominance by environmental factors (or 'press') over the dwindling personal resources of the dying resident. Viewed in this light, social death is a concept to which we shall return later in this essay, and particularly in chapter 5.

It is unlikely that many gerontologists would argue against the inclusion of mortality in the list of outcome or output dimensions for a residential home, although there are few explicit arguments in favour (recent exceptions include Manard, Woehle and Heilman, 1977; and Noelker and Harel, 1977). There have, however, been a large number of previous studies which have examined the effects of a variety of social and personal characteristics and events upon mortality rates in residential care settings.

Although the evidence contained in much of the literature is ambiguous with respect to causality there can be no questioning the high mortality rate in the period immediately following entry into a residential home (Carp, 1966; Lawton and Yaffe, 1970; Lieberman, 1969, 1974; Liebowitz, 1974; Markson and Cumming, 1974; Wittels and Botwinick, 1974). The mortality rates are particularly high during the first three months. Of course, there are many factors which will affect the impact of residential relocation on the well-being and survival of the ageing person. Schulz and Brenner (1977) recently reviewed the so-called 'relocation literature' and set out a theoretical model which brings together a number of personal and social factors under an umbrella concept of *control*. Loss of control has been found to be partially responsible for early death (Schulz, 1976; Schulz and Alderman, 1973). Graney (1977) addresses a related question, concerning the social factors that influence the sex differential in mortality. He concluded that this differential will gradually disappear as a result of more equalised social and economic opportunities for women. Whilst his study looked at the elderly in general, and did not focus on the institutionalised aged, Graney's conclusion has implications for the long range planning of care services for this section of the population – for the present range and character of these services has been very much influenced in the past by the greater longevity of women. The body of available evidence would therefore suggest that it is both personal *and* social (environmental) factors which influence survival rates amongst the institutionalised elderly. We must therefore treat with some caution the conclusion of Manard *et al.* (1977, p.74) that 'people die because they are sick, and not because they lack nursing care'. Callahan (1979) lists the prolonging of longevity among his most important objectives of long-term care. We return to the impact of environmental factors on well-being (broadly defined) in chapter 5 and take a further look at personal characteristics in chapter 6.

3.1.2 Morbidity[2]

Like mortality, morbidity can be regarded as an output in the sense that variations in it are in part attributable to variations in inputs and quasi-inputs. If persons were randomly distributed with respect to morbidity-generating characteristics between homes, a production model would allow the assessment of the degree to which observed variations in morbidity (and mortality) were caused by input and quasi-input variations. However, random distribution is not a reasonable assumption and difficulties may therefore arise from the fact that we are unable to take sufficient account of the factors affecting life and health expectancy without careful (and expensive) medical examination. On the other hand, these omissions will raise difficulties of rather less consequence if one uses the term morbidity to refer to functional or social health, rather than biological health. For example, physical incapacity has been shown to be sensitive to the presence of physical and social prostheses and the degree to which residents are encouraged to use their capacities (Kushlick and Blunden, 1974; Lawton and Cohen, 1974; MacDonald and Butler, 1974).

One must be careful to distinguish between three interrelated, but nevertheless distinct, morbidity or health concepts: self-rated health, functional health, and what we may term 'objective health'. All three concepts may lay valid claim to inclusion in a multidimensional output variable, but there are dramatic differences between them when one considers their respective justifications for inclusion and the ease with which data can be captured to indicate them. Measures of self-rated health have become increasingly popular in gerontological studies in recent years, a popularity due in no small way to the considerable ease of assessment ('How would you rate your health?') and the apparent importance of self-rated health in the determination of psychological well-being. (See Larson, 1978, p.119 for a review.) Most researchers are agreed that a measure of self-rated health would be a highly unreliable indicator of physical or mental status. What is not clear, however, is whether the concept stands as an important piece of gerontological information in its own right or whether it is merely a component of morale. Some researchers employ morale indicators which include a self-rated health item (for example, the unrevised PGC morale scale — see section 2.2.7 above), whilst others prefer to keep the concepts definitionally independent (Palmore and Luikart, 1972).

In terms of the dual criterion of theoretical validity and practical measurement, measures of self-rated health and of 'objective health' are poles apart. 'Objective health' is essentially biological health as rated, perhaps, by an experienced physician, possibly with the aid of a fully equipped pathology laboratory. The concept is very difficult to define and measure and, whilst valid as an outcome indicator in its own right, these difficulties have led researchers to favour measures of functional or social health — the well-being of an individual in his normal social context (Fanshel, 1972, p.319):

A person is well if he is able to carry on his usual daily activities. To the extent that he cannot, he is in a state of dysfunction, or deviation from well-being. . . . Clearly, we have described health as a social phenomenon.

A social or functional perspective on morbidity has the appealing virtues of being both valid and operational. It is not surprising, therefore, to find a long and developmental series of indices and scales for its measurement, many of which have recently been the subject of review — physical function instruments by Wright (1974, 1978), and mental function instruments by, for example, Pyrek and Snyder (1977) and Challis (1978).[3]

As the human body ages there is a deterioration in both physical and mental function. Biological ageing or senescence is a gradual, individual, and inevitable process, and involves the deterioration of the major organs of the body, the nervous, circulatory and digestive systems, and the ability to resist disease. Reliance on physical function, or change in physical function, as an outcome measure in a model of old people's homes must therefore take careful account of this natural and inevitable deteriorative change. With this in mind, there would appear to be two approaches to outcome assessment in a production model of the form described in this essay. Firstly, one can take *compensation* for ill-health or disability, rather than ill-health or disability *per se*, as the relevant outcome dimension. Secondly, one can attempt to identify and compare the factors which accompany different rates of deterioration in order to determine those that are beneficial and those that are detrimental. Quite a number of policy documents stress the former compensation approach to outcome measurement (see Challis, 1978, or Wright, 1974, for partial reviews), whilst the latter, Markov-type, approach is being successfully applied by Wright (1974, 1978).

As well as these physical changes, ageing is also characterised by a deterioration in sensory acuity (Brophy, Ernst and Shore, 1977, p. 1):

Sensory change that accompanies ageing is basically one of decline in sensitivity and affects the various modalities differently. There is an enormous variation among aged individuals as to the type and extent of sensory loss that they experience. . . . The degree of handicap that sensory decline imposes upon an individual also varies widely.

It is not clear how far sensory impairment and decline is determined by personal factors and how far by environmental factors, particularly within the old people's home. Once again, it is the *compensation* for sensory loss that is the important output of residential care. A study of hearing impairment amongst the residents of twelve homes in North Yorkshire indicated that the impaired were rated by staff as 'More confused, socially isolated and paranoid than their less impaired peers, but this probably represented stereotyping rather than residents' actual behaviour' (Martin and Peckford, 1977, p.2). In other words, if the inference of these two researchers is correct, residents with marked sensory impairment will be given other labels which represent *reduced* compensation for impairment. Brophy *et al.* (1977) have developed a conveniently short instrument for the assessment of sensory loss – in hearing, vision, smell, taste, tactile sensitivity, dexterity and balance. It would seem to be possible to use this type of instrument as a basis for an output dimension measure, provided one recognised the need for assessing the degree to which the caring environment helped the resident overcome his impairment.

The third aspect of morbidity is mental function or health. Generally, mental or psychological change in old age is less visible and less well understood than either the physical or sensory changes. We have already discussed some of the changes in personality as an individual ages and these 'personality developments' have been used to generate and subsequently validate our central output concept of psychological well-being (see chapter 2). In addition, there are changes in intellect, although not all dimensions of intelligence necessarily change with age. Evidence on the observed changes is not unambiguous but it seems that there are declines in memory and drive, and the abilities to categorise and to feel emotions. Rigidity, the opposite of creativity, tends to increase with age. Many of these changes may, however, be more representative of the influence of social factors than of developmental processes. As with physical function and sensory acuity, there have been a number of attempts to develop scales and indices for the measurement of psychological function and its decline. Also in common with these other two dimensions of morbidity, there are a number of recent reviews of these various measurement instruments and we do not therefore attempt to review them here (Challis, 1978; Copeland *et al.*, 1976; Pitt, 1974; Pyrek and Snyder, 1977; Snyder *et al.*, 1978). In the residential context researchers have tended to focus on anxiety, depression and, most frequently, confusion. Lipman and Slater, working from the Welsh School of Architecture, pulled together a number of previous mental status questionnaires for use in their study of the architectural design implications of residential homes for the elderly. They found that a very simple rating of resident confusion by the matron of the home (rational/moderately confused/severely confused) was related significantly to scores obtained from their carefully developed 21-item confusion assessment schedule. Confusion scores were significantly related to a number of architectural and environmental characteristics (Lipman and Slater, 1975, 1977a). A few years earlier, Meacher's (1972) study of the elderly mentally infirm had shown how confusion is often an adaptive response to incongruence between the environment and the resident, and a smaller study of ten old people's homes in Cheshire suggested that resident confusion was higher in environments providing more activity (Townsend and Kimbell, 1975). However the relationships between environment, personality disorder, depressive states, and confusion have generated a large literature, as has their measurement (Challis, 1978). It is not dealt with here. Whilst we would have a few methodological reservations about some of the studies that have been performed, there is no denying the weight of theoretical and empirical support for treating confusion as an output variable.

Central to our general discussion of the output concept is a comparison of the welfare consequences of intervention and non-intervention. In the case of morbidity, this comparison will be particularly problematic in view of the deteriorations in physical, sensory and mental function that constitute the ageing process. However, research efforts to increase our understanding of these deteriorative processes and the factors which influence them will at the same time make the output measurement problem a little more tractable.

3.1.3 Other dimensions

Any feature employed by the resident and regarded by him as of value in its own right is potentially an output, however many of them contribute (and with whatever importance) to his more general assessment of his psychological well-being. Indeed, the justification as far as the resident is concerned for experiencing these features is that they *do* contribute to his global well-being. This fact is implicitly recognised in some of the American literature, but is of practical significance only in as much as it is feasible to attempt the hierarchical approach to psychological well-being discussed, for example, by McKennell (1974). Hall and Ring (1974) have implemented the hierarchical approach in a general population and consider a large number of the features to be important.

However, as argued above, the recipient's perception of his welfare is not what directly determines the need judgment. The 'need' judgment is the outcome of many factors and separate decisions, contributed to by many — including recipients, their significant others, professionals and politicians in local and central government. To the degree that the need judgment is made within a clear intellectual framework, it is that of the policy paradigm — in this case the social welfare paradigm — which provides an operating ideology with a pervasive influence on value choices, perceptions of material fact, assumptions about cause and effect, and expectations about the consequences of alternative interventions.

The social welfare paradigm treats as consequences to be valued in their own right those factors which may be treated as unimportant by the resident, and to other factors it may impose different weights from those of residents. Probably central and local government applies a greater weight to the prevention of personal disaster because of a fire in the home than does the resident. They act as if to be burnt to death in an old people's home is a far more serious affair than to be burnt to death in one's own home. No doubt this is because someone who is a resident in a council home is more clearly a council responsibility than is someone, of equal infirmity or confusion, living alone in their own home with or without the support of substantial state inputs of day and domiciliary care. Indeed, several types of input are quite clearly accorded importance in their own right by the social welfare paradigm, irrespective of the degree to which the psychological well-being of residents is affected by them; in particular, some that are related to the most basic categories of Maslow's typology of needs, such as nutrition, cleanliness and warmth. A comprehensive listing of the outcome dimensions suggested by the social welfare paradigm has been recently provided by Challis (1978). He suggests seven dimensions in the context of community care of the elderly: nurturance, compensation for disability, independence, morale, social integration, family relationships and community development. There are, of course, an abundance of alternative dimensionalities and typologies, including the interesting model of Golant and McCaslin (1977) which builds on a competence-independence dichotomy. However, when it comes to the practical application of such classifications of output for policy-making purposes, most researchers depend on the major output dimensions outlined above — psychological well-being, mortality, functional status and mental status.[4]

3.2 Outputs enjoyed principally by residents' significant others

Residents' 'significant others' — their concerned relatives and friends — are major beneficiaries from residential provision. Benefits of two kinds may be distinguished — those flowing during the process of, and immediately subsequent to, entry of the aged relative or friend to the home, and those experienced in the period of residence as a whole. These benefits are not separate; they merely have a different incidence. At first residents' significant others express feelings of relief from the strain and responsibility of caring for a dependent and often sick elderly person, but feelings tinged with doubt, guilt and loss. Later, when residence of their aged relative or friend in the home has been fully accepted and adjusted to, the benefits and disbenefits to significant others flow mainly from their perceptions of the quality of care in the home and the quality of life of the residents. Comparisons of the costliness, desirability, and social efficacy of alternative modes of care for the needy elderly have all too often ignored the feelings of strain and responsibility of significant others, and the social and economic restrictions forced upon them. Widely recognised as important, these factors are rarely subjected to the detailed examination they clearly deserve in a practical context.

An immediate benefit of the admission to a home of a dependent person is relief of relatives from strain and responsibility (Cartwright, Hockey and Anderson, 1973; Davies and Duncan, 1975; Isaacs, Livingstone and Neville, 1972; Karcher and Linden, 1974). Many dependent elderly persons in the community live with a sibling or child, themselves often of an age where such additional burdens can be intolerable. The studies mentioned above, and others, have identified many aspects of strain or burden — adverse influences on the mental and physical health of the carer, interference with social and leisure activities, disruption of the household routine and of normal intra-family relationships, and overcrowding of the residence. The middle-aged single woman, frail elderly relatives and spouses, and families with children in housing inadequate to accommodate grandma as well as others, have been particularly the subject of concern. From an economic point of view, a family's responsibility for an elderly relative severely restricts opportunities for employment and imposes an additional financial burden. Strains may lead to intolerance, manifested perhaps through physical ill-treatment or by making life unpleasant for the elderly relative, and significant others may additionally experience tension brought on by feelings of inadequate provision of care (Davies and Duncan, 1975). Admittance of an elderly person to an old people's home thus lifts the burden of care, protection and economic support from the shoulders of children, siblings and friends and removes the concomitant strains and tensions. At the same time, however, residents' significant others may have feelings of guilt because of their failure to care or because they discharged their caring duties so readily (Stevenson *et al.*, 1978), and feelings of loss from the removal of various psychological comforts. Linn and Gurel (1972) found that family opposition to nursing home placement was related to the elderly patient's estrangement and isolation from family and community.

Another aspect of the output question concerns the general psychological well-being of residents' significant others as influenced by, for example, the removal of strain and the feelings of guilt elucidated above, as well as perceptions of the quality of care in the home and of the quality of life of residents. Family ties and relationships generally get closer as one moves from middle to old age, sibling and filial concern for the elderly person being particularly strong (Cicirelli, 1977; Seelbach and Sauer, 1977; Shanas *et al.*, 1968). The satisfaction of significant others with the residential environment and with the individual resident's position within it will thus be an important benefit of residential care. The most visible and tangible element is the quality of care provided in the home. Greenwald and Linn (1970) questioned the wives of new admissions to a small sample of American nursing homes. The most common complaint was of inadequate services, followed by poor food and improper diet, lack of therapy or recreation, infrequent visits by a physician, lack of medication, absence of 'convenience items', and over-sedation.[5]

As well as quality of *care*, the benefits and disbenefits to significant others will be influenced by the quality of *life* — that is, the morale and general well-being of the residents — as *reported* by residents and as perceived by themselves during visits to the home. All life events of the resident within the home have a potential influence, but the event with the greatest impact is clearly death. Bereavement can take three forms (Atchley, 1977, chapter 10): physical, emotional, and intellectual. Zach (1978) reports a Welsh study which found the mortality rate of widows in the first year after bereavement increased ten-fold, and Kalish (1976) documents a wide range of physical reaction from frequent sighing to stomach upsets. In the first six months of widowhood, the likelihood of seeking psychiatric help increases dramatically, depression, anxiety, anger and grief being the most common symptoms (Parkes, 1972a). The final aspect of bereavement — the intellectual aspect — concerns the idealisation or 'purification' of the deceased, and is of little significance in the present context (Lopata, 1973). Whilst resident mortality has received most attention in the literature, it is clear that all dimensions of well-being previously discussed in this and other chapters make a secondary appearance in the production of welfare model through their ability to confer benefits and disbenefits on residents' significant others.

The social welfare paradigm treats some client states and inputs as having an importance that is quite independent of their contribution to the psychological well-being of residents or significant others. Because many of these are inputs, they are more easily measured than psychological well-being, and so more adequate account has been taken of them in research, particularly in British research. We have devoted little space to them here not because we think them to be un-important, but partly because more account has been taken of them in other literature, and partly because we judge that some of them bulk large in the literature of the policy paradigm because they are *assumed* to influence the psychological well-being of residents. If they bulk large for that reason, they must be treated as inputs in empirical studies embodying the production relations approach: their importance is based merely on an hypothesised set of consequences whose existence it is the business of a production relations study to test. Therefore there are some characteristics of residents and of the home that are discussed as inputs in the next three chapters, although they have some-times been treated as if they were outputs in previous research and have been discussed in policy documents in a way that does not indi-cate that they are of importance in their own right. Similarly, the benefits and disbenefits to significant others are many, and some are subtle; but they have been too neglected in the literature for our discussion of them to have much depth.

Part three

Inputs and the production process

The three chapters of Part three discuss inputs and the process of the production of welfare in residential homes. Our discussion is arranged around three simplifying dichotomies. We first distinguish *resource inputs* from other inputs. Resource inputs are the tangible factors entering the production process, inputs which probably receive most of the attention in the policy literature. They are discussed in chapter 4 under the usual headings of labour and capital. This first distinction, between resource and other factors, is maintained in order to highlight the respective foci of economic production models and gerontological and psychological studies.

Our second dichotomy is to distinguish within the 'other inputs' group, between what we may call the *non-resource inputs* and the *quasi-inputs*. Both sets of inputs are intangible influences upon output, and the distinction that we draw between them is that the former are largely *within* the domain of control of the 'producer' (in this case, the director of social services, the matron, or the resident perhaps), whereas the latter are largely exogenous influences upon output in the sense of being *outside* the producer's domain of control. (By exogenous influences we mean influences which are not substantially caused by other factors dealt with in the argument.) These exogenous quasi-inputs are accepted by the producer as parameters of the production process. It is not our intention in this book to attempt to draw a thick dividing line between the endogenous and the exogenous influences upon output. Endogeneity is a concept — and in many respects an *empirical* concept — which is strictly defined relative to the time-scale of an investigation or policy initiative. Furthermore, the social welfare and gerontological literatures are as yet not sufficiently well developed to permit of any definitive empirical classification of endogeneity/exogeneity of influence. Our discussion of the non-resource and the quasi-inputs may however cast some light on the question of endogeneity,

67

and therefore policy control, of important influences upon resident well-being.

Our third and final dichotomy is the basis for our allocation of non-resource and quasi-inputs to chapters 5 and 6. Roughly speaking, these factors fall into two broad groups. Firstly, there are those influences which are brought into the production process by the residents themselves — such as physical well-being at entry, experiences during various phases of adjustment to life in the home (entry into it and adjustment to its milieu), and some rather more durable characteristics attributable to personality and life experience. Some of these factors will exhibit variations which are correlated with variations in resource inputs and which have a direct influence upon outputs. Resident well-being at the point of entry (physical ability, confusion, sensory acuity, affect, and so on), for example, will have this characteristic. Secondly, there are those quasi-inputs and non-resource inputs which arise out of the interaction of resource inputs with resident characteristics and behaviour, staff attitudes and broad societal norms, principal among these being the social environment of the home, a shorthand term for the myriad of dimensions, practices, controls, activities and mores obtaining therein. Chapters 5 and 6 discuss non-resource and quasi-inputs and some of the leading studies of approaches to measuring salient aspects of each, and their relation to dimensions of final output. Chapter 5 focuses on social environment and chapter 6 on personal (resident) characteristics.

Chapter 4

Resource inputs:
labour and capital

For the purposes of this chapter we shall distinguish two broad categories of resource inputs — manpower and capital, the former comprising
all human, and the latter all non-human, resources used to produce the
various outputs discussed in Part two. Clearly, it will be difficult to
separate these influences from the social environmental influences to be
discussed in the following chapter. Indeed, our classification scheme
for residential environments in that chapter will include various aspects
of resource input influences as special subgroups. In this chapter, therefore, we particularly concentrate on the problems of measuring the
resource inputs, and detail some of their expected and established influences upon dimensions of output. A concluding section briefly considers
a third category of resource inputs — the so-called 'consumables'.

4.1 The manpower input

The manpower input into a production process has three basic components — the number of staff, whether paid or unpaid, in each of the
various staff categories distinguished; the number of hours worked by
each of them; and the nature and quality of the services rendered
during these hours (what some economists have tended to naively
label the 'intensity of effort'). In this section we arrange our discussion
around these three components. We shall see that the first two components — the number of staff and the hours worked — present few
problems of interpretation or measurement for the researcher. In
contrast, the third is difficult to describe without referring to its
effectiveness, and has so many facets that we cannot hope to adequately cover them all here. The numerous and oft-voiced issues concerning the education, training, secondment, support and supervision of
residential staff are all relevant to the discussion of the quality of the
manpower input. The importance of this third component cannot

be overemphasised in a residential care context, or indeed in any human service context, but only recently have economists turned their attention to the 'intensity of effort' and other quality variables in their studies of more conventional production processes. This has the unfortunate consequence that, whilst our basic production model and nomenclature have their roots in the economist's theory of the firm, much of the 'manpower economics' literature and many of the production studies are of little relevance.

We now discuss these manpower components in some detail. We first distinguish the various *types* of manpower in residential care, and list some of the corresponding tasks within the home. Second, we briefly consider the *numbers* of staff employed in the home, how these numbers are influenced by home and resident characteristics, and some related issues. Finally, we look at the effectiveness of their performance, focusing particularly on staff attitudes and, to a lesser degree, on training and support.

4.1.1 Types of residential manpower

The most common breakdown of residential staff is into three, or possibly four, major groups: supervisory, care, domestic and office and secretarial staff. This classification was used, for example, in the Residential Census of 1970 (DHSS, 1975) and has been the basis for most central and local collections of manpower information. Of course, classifications are useful only to the extent that they reflect real divisions in the roles and tasks of residential staff. Valerie Imber (1977, p.1) followed up the Census collection with a detailed study of staffing in a dozen local authority old people's homes to examine:

> the extent to which the labels used in the classification covered homogeneous groups of staff, . . . to discover whether a distinction could be drawn between domestic and care staff, . . . [and] to examine the feasibility of distinguishing two types of care staff – those who provided nursing care and those who provided the social care which is regarded as the major function of residential homes and distinguishes them from either nursing homes or hotels.

Her careful statistical analyses revealed that the distinction between supervisory, care and domestic staff was meaningful, with domestic staff keeping the home clean and tidy and care staff providing similar services to residents and attempting to provide for their social and psychological needs. Imber's detailed listing (ibid., p.26) of tasks performed by these groups was as follows:

(i) Supervisory staff – 'administering drugs, changing dressings, reading to residents, playing games with residents, organising social events, and paperwork'.[1]

(ii) Care staff — 'washing clothes, washing residents, dressing residents, making beds and taking residents to the toilet, sluicing'.

(iii) Domestic staff — 'preparing food, cleaning, tidying and washing up'.

A re-analysis of Residential Census data for 200 old people's homes provides further evidence of the validity of this classification schema. Variations in the number of staff in each of the three major categories, and in the corresponding staff-resident ratios, were found to respond in markedly different ways to variations in resident characteristics, aspects of home design, and the provision of 'peripheral services' (Knapp, 1979). We shall return to these variations in the next subsection.

As well as these conventional, and in many respects essential, man-power inputs to residential care, there are a number of other people whose input into the caring process should not be ignored. These other manpower groups are separated only because their input is less regular, is arguably non-essential in some cases, and is frequently peripatetic. The most common of these is the input of medical and nursing exper-tise. At a time when the overall and average dependency of residents of old people's homes is increasing at a considerable rate, the medical and nursing input must necessarily increase correspondingly, and general supervisory and care staff 'are not expected to provide the professional kind of health care that is properly the function of the primary health care services' (DHSS, 1977, paragraph 3). There are a number of arguments for and against a resident keeping his own general practitioner after entering a home (Greenfield, 1976). On the one hand, the resident's own GP helps maintain links with the com-munity and with significant others, and can reduce the risk of institu-tionalisation and regimentation. At the same time, however, this practice can be very inconvenient and doesn't allow an overall medical policy for the home to be established (No study seems to have been exa-mined what are the effects of this arrangement on the degree of effec-tiveness of access to such prostheses as hearing aids, spectacles and zimmers.) Unskilled nursing care is usually provided by the care staff of the home, but the increasing age and frailty of residents now ad-ditionally necessitates a skilled nursing input. Departmental recom-mendations provide for outside professional nursing assistance from district nurses and other primary health care nurses employed by Area Health Authorities. In general, British old people's homes are not expected to employ full-time medical or nursing staff, nor are they usually of sufficient size to warrant such an input. However, some are now doing so in order to cope with increasing frailty of residents. It is interesting that some health authorities see the provision of nursing care to be sufficiently unambiguously a health service responsibility to finance the provision of nursing staff in local authority homes out of joint financing moneys. Similarly joint finance money has been used to pay for physiotherapists serving old people's homes. (Compare the American position as reported by, for example, Manard, Woehle and Heilman, 1977.) Additionally, most American homes at least claim to provide, and are being required to do so by State regulation, specialised health care services such as dental care, chiropody, speech therapy, remedial therapy and psychiatric aid. Almost invariably, these will involve occasional visits to the home by suitably qualified specialists.

A number of the larger American nursing homes employ an 'activities director' – less specialised than trained recreational or occupational therapists, but more common (Manard *et al.*, 1977). It is the variety and range of manpower inputs into better American facilities that is most interesting for British practice. We shall have to return to the lessons they may have for us. The findings of the Wessex group that the provision of recreational material can substantially raise resident engagement levels and that engagement is particularly enhanced by the presence of an activities organiser lends support to requests for such 'psychological staffing' (Lunt, Felce, Jenkins and Powell, 1977; and see McClannahan and Risley, 1975). Other manpower inputs to residential homes include community-based social workers, chaplains, voluntary visitors (as opposed to voluntary workers who are included in the above categories), residents' significant others, and even gerontologists (Stathopoulos, 1977). They are most likely to have their influence indirectly, through their effects on the social environment.

Clearly, the number of staffing categories that can be distinguished is almost infinite. In a practical research context one must therefore balance two countervailing needs: the need for a simple breakdown to ensure generality and computational feasibility, and the need to distinguish manpower groups whose roles and tasks are sufficiently different for their impact upon outputs to be qualitatively and quantitatively different.

4.1.2 The number of residential staff

The easiest component of the manpower input to measure, in principle at least, is the number of staff in the home. Most published statistics work in 'whole time equivalent' staff member units. National surveys of local authority, voluntary, and private homes revealed considerable variation in staff-resident ratios between homes and between areas (Carstairs and Morrison, 1971; DHSS, 1975; Williams Committee, 1967). Part of this variation can probably be explained by reference to certain historical traditions, practices, and 'accidents of policy', but three recent studies suggest that much the greater part of the

variation is attributable to variations in resident and home characteristics, and in the services offered by the home to its residents and to the
community in which it is situated (Battelle Health Care Study Centre,
1977; Knapp, 1979; McCaffree *et al.*, 1977). The explanatory power of
these factors should not surprise us, for one of the most important
derivatives of the production function between inputs and outputs is
the employment, or input-demand, function. The employment function
attempts to model the process whereby a particular level of the manpower input is decided upon by referring to the desired and actual
levels of output, the relative costs of the inputs, the levels of employment of other inputs, and other relevant factors.

Our own study used data collected in the Residential Census for 82
purpose-built old people's homes and distinguished four staff groups:
supervisory and office staff, care staff, domestic staff, and night staff
on duty and on call. For each group, the number of whole time equivalent staff and the corresponding staff-resident ratio were regressed (in
turn) on selected sets of home and resident characteristics. Although
the Census data had not been collected for the purpose of examining
variations in staffing levels, the estimated relationships proved to be
both powerful and plausible. For example, the employment of care
staff was strongly positively related to the degree of resident dependency and to the provision of day care, and influenced to a lesser
degree by certain features of design (average size of sitting room and
dining room, provision of room for residents' private use). The number
of care staff is given by:

$$
\begin{aligned}
-2.64 + \ & 0.31 \quad \text{x number of resident places normally in use} \\
- \ & 0.09 \quad \text{x average size of dining room} \\
- \ & 0.17 \quad \text{x average size of sitting room} \\
- \ & 1.13 \quad \text{if there is room set aside for residents' private use} \\
+ \ & 2.30 \quad \text{if there is additional provision for day care} \\
+ \ & 6.25 \quad \text{x proportion of residents of heavy dependency} \\
+ \ & 11.13 \quad \text{x proportion of residents of appreciable dependency} \\
+ \ & 2.76 \quad \text{x proportion of residents of limited dependency}
\end{aligned}
$$

In contrast, the number of domestic staff was unaffected by the dependency of the residents but influenced by a dozen different design features, ranging from the incidence of lavatories and single rooms to the
provision or otherwise of a laundry. The number of whole time equivalent domestic staff was given by:

$$
\begin{aligned}
-5.50 + \ & 0.28 \quad \text{x number of resident places normally in use} \\
- \ & 0.003 \quad \text{x (number of places) squared} \\
+ \ & 0.69 \quad \text{x number of residents per W.C.} \\
+ \ & 0.15 \quad \text{x average size of dining room} \\
+ \ & 0.10 \quad \text{x average size of sitting room}
\end{aligned}
$$

   − 3.54 if there is sufficient sitting space at one time
   + 3.00 x number of non-self-contained buildings
   − 1.38 if room set aside for residents' private use
   − 3.63 if home is seriously inadequate (fabric index)
   + 0.82 if additional space for day care
   + 0.94 if room set aside for laundry

Full details for this and analyses for other staff types are given in Knapp (1979).

In contrast to our British study, the research conducted by the Battelle Centre at Seattle collected information from only a small sample of homes − twelve homes in their first study of 1974 (McCaffree *et al.*, 1977), and sixteen in their second study three years later (Battelle Health Care Study Centre, 1977). Their principal interest was the influence of residents' characteristics (dependency, physical health and mental status) upon 'employee contact time' for each resident and upon labour costs. Home characteristics were included in the later study but only to a limited degree. The studies differed in other ways from the British study − the homes were *nursing* homes, some of them certified to provide skilled nursing care; some of them were proprietary, profit-seeking, institutions; in the first study only homes which were perceived by administrators to be 'efficient and effective' were included, whilst the second employed a stratified sample of homes with 'average (typical) staff mix and ratios'; and, of paramount importance, the analyses were conducted at the level of the individual resident or patient and only occasionally at the home level. For these and other reasons, the results of the studies by Knapp and by the Battelle Centre are not directly comparable. Nor can we draw immediate inferences about British old people's homes from the Battelle findings for American nursing homes. We briefly report their findings here, however, because they represent the best that are currently available and because their findings should influence future research into this problem.

Three categories of care staff were distinguished and examined in relation to resident characteristics and demands:

(a) nursing aides and orderlies;
(b) licensed nursing care personnel ('registered nurses and licensed practical nurses'); and
(c) non-nursing care personnel (occupational, physical and speech therapists, activities and social services personnel, physicians, and volunteers).

Several types of multivariate analysis were used to identify and qualify the contribution of residents' characteristics to explaining the variability in employee contact time with each resident. Without going into detail, the analyses suggested that the following characteristics influenced the amount of contact time by *nursing aides and orderlies*: disease of the nervous system; degree of help required with dressing, transferring, feeding, and bathing; incontinence; and certain mental status characteristics (unresponsive, withdrawn, disoriented, forgetful, wanders). Contact time with resident by *licensed nursing care personnel* was affected by: disease of the nervous system; number of activities (transferring, feeding, bathing, dressing, incontinence) with which help is required; number of medications required; number of non-oral medications; and mental status characteristics (unresponsive, withdrawn, disoriented, forgetful, wanders). Four categories of non-nursing care personnel were distinguished and examined separately in an analogous manner to nursing personnel and aides. The influential residents' characteristics were relatively few in number and their collective influence was actually pretty slight. (See McCaffree *et al.*, 1977, pp.79-81, 105-10). They concluded (ibid., pp.109-10) that:

> The probability of receiving non-nursing services was significantly related to the residents'/patients' level of dependency in activities of daily living. . . . Residents/patients whose status was being maintained or had been stabilised were less likely than persons in the process of being discharged, dying, or whose health state was being stabilized, to receive physical therapy, occupational therapy, and social services.

Summarily, we can see that a number of residents' disabilities and characteristics and a broad range of home design features have an apparent impact on the staffing levels of old people's homes and nursing homes. There are thus a number of associations between the major elements of our production of welfare model working in a number of causal directions. Variations in the combinations of both resource and quasi-inputs in the residential setting affect the outputs of welfare for residents and residents' significant others. The dominant thesis of this essay is valid: the production model has enough correspondence with the causal process in homes to provide an illuminating way of conceptualising them. Foremost amongst those outputs is the improvement or maintenance of residents' well-being measured along the dimensions discussed above. The discussion of the present subsection has given us two further causal associations. Firstly, staffing needs and deployment are partly determined by residents' characteristics − a causality in no way inconsistent with the production thesis. Secondly, staffing needs and deployment are partly determined by the physical structure of the homes; that is, the variable manpower inputs are adjusted to compensate for, or to complement, variations in the fixed capital input.

A number of writers have stressed the importance of staff numbers, or staff-resident ratios, for the determination of either the quality of care (an intermediate output) or the quality of life of residents (final output). Linn (1974) found that the number of staff hours was related to the quality of care, and Anderson, Holmberg, Schneider and Stone (1969) and Linn (1974) also found that the number of staff hours *per patient* had a similar effect. Curry and Ratliff (1973) argue that staff-resident ratios will be a determinant of institutional milieu, and hence of residents' well-being. As the staff-resident ratio decreases, more formal and less personal procedures of care are adopted, so that the environment becomes 'more total' in the Goffman sense. Residential home staff feel that they should have more time to talk to residents (Neill, McGuinness and Warburton, 1976). The absence of staff forces senior and direct care staff to devote more time than intended to domestic activities and less attention to residents psycho-social needs. However, there is no scarcity of evidence that in some related institutions the staff-resident ratio itself has little effect on resident management practices (Grant and Moores, 1977; Harris *et al.*, 1974; Raynes *et al.*, 1979; Tizard *et al.*, 1972). Related is the evidence that the presence of more members of staff does not necessarily improve the interaction with residents, since staff tend to talk with one another, although some of this may be discussion from which residents gain (Morris, 1969; Thormalen, 1965; Tizard, 1964). What seems to be more generally the case is that any one resident is spoken to more often as a member of a smaller than of a larger group. Lipman and Slater (1977a) take a quite different line. They recommend that the range and scope of staff-resident interaction should be *limited* in order to maximise the opportunities for resident initiative and to reduce resident dependence upon staff. Their design recommendations for residential homes thus attempt to reduce the number of 'chance' resident-staff interactions and to minimise staff surveillance.

The conflicting opinions that emerge from even such a small number of studies serve to emphasise the hazards of relying upon input indicators when assessing residential care. Although empirical research must distinguish between the effects of the number of whole time equivalent staff, the total number of staff *per se* (residents' confusion may well be exacerbated if the number of different staff in frequent contact is excessive), the *effective* number of staff (or staff hours) during peak periods of the day (King, Raynes and Tizard, 1971), the effects of staff absenteeism during periods of epidemic illness among residents, and probably also the rate of turnover of residential staff, particularly those in closest contact with residents (Molberg and Brothen, 1977; Sinclair, 1971), an assessment of how they affect the quality of life must put them into a context of more complex argument.

4.1.3 The quality of manpower services

The quality of the care services that residential staff render to the elderly residents during their working hours is clearly the crucial component in any discussion of the manpower input. It is also the most difficult component to conceptualise, define and measure. It is important not to skirt the issue, however, if we are to reproduce the production of welfare process in a way that is both accurate and useful. We cannot design systems of care which aim to maximise the quality of resident life without imputing to each input its proper contribution to the production process. Conceptually, it is very difficult to distinguish between the quality of manpower and the quality of care services for the former can only really be defined by reference to the latter. It is then possible to distinguish a number of approaches to the problem of measuring manpower quality.

(A) Attempts have been made to measure the quality of care *per se*. Quality of care measurement generally concentrates on a handful of inputs and quasi-inputs, such as staff-resident ratios, the number of residents per room, the state of repair of the home, and the activities available.[2] The measures are a *mélange* of variables of quite different degrees of causal priority in the production of welfare. They appear to be of both doubtful validity and limited utility. They cannot be employed in *place* of quality of life or final output indicators, for the production of residents' welfare or quality of life is a very complex, individualised process. But they are also of little use in conjunction with a final output indicator, for the quality of care scales so aggregate the various inputs and quasi-inputs as to be quite useless for policy-making purposes. The first attempt to assess quality of residential care was probably made by Townsend (1962) and at the time his approach represented a significant departure from all that had gone before. Our better understanding today of the process of residential care and the generation of residents' welfare does however render the approach obsolete. As used in most studies, the measures are a rag-bag of variables purporting to reflect influences on the quality of care, not a set of indicators whose properties as measures of important aspects of caring behaviour are known, and systematically cover the most important dimensions of caring behaviour.

(B) In discussing the types of residential manpower in an earlier subsection, we listed some of the tasks performed by care staff, by domestic staff, and by other groups. Indirectly, a listing of tasks in this way gives some indication of the quality of caring services that staff are able to render to residents. There are two strands to this argument. Firstly, a listing and 'frequency distribution' of the tasks performed by each staff member or group of members gives an indication of the caring services rendered to clients. For example, a predominance of 'social tasks' over domestic chores may allow one to make inferences about the quality of caring by care staff, and a comparison of the extent of this predominance between two homes may allow further inferences to be drawn. Imber (1977) listed twenty 'staff tasks' and recorded the frequency with which each was performed. Forms completed by matrons (for all staff) indicated that 81 per cent of residential staff in Authority A never read or wrote letters for residents, or did so less than once per week, that 81 per cent played games with residents less than once per week, or never, and that 88 per cent organised or took part in social events with the same frequency. The corresponding percentages for staff in Authority B were 88 per cent, 79 per cent and 92 per cent. A comparison of this form may be meaningful in assessing the quality of the manpower input and may be a reasonable basis for a quality measure. The second strand to the argument concerns the *opportunities* for staff 'to individualise care for all residents' (Walton, 1978). Without adequate administrative and domestic support, care staff will be unable to concentrate their efforts on primary care functions. A number of the staff interviewed by Elizabeth Patterson (1977), in her ethnographic study of six British old people's homes complained that they had insufficient time to devote to 'doing proper care' and as a result 'staff came to view residents as the objects upon which the lists of duties had to be performed in a given time' (ibid., p.354). What is particularly worrying is that staff opportunities for 'proper care' will become progressively fewer as residents' dependency increases and more complex tasks are required. As Walton (1978) argues, it is necessary to combat the 'survival syndrome' whereby the major emotional and physical resources of the staff are expended merely to survive the day, leaving 'no mental surplus to develop a long term perspective, or to alter the existing situation'.

(C) Some of the quality of care measures that have been applied in residential settings have distinguished one or more separate 'ambience' or 'regime' dimensions. Our production of welfare model includes as one of the most important quasi-inputs the social environment of the home. A third approach to the assessment of the quality of manpower (caring) services might therefore be to examine the social climate within which the services are rendered to clients, particularly since climate will be partly fashioned by the staff themselves. Such an approach would, however, cloud over too many important issues. There are many more facets to the manpower input quality dimension than the creation of the caring milieu, and the social climate of the home is a product of a number of other factors in addition to the characteristics of residential manpower. It is thus preferable to maintain the distinction between the two concepts and to examine separately their respective impacts on the welfare of residents and the outputs of the home generally. However, the causal processes that determine the quality of the labour input — and therefore, *inter alia*, features of the social climate — should be analysed even though the over-ready identification of the one with the other in much of the literature makes it difficult to find criteria of the quality of labour input (its 'marginal productivity' in the typical resident's own production of welfare) that are completely independent of social climate.

The literature is disappointing. Given its significance, it is surprising that a better attempt has not been made to develop more sophisticated theoretical argument about the determinants of the quality of the labour input in old people's homes. In particular it is surprising that a more impressive attempt has not been made to relate the quality of the input of the direct care staff to (a) organisational characteristics of the home and the sections of authority that most affect it; and (b) variations in the personality and social characteristics of the care staff. However, such attempts have been made in other types of institution.

We can venture with some confidence one generalisation. As Kushlick stresses, it is the workers having most direct and continual contact with residents whose quality of work is vital. The principal theoretical task is therefore to explain variations in the quality of input of the direct care staff. It is to this we turn in discussion of two topics: the characteristics of homes and their environments as formal organisations; and the characteristics of care manpower as predictors of their marginal productivity in the resident's own production of welfare.

4.1.3.1 Characteristics of homes and authorities as formal organisations

Some American literature has drawn on the conceptual framework provided by the application by the Aston group, and others, of Weber's theory of bureaucracy to the study of the determinants of the quality of caring, notably Raynes, Pratt and Roses (1979), whose argument we draw upon freely in the paragraphs of this section. What distinguished the approach of the Aston group was that, whereas the treatment of bureaucracy by Max Weber and most later organisational theorists was based on the development of one or more ideal types, the Aston group treated bureaucracy not as a unitary concept but as multidimensional. Secondly, the Aston group treated bureaucracy as a variable not as a characteristic — organisations, they argued, showed the differentiating characteristics associated with the theory of bureaucracy to a greater or lesser degree. It is these dimensions that some of the literature on residential homes and institutions treat as causal variables in their theory of the determination of the quality of caring.

Raynes *et al.* discussed four such characteristics: *centralisation* (the extent to which authority is delegated); *formalisation* (the extent to which rules and written regulations constrain the manner in which tasks are carried out by workers); *communication* (the level of contact that staff have with other groups involved in the care of the residents); and *specialisation* (the degree to which the task of caring for people is split up into tasks and shared out between staff).

Centralisation. Numerous studies of a variety of contexts, including health care institutions (Hall, 1967; Paulson, 1974), argue that centralisation diminishes the degree to which organisations achieve their perceived goals. In residential settings for mentally retarded children King *et al*. (1971) had found that the resident orientation of care was most noticeable where those in daily charge of living units most frequently participated in the aspects of the decision-making process they studied. Holland (1973) found that where the unit directors perceived decision-making to be decentralised, resident management practices (measured by the Resident Management Practices scale of King and Raynes, 1968) tended to be more resident oriented. Tizard *et al*. (1972) found that where the staff of residential nurseries perceived themselves to have more authority over aspects of day-to-day management, such staff more frequently used stimulating 'informative' speech. Decentralisation of care varies within as well as between settings as Holland (1973) and Raynes *et al*. (1979) showed. More generally, the classic paper by Aiken and Hage (1966) showed that workers tended to feel alienated in organisations with a high degree of centralisation.

Raynes *et al*. found that, allowing for the effects of variations in IQ and the scale of the living unit, their index of centralisation was negatively correlated with their index of resident-orientated management practices (a revised version of King-Raynes Resident Management Practices scale), whose relationships with the dimensions of institutionalism implicit in Goffman's ideal type we have discussed elsewhere (see chapter 6). Again, the authors found that centralisation was negatively correlated with their index of the prevalence of informative speech. Raynes *et al*. argued that a feeling of some control over their work-life may well be a direct cause of stimulating care giving. They found some evidence that a high proportion of workers who feel that they have no say in any matters immediately relevant to their job may well 'take it out on the residents', thus supporting an argument put forward by Alutto and Acito (1973).

Tizard *et al*. (1975) had argued that it was a necessary condition for the performance of certain staff roles for the building's head to have freedom to make decisions about matters which in other organisations are decided centrally. This was investigated by Raynes *et al*., who asked supervisors about their participation in decision-making about such matters as the times residents arose in the morning and retired at night; the admission and discharge of residents; the planning of residents' activities; the hiring and firing of the direct care staff;

arrangements for days off and vacations for direct care staff; and the planning of programmes for residents. Differences in the degree of centralisation perceived by care managers were correlated with differences in the resident orientation of the management practices. It seems that the supervisor's authority affects resident-wide treatment policies, although Raynes *et al.* failed to find an effect on their informative speech index, implying that the influence of a supervisor's authority on individual styles of care were less.

Formalisation. Aiken and Hage (1966) found that the presence of rules and regulations was associated with a dissatisfaction with work tasks and with co-workers, these being highly correlated with one another. Grusky (1959), they noted, found that the absence of formal rules in a therapeutically oriented prison legitimised relatively individualised relationships between staff and inmates and also that Blau (1970) had argued that formalisation of procedures impeded flexibility of practice. They found partial support for the hypothesis that more formalisation according to the perception of the care workers, was likely to be detrimental to caring behaviour. No doubt partly because the codification of the duties of care staff studied by Raynes, Pratt and Roses emphasised custodial aspects of their work, formalisation appeared to have an adverse effect on the prevalence of informative speech, although there appeared to be little correlation between resident orientation and resident management practices. However, on balance they judged that the evidence about whether formalisation at the level of the care staff was detrimental to the quality of their labour input was inconclusive (Raynes *et al.* did not examine the inference of formalisation at the level of their buildings' heads).

Communication. Perrow (1972) shows the way in which communication between personnel of the same status level is of particular importance to the effectiveness of work in non-routine task situations. The resident-oriented provision of care is one such situation. Such care, Raynes *et al.* argue, could best be maintained by frequent contact between care workers in different shifts, and by communication between direct care staff and other personnel involved in the planning and implementation of programmes and activities for residents. The importance of communication for effective care seems to be established in studies of such institutions as mental hospitals and there is evidence supporting the general argument that increased frequency of group discussion increases subordinates' support for new activities. Most of the literature on residential institutions reflects the assumption that communication has positive effects on the quality of care (see for instance Stanton and Schwartz, 1954; and Perrow, 1972). However, Raynes *et al.* found that the frequency of contact of care staff with staff on other shifts was unrelated to the resident orientation of management practices or the prevalence of informative speech with residents. Again, higher levels of contact with professionals appeared not to have a directly beneficial impact on care-giving. What they did find was that contact with the unit director was associated with resident oriented management. These results could be explained in several ways. Perhaps the nature of communication is more important than its frequency. Again, it is easy for those whose contacts are mainly with professionals to overestimate the consequences of what Kushlick described as the 'hit and run' workers. Again, Raynes *et al.* were able to find only conflicting evidence about the consequences for the quality of care-giving of supervisors' communications with others. The frequent meetings of unit directors with care staff, and also with workers on other shifts, did appear to be associated with resident oriented management practices, though not with the prevalence of informative speech between care staff and residents. The authors argued that there were a number of ways in which such communication could have a positive effect on care practices: for instance they permit the discussion of programmes to implement resident-oriented care and the problems and progress of staff in achieving it, and reduce the degree of inconsistency in handling of individual residents. However, it is at least possible that resident oriented management practice is merely a correlate of such communications.

Specialisation. Henry (1957) argued that where all caring tasks are carried out by the same person, workers tend to be more highly motivated and can plan on an individual basis all aspects of the client's care. Moreover, in such circumstances, the worker tends to have a single supervisor and so communication is easier and the worker feels supported. Evidence from the study by King, Raynes and Tizard (1971) appears to support that argument. King and his associates found that the clearer the division of labour between direct care staff and buildings' heads, the more institutionally oriented the care tended to be. But Raynes, Pratt and Roses found no association between the extent to which the buildings' supervisors devoted their time to activities directly involving the staff with residents and the resident orientation of management practices, although there was such an association with the prevalence of informative speech. However, Raynes *et al.* did find that greater role specialisation between the staff status groups reduced the prevalence of informative speech. From such results, Raynes *et al.* inferred that a characteristic style of a daily activity like speech is more likely to be influenced by direct example than by differences in the wider structural properties of the organisation. Therefore, where the supervisor's role is more heavily weighted with activities which do not directly involve them with the residents it is less possible for them to provide a role model for care-taking.

So we may hypothesise first, that each of the dimensions may contribute in some way to the quality of care-giving by direct care staff, though the dimensions should not be considered independent of one another, since they reflect control devices that can sometimes be used as alternatives to one another and sometimes to reinforce one another. The influence seems to be felt through what Raynes, Pratt and Roses identified as staff morale. The morale may operate both directly and indirectly, since there is literature that suggests that morale influences turnover (Minge and Bowman, 1969; Molberg and Brothen, 1977) and so also such factors as the continuity of relationships. The maintenance or raising of the morale of care staff must be viewed as a process through time, the involvement and responsibility stimulating interest and a creatively individualistic attitude towards tasks. Perhaps those with authoritarian personalities are more likely to stay in an excessively controlled environment.

Second, it seems likely that the characteristics of organisations as they appear at different levels of the hierarchy have real and separable influence. Indeed the organisational characteristics of different levels influence different aspects of care-giving. For instance, the organisational factors that affect the managerial level tend through their influence on the manager's behaviour to influence the resident-wide treatment practices, while organisational factors influencing direct care staff directly have an effect on actual staff-client interaction. Certainly the larger British old people's homes have a hierarchical structure to which these arguments have salience. Moreover, they are set on a context of local authority managements which are very different from one another. Any attempt to sort out the influences of organisational characteristics on care-giving must therefore extend beyond the organisational boundary of the home itself.

However, it would be naive to argue that once the influence of organisational structure and the quality of the labour input is understood it is easy to choose how to change that structure; or even in what direction to seek to change it. Such choices demand also that we consider why the organisational structure is as it is. Contingency theory shows that this variation is not just random but is in part an adaptive response to the organisational environment (Kast and Rosenzweig, 1973; Lupton, 1971). Contingency theory has made some progress in identifying the types of situational factor that make alternative organisational structures more or less conducive to good organisational performance. Among the 'contingencies' (situational factors in the environment) whose effects have been explored are market environment, mode of technology, organisational size, geographical location, culture, professional and bureaucratic ideologies, and the existence of elected representatives to whom organisations are subordinated. In particular, Greenwood (1978) has investigated the degree to which strongly politically organised local authorities cause adaptations of their organisational structure to avoid scandals of maladministration (like the inequitable or unthinking treatment of clients with similar rights) or malpractice (for instance, financial corruption or illegal behaviour). He argues that the organisational devices used to minimise the risks are precisely those that may well influence the quality of care through their effects on morale: *standardisation* (an emphasis on rules and procedures), *formalisation* (use of forms and documentation to record behaviour and decisions), and *centralisation*. However, since the type of service or function affects the extent and nature of the risks, and other contingencies also affect the choice, how demands of political accountability influence organisational structure differs between the parts of an authority.

Greenwood found that social services departments tend to control activities associated with external relations of departments, including relations of social workers with clients. He inferred that this was because external relations tended to have the greatest potential for political embarrassment. In contrast with, for instance, planning or finance departments, the method of control was not standardisation but formalisation. No doubt this was in part due to the influence of social services departments on a professional social work ideology whose values are rather different from other local government ideologies, and the nature of the tasks performed. Moreover, since the social problems that generate need for social interventions are not usually entirely preventable for the department, the political support for the department depends more on its ability to justify its actions after the event than on its efforts to control future demands. Thus, argues Greenwood, one of the reasons why social services departments control external relations by means of documentation (formalisation) is that formalisation is the form of control most appropriate for retrospective defence. Greenwood found that where the activities of other departments involved political risks, they too were subject to control; and he was able to cite evidence that the type of structural controls chosen are also ones most appropriate to the set of environmental contingencies they face. Thus, public bureaucracies may be more discerning in the application of structural control than is popularly believed and 'certainly the "red tape" image of public agencies is inconsistent with the degree of specificity identified here' (Greenwood, 1978, p.417). However, bureaucracies may be less sensitive to the technological requirements for providing services that at best justify the needs of clients than to the requirements imposed by political accountability. It remains important both to assess how far the characteristics of the residential home's organisation, particularly the control mechanisms it uses and to which it is subject, is compatible with providing care most effectively; and also to assess in what ways the legitimate needs for control that arise because of such contingencies as political accountability can be reconciled with more effective caring.

The body of argument about the influence of organisational characteristics is vague in several respects, and so provides only a limited basis
for policy-making. First, the arguments developed by Raynes, Pratt and
Roses (1979) were based on an empirical study whose measurement of
organisational characteristics was not as thorough as that used, for
instance, by the Aston group. Second, the dimensions of organisational
diversity around which Raynes *et al.* built the argument are a small
proportion of those developed by the Aston group and others, and
indeed cover only some of the main dimensions. It is not obvious that
the others are less relevant. The same can be said for Greenwood's
argument: only a few dimensions related to his focus on political
organisation are measured. The investigation of the consequences of
a wider range of contingencies may make other dimensions seem
relevant. For instance, the settlement patterns of the population and
the scale of the authority may both affect specialisation, another of
the main dimensions distinguished by Pugh *et al.* (1968). Third, although the studies acknowledged the multidimensionality of care-
giving, it is not obvious that the dimensions studied adequately cover
the range of resident-affecting variation in the quality of care-giving
input. Fourth, none of the studies have been of British old people's
homes; and although they suggest plausible causal arguments, only
by empirical investigation can the validity of these arguments be tested
and the relative importance of these and other causal arguments assessed. Fifth, we need to understand the relationship between resources
and the other factors; the resource causes and effects of formal organisational characteristics, and the contingencies that influence their
choice by authorities; and the way in which these factors work on
causing interactions at different levels of resources. There seems to be
no empirical research concerning these.

4.1.3.2 Characteristics of care manpower

The other main approach to the explanation of manpower quality has
been to look at levels of *training, education, and experience* of the
home staff, for there can be little justification for training residential
staff if they do *not* improve the standards of care and the quality of
life of residents. It is widely recognised that there is a severe shortage
of qualified care staff in British old people's homes, although opinions
differ as to the desired level or orientation of training (British Association of Social Workers, 1977; DHSS, 1976b; Ward, 1977). A recent
Government memorandum (DHSS, 1977, paragraphs 32, 33) stated:

> The effective and successful running of old people's homes depends
> to a large extent on the degree of knowledge and professional skill
> of the head of the home. .... Although nurses often have a

considerable contribution to make when they hold senior posts in old people's homes, they will need additional training and experience to acquire the range of skills needed for management in residential care. ... All staff engaged in the residential care of the elderly are likely to need some form of training to equip them for the wide range of tasks involved. Suitable training can not only significantly increase knowledge and enhance existing skills but also enable staff to extend the services provided by visiting professionals.

Some of the British discussion of social environments in old people's homes suggests that a head with a nursing background often promotes a model that puts less emphasis on residents' psychosocial needs (D. Harris, 1977). Despite this consensus regarding the efficacy of suitable training for residential staff, there is very little empirical evidence to draw upon. King, *et al.* (1971) found that scores on their child management practices scale (an indicator of environmental milieu in children's homes) were related to the training of the living unit's head, but Kart and Manard (1976) found no evidence of a relationship between the proportion of 'highly trained professionals' in American nursing homes and either the quality of care or the level of final output. This virtual absence of empirical evidence is disappointing but the wealth of qualitative and anecdotal evidence from social work administrators, educators, teachers and supervisors serves to emphasise the pressing need for better trained residential staff. Another aspect of the training question that is also emphasised is the support given to care staff. Without adequate support the knowledge and skills acquired in training can very easily become redundant. Such support can 'facilitate understanding of the residential task ... maintain focus on the task ... mitigate stress ... find solutions to problems encountered in daily living ... [and] assist professional development' (Payne, 1977, p.14).

One of the essential purposes of social work training, and one of the central aims of most organisations concerned with the elderly, is to foster positive *attitudes towards the elderly* and to help dispel the negative stereotyping of the elderly that otherwise dominates. It may therefore be valid to assess the quality of manpower services in terms of staff attitudes towards the residents and towards the elderly in general. The Personal Social Services Council review of residential care succinctly sums up the importance of positive attitudes (PSSC, 1977, pp.51 and 50):

the attitudes staff have and reveal towards residents set the tone for the pattern of life in a home. They also call forth corresponding attitudes from residents towards them and each other.
Personal relationships flourish or flounder on the attitudes of people. ... The pattern and activity of daily life will reflect the

success of personal relationships — both those between staff and residents, and those between staff themselves.

Residential staff's attitudes towards their work and towards the residents as individuals will determine the general atmosphere and regime of the home, the attitudes the elderly hold about themselves and about the home, the quality of the care services rendered to the residents, the degree of 'individualised understanding', and, ultimately, the quality of life and general outputs of the home (Brearley, 1977; Patterson, 1977; Romaniuk, Hoyer and Romaniuk, 1977). Attitudes are known to be related to the residential task and position in the home, to the amount of education and training, and possibly also to age and length of experience in residential and social care (Gubrium, 1974; Kosberg, Cohen and Mendlovitz, 1972; Patterson, 1977).

There have been only a few comprehensive studies of the quality of manpower in residential facilities for the aged. The most recent, and probably the most thorough, was the nursing home research of Baltz and Turner (1977). These two authors developed a 'nursing home aide screening device' to be used in the selection of residential staff. The instrument was constructed from a number of related instruments and scales and tested against supervisor rating of 93 presently employed female aides. The ratings were simplified so that aides were described either as successful ('the kind of aide I would like to rehire') or unsuccessful, and were made by at least two supervisors for each employee. In all there were forty items on the screening instrument which distinguished significant differences between successful and unsuccessful aides. Summarily, the analyses revealed that successful aides were older, had received much more training in health care, had accumulated more health care experience, held positive attitudes towards death and illness, had visited nursing homes more often, and scored significantly higher on all four traits of a personality instrument (ascendency, responsibility, emotional stability, and sociability). The authors point out a number of methodological drawbacks in their research, and these should be borne in mind. From the point of view of this essay, the most important drawback — one that makes the study more interesting for the question it tackles than for its findings — is that the Baltz and Turner study focuses on nursing aides, a group of employees not often found in British old people's homes.

One would expect to find relationships between the personality, attitudes, and training of care staff and the quality of the labour input. In fact, the evidence is ambiguous. However, throughout social science, it has proved difficult to link personality, attitudes and behaviour without developing a precise theory of the way contextual factors affect the processes. As is argued elsewhere in this essay, the pressure of social environment often seems to overwhelm personality as a determinant of behaviour (Zimbardo, Haney and Banks, 1975; Milgram, 1965; Mischel, 1973). This is particularly so when the variations between units in the incidence of care staff with differences in a characteristic are not great. Perhaps the proportions of care staff trained and the personality variations have therefore been less important than would have been expected from the emphasis given to them. More important may have been cultural or age differences that reflect varying labour markets — differences, that is, that are not due to random variations among individuals within homes, but are the systematic effect of powerful and general factors influencing the characteristics of the staff of the home as a whole.

In the final analysis the quality of the manpower input (as reckoned through the quality of caring), cannot be divorced from the quality of a resident's life. Only by looking at the influence of the various characteristics of the manpower input on the outputs of the residential home, particularly the well-being of residents, can we accurately and reliably assess the true quality of the services rendered by residential staff.

4.2 The capital input

In conventional economic usage, capital is the hold-all term used to denote all physical, man-made aids to production. In the residential care setting there are literally hundreds of capital items, ranging from the building itself to the cutlery utensils in daily use and bedpans. Correspondingly, perhaps, there have been many studies of the physical structure, design and facilities of residential homes for the elderly — a depth of interest which partly reflects the fact that the capital input is the most visible and tangible aspect of residential care, and the one that has historically aroused most indignation and discontent. For instance, some argue that design can create a living situation which offers residents a choice about how to spend their time or one that effectively forces them into a fixed pattern of life. (Cheshire County Council, Social Services Department, 1976). Others argue that residents can be confused by endless corridors, complicated shapes and colours and repetitive design elements (Olsen, 1978). In this section we are predominantly concerned with residential home design and its impact upon life in the home and resident well-being. At the end of the section we briefly discuss certain 'summary indicators' of the capital input, but on the whole our focus will be on certain constituent features of design and structure.

4.2.1 Indicators of residential home design

The first British study of residential home design, and one of the first to appear in the international literature, was conducted by Peter

Townsend nearly twenty years ago. Townsend (1962) examined eleven dimensions of the physical environment selected to represent those that significantly influenced life in the home and those that had been stressed in successive Ministerial and Departmental guidelines. For each of the homes in his sample he compiled indicators for the number and condition of WCs, baths and hand-basins, the proportions of single and double bedrooms, the availability of a lift service and the proportion of beds served by it or situated on the ground floor, the number of beds with wooden frames, the number of interior sprung mattresses (as opposed to mattresses filled with hair, flock or straw), the exclusivity of a resident's use of certain bedside furniture, and the sizes of dining and sitting rooms. Townsend found considerable variation in residential home design, with most homes falling a long way short of Ministerial guidelines. This evidence on home design and facilities provided one important strand in his vitriolic attack on the whole concept of 'total care'.

Whilst his recommendations regarding the role of residential care in the system of services for the elderly were not taken up, Townsend's approach to the assessment of physical structure proved influential amongst academics and administrators alike. Most subsequent surveys and censuses have adopted some or all of his *design indicators* (Williams, 1967; Harris, 1968; Sumner and Smith, 1969; Carstairs and Morrison, 1971; DHSS, 1975; Scottish Education Department, 1976).

In the next few pages, we discuss residential home design under fifteen heads, corresponding to those features of design and structure which have been the subject of attention in the above-mentioned studies, in the American literature on residential care of the elderly, and in the Ministry of Health and DHSS recommendations of the last thirty years. Each head distinguishes a particular feature, for which there may be a number of alternative and complementary indicators. In each case we shall be concerned with the problems of measurement (which are generally few), the institutional and individual correlates of differences in design and scale, and the apparent significance for the process of production of welfare. We shall have cause to refer to a large number of research studies, most of them conducted in the USA or Canada. Of British work in this field, the most useful for present purposes has been the series of studies conducted by the Welsh School of Architecture under the direction of Alan Lipman (Barrett, 1976; Harris, 1977; Harris, Lipman and Slater, 1977; Lipman and Slater, 1977a, 1977b; Slater and Lipman, 1977). Our own reanalyses of Residential Census data are also relevant although we do not reproduce all of the detailed findings here (Knapp, 1977c, 1979).

(a) Ownership and original function

The conventional breakdowns of ownership and original function in the British context distinguish between local authority, voluntary and private homes, on the one hand; and between purpose-built homes, converted private dwellings, former Public Assistance Institutions (PAI) and the remainder, on the other. Although the available evidence is scant, there do appear to be differences in staffing, in caring practices, and in many aspects of design attributable to differences in ownership and original function (Carstairs and Morrison, 1971; DHSS, 1975; Hobman, 1978; Knapp, 1977c; Robb, 1967; Townsend, 1962; Williams, 1967). In the USA, where the differences between the local authority or voluntary home and the profit-seeking private home are perhaps greater, there has been research to examine quality of care differences between the two. The evidence is ambiguous: Anderson et al. (1969) found that non-profit nursing homes provided more physician hours per patient than private homes and that the original function of the home was also a determinant of quality of care, and Beattie and Bullock (1964) discovered that social milieu and attitudes of staff were much better in non-profit homes. On the other hand, Levey et al. (1973) found no relationship between quality of care and ownership. As we noted earlier, however, quality of care indices are of questionable utility, particularly when used instead of, rather than in conjunction with, quality of life measures.

(b) Size of home and size of living unit

The aspect of physical design most frequently discussed in the policy and research literatures is the size of home or size of living unit. 'Size' is generally measured in terms of the number of places or number of residents, although architects also look at the scale of the building itself, measuring the height or wall surface of the home or counting the number of floors.[3]

Central government thinking on the 'optimal' or desired size of a residential home has swung from Aneurin Bevan's vision of 25 to 30-place homes in 1948, up to a size of 60 places in 1954 (Ministry of Health Circular 3/55), and back to an intermediate scale of 30-50 residents in 1962 (Local Authority Building Note No. 2), a size reiterated in the revised Building Note of 1973. The criteria used to reach such specifications are not altogether clear, but it seems that administrators were anxious to strike a balance between the lower unit costs of the larger homes, and the more domestic atmosphere of the smaller buildings. Assumptions about scale economies for larger homes have recently been proved largely correct in terms of both construction and operating costs (Wager, 1972; Davies and Knapp, 1978; and Knapp,

90

1978b). However, official concern about domesticity has been
on a relatively naive model of residential care, for architects and other
have long emphasised that it is not the size of the *home* that is important, but rather the size of each individual *living unit* or grouping of
rooms (Goldsmith, 1971). Lipman and Slater (1977a) recommend that
if the 'optimum' size of 25 places was exceeded, the number of residents in a home should be limited to approximately forty who are
accommodated in 'family groups' of some eight individuals.

In April 1975 the DHSS commissioned a study of the 'group unit
design' and a report was published in the summer of 1979 (Thomas,
Gough and Spencely, 1979; and see DHSS Circular LASSL (79) 10).
The report (Thomas *et al.*, 1979, paragraph 2.2) concluded that

> While the group unit design does make possible flexible care for
> groups of people with different needs, the design implications
> of the principle have not yet been fully explored . . . and the range
> in the total spectrum of care which the group unit home can appro-
> priately encompass remains an open question.

Home or living unit size has been examined in relation to factors at
various points along the causal chain of production. Our own study of
a sample of 200 homes, using Residential Census data, found home
size to be significantly related to a large number of internal design
features and structural characteristics (Knapp 1977c). Larger homes
were generally more 'institutional' in character, although this was by no
means pervasive through all the characteristics examined (ibid., p.210).
Moving one link along the causal chain we find a large body of (contradictory) evidence regarding the relationship between size of home and
quality of care. Empirical associations have been found to be positive
(Anderson, *et al.*, 1969; Beattie and Bullock, 1964), to be negative
(Linn, 1974; Townsend, 1962) and to be non-existent (Gottesman,
1972; Levey *et al.*, 1973).

Quality of care, as we have argued above, can be no more than an
intermediate indicator of output, and even here it plays a rather
dubious role. However, what is interesting is the steadily growing
evidence to suggest that size of home is related to social milieu. Much
of the *a priori* argument in the early 1960s stressed the importance
of the small, 'domestic' home, but only recently have the hunches
implicit in these recommendations been put to the test. For example,
Curry and Ratliff (1973) argued that as the size of home is increased,
the number of staff increase proportionately less, so that more formal
caring procedures would be adopted, thereby increasing resident
isolation and dissatisfaction. Kasarda (1974) described how the internal
order of an organisation would be shaped to a considerable degree by
its size. Increasing size in residential care may necessitate an increasing
commitment of resources to clerical, administrative and other im-

personal activities, so adversely affecting the morale and general well-being of residents (Kart and Manard, 1976).

Finally, towards the end of the causal chain, there are a small number of studies which have considered the relationship between size of home and residents' well-being and behaviour. Greenwald and Linn (1971) found that activity and communication between residents declined as homes got larger. Lawton, Nahemow and Teaff (1975), in a study of 154 federal housing projects for the elderly in the USA, established a similar negative association between community size and friendship scores, housing satisfaction, and activity participation. Curry and Ratliff (1973) attempted to explain such findings in terms of self-selection biases, arguing that residents of larger homes had significantly more relatives outside the home, and more contact with them, than did residents of smaller homes; and therefore experienced greater isolation within the home. The argument is ingenious and plausible, but has little validity in the British context, where residents rarely face a choice of homes. Resident psychological well-being is probably only indirectly influenced by home or dwelling unit size, so that the empirical associations reported in the literature are really only convenient summary indicators of a more complex process involving specialisation, staff morale, and other factors discussed in relation to the 'quality' of the input of care staff. The ambiguity of the results lends support to this interpretation (Lawton, Brody and Turner-Massey, 1978; Lawton, Nahemow and Teaff, 1975; Schooler, 1970b). So also do investigations for other types of institutions. The importance of social and physical 'niches' in the home to the well-being of residents is a much more interesting question. For instance, the whole of a resident's life can be illuminated by a genuine friendship with another resident or a warm relationship with one or two staff members.

(c) General home design

Under this heading are grouped features of design which have generally not been singled out for special consideration in the succession of Building and Design Notes since 1948. Nevertheless the social and psychological ramifications of alternative designs can be far from inconsiderable, as has long been recognised by architects, planners and administrators.

Both Barrett (1976) and Hitch and Simpson (1972) emphasise the importance of forging a domestic, private home-like, atmosphere in the home, particularly by careful planning and design. The latter authors in fact found that a domestic atmosphere resulted in significantly more desirable behaviour among residents than did non-domestic, institutional environments, and Barrett used domesticity as the key to the derivation of his seventeen design indicators. In this physical design context, domesticity can possibly be best fostered by grouping resident rooms into a number of self-contained units within the home. Lipman and Slater (1977a) strongly oppose centralised accommodation, which subjects residents to staff surveillance and attention, which may encourage depersonalising and dehumanising caring procedures (queueing for meals, block treatment at various activities, large and impersonal dining and sitting rooms), and which generally emphasises the institutional nature of care. The key to the proposals of Lipman and Slater is their assumption that an objective of residential care should be the promotion of residents' independence. Thus, residents should be able to experience 'complete activity cycles' in all aspects of daily living – not only the consumption of meals, but also their purchase, preparation, and clearing away. Whilst not all residents would be capable of performing all these tasks, it is important to reduce dependence amongst those who can, and decentralised accommodation would appear to be one way of achieving this. Many other design ramifications follow from this dependence/independence stance – for example, bed-sitting rooms should be large enough and sufficiently well appointed as to enable residents to engage in the day-to-day activities customarily pursued outside the home.

On the basis of his interviews with designers and residents and his literature survey, Barrett operationalised the domestic-institutional classification with the following ordering:

- Domestic.
- Small family - less than 10 beds per group, sitting and dining room.
- Large family - more than 10 beds per group, sitting and dining room.
- Small communal - less than 10 beds per group, sitting room.
- Large communal - more than 10 beds per group, sitting room.
- Small institutional - less than 10 beds per group.
- Large institutional - more than 10 beds per group.
- Large institutional with no WCs per group.
- Institutional.

(Of course, whether or not the climate created is familial, communal, or institutional depends on much else other than design features.) He further considered doubling the number of gradations by distinguishing groups/homes according to the presence or absence of WCs within each group of rooms. However, his survey sample of plans showed that all groups classified as 'familial' possess WCs, so that the additional data collection expenses would hardly be warranted. For each home, Barrett recommends calculation of the proportion of residents living in room groups of each of the above seven kinds.

One aspect of general home design sometimes mentioned concerns the entrance/exit points for the home, whose number and location will partly influence the extent of residents' interaction with the community.

Entrances should be sited close to bus stops (or vice versa) and, if entrances are to be spacious and fitted with seats for residents, should afford a good view of nearby activity areas (particularly pedestrian traffic routes). In the design of the main entrance, Lawton (1970b, 1975b) has stressed the need for security, for shelter from the elements, for community identity (the home should have its road number clearly marked), and for non-institutional appearance. Barrett (1976) similarly included the scale of the entrance area in his collection of important indicators of design, but found this aspect too difficult to operationalise along the domesticity dimension. He also looked at the number of entrance/exit points for residents but once again was forced to drop this from his final listing, this time because the number was almost certainly a function of home size. Ministry of Health fire regulations set out in 1965 specified the maximum distance between any room and the nearest fire exit so that the size and arrangement of the home would largely determine the number of such entrance/exist points. However, these regulations refer to fire doors and not to doors in daily operational use by residents. A single main entrance, often with the matron's office situated close by, will undoubtedly increase residents' awareness of surveillance by staff but will comfort those concerned with personal security and safety.

(d) Internal scale

The internal scale or size of the home is clearly closely allied to the external scale (subsection (b)) and to the scale of bedrooms, sitting and dining rooms, and corridors (see below), but at least a few authors have chosen to consider it separately. Lawton (1970b) describes how self-maintenance skills can be maintained if toilets, bathrooms, and dining facilities are situated close to popular sitting areas. Barrett (1976) takes this one step further, explicating spatial proximity by measuring the distance between the pairs of rooms. (Figures in brackets indicate the maximum distance in feet considered to be of domestic length — obtained as the mean of maximum walking distances in a sample of private house plans.) The pairs and distances are: (a) resident's bedroom and nearest sitting room (33.5); (b) resident's bedroom and nearest WC (17); (c) sitting rooms and nearest dining room (13); (d) sitting rooms and nearest WC (15); (e) dining rooms and nearest WC (20.5).

Spatial proximity of residents and residents' rooms has been found to be an important determinant of social interaction and peer friendship formation (Rosow, 1967; Lawton and Simon, 1968; Lawton, 1970b; McClannahan, 1973a). Generally, proximity facilitates friendship formation, although there is contrary evidence to suggest that restricted spatial range may foster conflict, whilst distance may foster interaction (Jones, 1975), implying the need for both closeness and distance for the maintenance of normal friendships.

(e) Corridors

The dimensionality and prosthetic attachments of corridors may well be important in the determination of the character and quality of life of the residents of old people's homes. Surprisingly, there are few studies of this facet of design. Osmond (1957) found that long corridors tended to cause anxiety among patients in hospitals. In designing specifically for the elderly, Barrett (1976) and Lawton (1975b) had this and related findings in mind when drawing up their recommendations. Barrett emphasised the length-width ratio, defining a corridor as 'domestic' if this ratio was between 4:1 and 2:1. A ratio of less than 2:1 was defined as a circulation space and not a corridor; a ratio of greater than 4:1 was 'institutional' in character. Corridor height will also determine the domesticity of a home but, in Barrett's sample of (recent) design plans at least, there was very little variation in this dimension. Alcoves and windows 'break up' corridors and were thus notionally assumed to terminate a corridor; fire doors closed only at night did not. Ministerial and Departmental guidelines and recommendations for design have focused additionally on the need to provide handrails, ramps and seats along the corridors of homes for the physically frail and the elderly. Such 'physical prostheses', which will also include fire doors that can be opened by even the most frail, and floor coverings which do not hinder the less confident (such as non-slip mats and floors that are not highly polished), will encourage resident mobility and independence and will generally improve the quality of institutional life.

(f) Bedrooms

Ministerial directives on bedrooms in the period since the National Assistance Act of 1948 have been almost wholly preoccupied with occupancy levels. In 1954, faced with rapidly increasing demand for residential accommodation, the Ministry of Health issued Circular 3/55 recommending that more multi-bedded rooms than had hitherto been available should be provided. Since that date, successive Circulars and Notes have expressed the doubtful value of 4-, 5- and 6-bedded rooms for the very infirm, and stressed the need for single bedrooms to be provided for all single residents. As a result clear patterns of design are discernible in the present population of homes. Analysis of the 1970 Census data shows that just under two-thirds of the variation both in the proportion of residents in single rooms and in the mean number of beds per bedroom (slight variants on the same theme) can

95

be accounted for by reference to the original function, age and size of home (Knapp, 1977c).

Some of the earlier gerontological literature took the number of nursing home patients or residents per room as either an indicator or an important determinant of the quality of care (e.g. Anderson *et al.*, 1969). Rather more interesting conclusions emerge from studies more firmly based in the environmental psychology tradition. Ittleston, Proshansky and Rivlin (1970), for example, conducted a very detailed study of the relationship between bedroom size and social interaction on a psychiatric ward. The number of residents using their rooms at any one time increased more or less proportionately to the number assigned to each room, but the range of residents' activities showed marked differences. In the larger rooms there was a predominance of isolated passive activity, whereas residents in smaller rooms favoured social activity involving their room-mates. These researchers thus concluded that there was a functional equivalent of privacy which does not require physical separation, whereby large, multiple-occupancy rooms provoke patient withdrawal. In the context of care of the elderly, researchers have had mixed success in establishing an association between bedroom occupancy and social interaction. Bader and Lawton (1969) with a very small sample found no change in interactions following a change from 4-person to single rooms, whilst with the slightly larger sample studied by Lawton, Liebowitz and Charon (1970) a similar change from 4-person to single rooms effected an increased range of movement and a decreased amount of staff-patient interaction.

Residents' preferences are certainly in favour of single rooms. Barrett's interviewees felt that single rooms should be available for *all* unmarried residents and that married residents should have the opportunity of a double room, and Goldsmith (1971) assumes as much in his appraisal of a home from the architect's viewpoint. However, as with any of the inputs entering the welfare production process, we cannot discuss influences and variations in isolation. The practices and attitudes of staff and the day-to-day rules of the home, can neutralise many of the welfare-enhancing qualities of single bedrooms. Single bedrooms are critical for a resident's identity (Patterson, 1977), but cannot ensure privacy if doors must be left open or unlocked, or if staff enter unannounced without respect for the resident's only place of 'personal territory'. The interdependence of home inputs is further emphasised by our findings of significant associations between bedroom size and staffing levels. A regression-based study of purpose-built homes found that homes with a higher proportion of residents in single rooms employed, and thus (on the assumption of rationality on the part of managers, administrators and matrons) *needed*, more supervisory and more night staff (Knapp, 1979). The numbers of care and domestic staff were not influenced by this proportion.

Certain other aspects of residents' bedrooms are discussed in other subsections — bedroom size has been discussed in subsection (c) above, and internal design, furnishings and fittings will be considered in subsection (m) below.

(g) Sitting rooms and sitting spaces

Whilst successive Building and Design Notes have been a little more reticent as regards size and design of sitting rooms than they have been as regards, say, bedroom occupancy levels or overall size of home, there have nevertheless been significant changes in the post-1948 period, with a pervasive trend among the newer purpose-built homes towards fewer places per sitting room. The number of residents per sitting room in a random sample of 200 local authority homes in use in 1970 was found to be related to original function, size and age of home, with 27 per cent of the variance being explained. This variation worked through to induce significant variations in staffing levels and staff-resident ratios in the purpose-built homes in the sample (Knapp, 1977c, 1979). With such variation in sitting room size, the social and psychological correlates of scale and design are of some importance, and yet, to the best of our knowledge, there have been few studies of these relationships. Most of these few have been conducted by Alan Lipman.

Lipman's earlier work was very much concerned with the 'microfeatures' of sitting room layout and particularly the association between seating arrangements and proximity and friendship formation (Lipman, 1967, 1968). He found that sustained verbal interaction established friendships, and that this was severely limited by regular occupancy of the same seats by residents and by fixed furniture arrangements. Staff usually directed new residents to chairs in order to form dyads or triads which they perceived to be compatible, and residents would then habitually occupy them and cause considerable disturbance should 'their' chair be occupied. Social exchanges, and especially those with affective content, were limited to these small groups of elderly people.

In later work, Lipman and Slater (1975, p.23) defined a friendly sitting space as one with a high proportion of supportive/acceptive interactions and concluded that such a space should be:

(a) small enough for all interactions to fall within the 'arc of comfortable conversation' or have chairs arranged to achieve such an effect; (b) infrequently visited by staff; (c) characterised by supportive/acceptive interactions between staff and residents; (d) without many 'gibberish-prone' residents; (e) populated by either rational or by severely confused residents; (f) populated mainly by rational residents.

However, no consistent relationship was found between most of a set of design variables — lounge size, whether the lounge was open-plan, the aspect from the lounge windows, the lounge's position in the home or in relation to staff-activity areas — and the level and proportion of supportive/acceptive interactions between residents in sitting spaces. They thus concluded that 'the nature of the interactions between residents is more clearly a function of the nature of the interaction between staff and residents than it is a function of specifically isolated design features of the home' (ibid., p.23). Nevertheless, in a later discussion of their findings, Lipman and Slater (1977b) considered it both worthwhile and appropriate to score individual seat positions and sitting spaces by reference to the number of adjacent chairs, the view of the TV and of activities inside and outside the home, the level (ground floor or otherwise), and the size of the sitting space. Employing these scores in their study of eight homes they noticed that the 'best' seats were occupied by a higher-than-expected proportion of rational residents and the 'worst' seats by a higher-than-expected proportion of confused residents.

Four characteristics of sitting rooms and spaces were examined by Barrett (1976), whose postgraduate research was supervised by Lipman: the grouping of rooms (discussed in (c) above), the size of sitting rooms, their shape, and the number of sitting spaces on circulation routes. His interviews with architects, planners, and residents suggested that a maximum of ten residents per room was considered institutional. He then calculated the number of residents per sitting room by dividing the total floor area by the recommended twenty-five square feet per person. As regards the shape of the sitting rooms, three aspects appeared to affect the 'degree of domesticity': (i) the number of alcoves and recesses (being purposeful in preventing residents from sitting around the walls and inducing them to gather in small groups); (ii) the proportions of the rooms (long narrow rooms are considered institutional; a length-to-width ratio of less than 4:1 was defined as domestic); and (iii) the presence of fireplaces (they are 'homely' and act as focal points). For each aspect of sitting room shape he derived an operational indicator. Finally he looked at the number of available places in sitting spaces on circulation routes (corridors, stair wells and entrance areas). These foster resident locomotive competence and general independence, and facilitate casual contact between residents.

The trends are thus fairly clear in both the literature and in Ministerial directives — sitting rooms should be small and dispersed, should allow small groups of residents to get together if and when desired, but should be flexibly arranged to increase the range of interactions. One further consideration regards the tidying of dayrooms. Both residents and social work staff would prefer that dayrooms *not* be tidied each and every day (Neill, McGuinness and Warburton, 1976).

(h) Dining rooms

As with lounges and sitting spaces, architectural research emphasises the desirability of small and dispersed dining rooms. In contrast to lounges and sitting spaces, however, dining rooms appear to be getting larger. A random sample of 61 post-1960, purpose-built homes for the elderly in operation at the time of the 1970 Census all had a single dining room, catering on average for 46 residents (Knapp, 1977c). One of the less attractive features of many institutional environments is the block treatment of residents, and nowhere is this more obvious in the modern home than in the dining room. Queueing, the lack of choice on the menu, and the fixed number of residents per table are all aspects of this enforced uniformity. Instead the large formal dining room should be abandoned and replaced by a number of small and dispersed dining areas, decentralised so as to minimise staff-resident interaction and increase residents' initiative and independence (Lipman and Slater, 1977a). Meals should be prepared close to each dining area to further foster independence and reduce block treatment, and also to avoid the practical but not insignificant problem of food getting cold as it is transported from a central kitchen, as was the case in one home recently appraised (Goldsmith, 1971).

(i) Bathrooms and toilets

The revised edition of Local Authority Building Note No. 2 issued in 1973 laid down minimum resident-to-facility ratios of 15:1 for bathrooms and 4:1 for WCs. By these admittedly limited criteria most homes in operation at that time were satisfactory, with post-1960 purpose-built homes revealing average ratios of just under 13:1 and 5:1 in 1970 (Knapp, 1977c). Resident-facility ratios have been laid down in most design recommendations and are clearly important in as much as 'readily available' amenities facilitate resident self-reliance (Lipman and Slater, 1977a). However, the location (dispersion) and design of these facilities is perhaps equally, if not more, important in determining the institutional environment and fostering residents' competence. Residents' dependence will be reduced if basins and WCs can be located in or near each bedroom, and preferably if provided individually (Goldsmith, 1971). Barrett (1976) sees this as a key determinant of domesticity in the old people's home. He focuses on the grouping of WCs, reporting interviewees' ideal design as being two adjacent WCs with separate doors onto a circulation route. His final indicator of this facet of home design was thus the proportion of WCs in the home that were available for residents and were non-institutional.

(j) Activity amenities

One of the reasons why local authority architects have preferred to provide a large single dining room in their newer purpose-built homes instead of a series of small dispersed rooms has been to provide a large activity room where concerts, parties and bingo sessions may all be held. This may be a high price to pay for such functions, which are commonly infrequent and poorly attended (Haringey, 1978; McClannahan, 1973a). Goldsmith (1971) argues that a large entertainments room should be provided in *addition* to a number of small dining spaces, but that there should also be available smaller rooms for individual or small group activities. Only 60 per cent of purpose-built homes have a room or rooms available for residents to interview or receive their visitors in private. Frequently residents are forced to receive daytime visitors in the entrance lobby or the television room.

Provision of space for residents' activities is only a start, however, for spatial arrangements, staff instrusions, apathy of staff and residents, and residents' choice will all determine the extent to which the space is used. Lipman and Slater (1977a), in keeping with their desire to promote residents' independence, argue that activity settings should mobilise residents' resources to counter symptoms of institutional neurosis, 'a disease characterised by apathy, lack of initiative, loss of interest, especially in things of an impersonal nature, submissiveness . . . ' (Barton, 1966), and to allow residents to fulfil their self-actualisation needs. Residents should be allowed to choose when to watch television, and when to change channels, and not have activity and dayrooms tidied daily by domestic staff. Therapy programmes, wherever possible, should not be externally initiated, as this too can produce dependence among passive residents and resentment among the more active.

One of the most detailed studies of activity participation and residents' interaction in nursing and residential homes was carried out by McClannahan (1973a) and reported in her unpublished Ph.D. thesis and in a number of articles. Building on the 'Living Environments' approach of Risley, Doke and others (see section 2.1, and see also the work of the Wessex group reported in that section) a number of alternative strategies aimed at increasing participation were employed and the effects noted. The mere provision of activity rooms and amenities was not sufficient to produce anything above the minimum amounts of participation, and residents needed to be encouraged with the help of various prompts (a public address system, posters and an amplified announcement at lunch). Prompting was kept distinct from cajoling. Failure to prompt meant that only half as many residents attended the activities. Other strategies included setting up a small store within the home, selling cosmetics, clothing, recreation materials, tobacco and confectionary, providing suitable materials and other prostheses for severely disabled geriatric patients, and offering small prizes and serving snacks at group activities such as bingo, art and table game sessions.

The activity amenity characteristics that apparently contribute most to residents' quality of life are widely available activity rooms and re-creation spaces, good location in relation to internal 'traffic' routes and bedrooms, a wide range of choice exercised within them by resi-dents, and a certain amount of prompting.

(k) General resources

Under this rather vague heading we include such diverse resources as minibuses, kitchenettes, sunshades and libraries. Although some earlier American research suggests only a modest relationship between such sources and the quality of care (Kosberg, 1971, 1973; Linn, 1974), residential staff and administrators have nevertheless stressed the need for certain items to enhance quality of life (Lawton, 1975b; Neill *et al.*, 1976). Barrett's look at overall design produced two general resource indicators – the number of institutional and of non-institutional rooms. Institutional rooms are simply those considered by residents and planners to be institutional in character – visitors rooms, sick or medical rooms, specialists' rooms, sewing rooms, and 'smoke rooms'. Non-institutional rooms include kitchenettes. The number of the former should be kept as low as possible, whilst a greater number of non-institutional rooms is to be welcomed.

(l) Staff accommodation

We are not in these paragraphs discussing the need for staff to have somewhere to escape to for a short break from the emotional demands of caring. Case study literature suggests that this is of great importance for monitoring staff morale. In the context of the welfare production process it is the location of staff accommodation relative to that of residents and relative to major internal 'traffic' routes that is of inter-est, rather than the extent and quality of staff accommodation *per se*. The latter will undoubtedly influence staff morale, recruitment and turnover, but it is not considered in this book.

There are oppoisng viewpoints as to whether the matron, super-visory, and care staff should have accommodation within the home. The constant presence of at least some members of staff will reduce the likelihood of serious fires, and will provide a source of on-call night staff. However, resident staff will find it extremely difficult to separate their professional and private lives, may become unnaturally insulated from the norms of community life, and may reinforce the Victorian image of the matron or warden as an inescapable authoritarian figure amongst residents. These thoughts are possibly in the minds of administrators in those local authorities that are currently trying to persuade resident staff to seek accommodation outside the home, purportedly to increase occupancy levels at a time of service contraction or standstill.

Lipman and Slater (1977a) and Barrett (1976) assert the need for resident and staff accommodation to be well separated within the home. Access should be restricted to lifts and stairs, or to corridor links, these barriers preventing casual staff-resident interaction (and hence surveillance and dependence) but not deterring the more persistent members. The principle of least effort will then hopefully ensure that staff-resident interactions are replaced in part by resident-resident interaction. Barrett proposes an operational measure of the position of staff accommodation in relation to resident accommodation, although based on somewhat less extreme separation. Separation, in his view, should be defined as concealment: can supervisory accommodation be seen from resident bedrooms? His recommended indicator of concealment is the number of resident bedrooms from which staff accommodation is concealed, weighted by the total number of bedrooms (or resident places).

(m) Micro design

Practically every sociological treatise, architectural appraisal, Ministerial Design Note, and gerontological study has touched upon one aspect or another of 'micro design'. Detailed description and layout of residents' bedrooms, of corridor design, and of bathrooms, comments on floor coverings, the height of baths and basins, the position of light switches, the importance of slowly closing lift doors, the danger of raised thresholds on doors are just some of the micro design recommendations put forward. In an attempt to bring some order to this amorphous collection we shall follow Lawton (1975b, pp.213-17) in listing the various recommendations as they impinge upon fourteen self-maintenance skills.

1   Toileting — enough room for wheelchair turning; outward opening bathroom door; provision of bath *and* shower; low bath height; toilet paper at side; non-institutional design. (See also subsection (i).)
2   Grooming — full length mirror to increase self-concept, remind him of his social self, and improve his self-grooming. (See also

Lawton, 1970b.)
3   Housekeeping − storage space needed; view from windows; easily opened windows.
4   Eating − tables for four; choice of location. (See (h) above.)
5   Sleeping − separate bedrooms, L-shaped room (to hide bed); pictures and pegboards. (See also (f) above.)
6   Body comfort − heat control, air conditioning.[4]
7   Walking − locomotive prostheses in corridors; ramps not steps; clear contrast between step treads and risers; short hallways; smooth-paved main walks (McClannahan, 1973a).
8   Work − space for crafts, sheltered workshop.
9   Orientation − definite street address; non-institutional exterior design; large map with local amenities marked.
10 Life-enriching activity − at least one centrally located community room; resident kitchen near community room; seats in the entrance lobby; small-group activity rooms. (See also (j) above.)
11 Aesthetics − pleasant decor for all common space − clutter *is* desirable; warm exterior materials; consistency of building structure with other neighbourhood buildings.
12 Social behaviour − concentration of paths near entrance; small social spaces dotted throughout home; 4- and 6-person dining tables; widely spaced dining tables; snack bar.
13 Outdoor activity − seating to suit all climatic conditions; seating with maximum view of everyday life; two-person benches; portable seats; benches at nearby bus stops.
14 Privacy − 'individual dwelling units are the main means for gaining privacy'; locks on WC, bathroom and bedroom doors (Lipman and Slater, 1977a).

(n) Condition of the home

As was made clear by Townsend (1962), some homes may be well-appointed with resources and amenities, and be well-designed inside and out, but the influences of these will be negated by a poor state of repair of the home and its grounds. Schooler (1970b) found that a condition-of-home factor was related to residents' morale in his study of American housing for the elderly. However, if we take the domesticity criterion stressed by Barrett, we must be careful not to make the home too aseptic or hotel-like, for such environments are neither domestic nor in many regards in the least bit similar to those which residents have left.

(o) Siting of the home

The Census of Residential Accommodation in England and Wales of 1970 asked matrons to indicate whether the home was well, moderately or badly sited in relation to amenities for residents (shops, church, pub, transport). The responses, though subjective and subject to certain response biases, revealed that newer, purpose-built homes were 'judged only slightly more likely to be well sited than older homes' (DHSS, 1975, p.5). In the period immediately following the National Assistance Act, local authorities were faced with rapidly increasing demand for residential care and capital expenditure restrictions, and were thus forced to convert former private dwellings into residential homes. These were frequently situated outside of towns and away from centres of activity. As time has progressed and capital restrictions gradually eased (until recently), authorities have been increasingly able to integrate new homes into local communities, although often not without resistance from private householders. In particular, plans for new housing frequently include a residential home and/or day centre. The need to site homes 'centrally' needs no emphasis: residents have much greater incentive to go out and become involved in community activities, members of the local community are more likely to come to the home for activities and day care, residents have much more to watch from the home and, if the residents can be accommodated close to their former homes, there is a greater chance of life continuity. Schooler's (1970b) study confirms the importance of these factors. Residents in housing projects located close to facilities (barber, bank, stores, public transport), friends and relatives scored higher on morale scales than residents of poorly located projects.

4.2.2 Summary indicators of capital

Two quite distinct 'traditions' appear to converge upon a single summary indicator of the capital input in the case of residential care. Firstly, we can distinguish the vast majority of conventional economic production studies which have adopted a single capital index for use in the complex manipulations of their modelling exercises of production processes. Secondly, we have a group of planners and architects (and a few students of housing policy) who have exercised considerable ingenuity in deriving unidimensional housing or residence indicators. In both 'traditions' the emphasis has been on unidimensionality, although for quite different reasons. Economists have been constrained by severe data limitations and to some extent blinkered by a need to quote capital-labour ratios and marginal productivity values. Housing quality indicators, on the other hand, have usually been constructed to allow the mapping of housing condition differences between and within areas, and occasionally to help explain variations in house prices or housing demand and supply (Duncan, 1971; Wilkinson, 1973).

In the present context, we would argue that summary measures of residential home capital would be both difficult to obtain and wasteful of valuable policy-related information. Relatively few attempts have been made to obtain summary measures of residential home capital or design. Two *theoretically* based procedures are apparent. Firstly, many of the quality of care indicators suggest aggregating various design features, but usually in an arbitrary manner (for a survey, see Kart and Manard, 1976). Secondly, the DHSS have themselves attempted to obtain classification of data collected in the Census of Residential Homes, 1970.[5] The internal structure of each home was put into one of four categories by comparing various characteristics of the home with the standards laid down in Building Note No. 2, 1973. The categories were:

(a) home comes up to Building Note standards;
(b) home is adequate, possessing all of fourteen listed characteristics, but fails to come up to Building Note Standards;
(c) home is inadequate, not being in categories (a), (b) or (d);
(d) home is seriously inadequate, having one or more of nine listed characteristics.

Regrettably, every one of the 3,365 homes within the Census was, on these criteria, either inadequate or seriously inadequate. This is an indication, not of the stringency of the categorisation criteria nor of the 1973 Building Note standards (which, of course, were not in force at the time of the Census of 1970), but of the nationwide unsatisfactoriness of residential accommodation. Because the DHSS 'Fabric Index' is thus only dichotomous and of course unidimensional, it is not really adequate for an analysis of the kind described in this paper.

There have additionally been at least two attempts to find an *empirically* determined dimensionality for residential accommodation for the elderly. Schooler's (1970b) factor analysis included a number of design variables and he was able to determine six meaningful dimensions of home environment which he then scaled independently (although whether on the basis of factor scores is not clear). Second, Knapp (1977c) reported an application of both factor analytic and principal component techniques to a random sample of 200 County Borough homes from the 1970 Census, but found that neither produced a dimensionality with any plausible theoretical interpretation. This general uninterpretability of the extracted factors and components outweighs the reasonably good 'fit' obtained and thus casts doubts upon the usefulness of an empirically derived dimensionality.

This lack of dimensionality, both theoretically predictable and empirically interpretable, coupled with the general uncertainty within gerontology of even the *direction* of influence of the design variables upon residents' morale and well-being, indicate that it woud be unwise to attempt to construct 'hold-all' indices of design.

As well as these various theoretically- and empirically-based summary indicators of home capital, or at least home design, there is the conventional cost-based indicator familiar to economists. The diversity of the capital equipment employed in those production processes more conventionally studied by economists and, of course, the very nature of economic science itself have been responsible for this concentration on the *cost* of capital. As our discussion in this subsection makes very plain, residential home capital inputs are no less diverse — and probably more so — than the capital inputs of, say, a manufacturing industry. However, the reluctance of economists — with precious few exceptions — to concern themselves with the problems and policies of the personal social services has left us with very little knowledge of the capital costs of social care and, more generally, has left these services with an embarrassing paucity of sound economic expertise. There have been numerous periods of capital expenditure constraint in British post-war history, yet only Wager (1972) and Thomas *et al.* (1979) have studied the construction costs of old people's homes in Britain, whilst on the other side of the Atlantic, where the private sector is rather more important in the provision of care services than in Britain, there is apparently a better appreciation of these principles. The recent papers by McCaffree *et al.* (1975) and McCaffree (1977) provide clear accounts of the assumptions, methodologies and costs involved.

4.3. Conclusion

In this chapter we have concerned ourselves with the two principal resource inputs into residential care — the manpower input and the rather more durable capital input. It is, of course, extremely difficult to divorce a discussion of these resource inputs from a detailed discussion of the non-resource or quasi-inputs, particularly the social environment or caring milieu of the home. Thus, our discussion in subsequent chapters will frequently touch upon the concepts discussed in detail in the present chapter. There is a third set of resource inputs into the welfare production process which we should distinguish. These inputs differ from the manpower and capital inputs in that they are not directly supplied by home staff, they are very much less durable, and they are generally rather more 'individualised'. Some of these resources are clearly 'consumables' (to use the economic jargon) — medications, surgical appliances, disposable items of linen or clothing, diet and various other minor items. There would appear to have been very little research on these consumable items, with notable exception of the dietary intake of elderly persons. There is a strong tradition of 'nutrition research' among British geriatricians and gerontologists, exemplified by the numerous studies conducted by researchers at University College Hospital, London (Exton-Smith, 1968, 1970; Stanton, 1971) and Queen Elizabeth College, London (Davies, Hastrop and Bender, 1975; Holdsworth, 1978). Studies of malnutrition and of diets in general, like studies of hypothermia, are fairly numerous in the British literature, and in both cases we face the problem of deciding where they fit into the production of welfare process. Our arguments of chapter 3 indicate that there are elements of nurture and nutrition which may legitimately be included in a listing of the outputs of residential homes, whilst others should be retained as inputs. Also in this third set of resource inputs are the numerous and various personal possessions of the elderly residents, loss of which can dramatically alter the course of the individual's life within the home (Sherman and Newman, 1977). These are discussed again in the next chapter.

In the next two chapters we concern ourselves with the non-resource quasi-inputs into the welfare production process for old people's homes. We first tackle the social environment of the home and then, in chapter 6, focus on individual characteristics and experiences and their impact on the well-being of residents.

Chapter 5

Social environment

5.1 The general environment of the home

Our point of departure in this chapter is a theory of differences in environments and their social consequences, rather than a theory of individual personality and its implications for what types of environment stimulate psychological well-being. The focus of the theory is therefore on the role perceptions of groups of varying power, their interactions, and the structural factors that influence accounting processes which in turn influence behaviour in interactive contexts. For this reason, some of the studies that we shall review make use of parallel instruments to collect data on perceptions of the environment of both care staff and residents. The theory is thus predominantly sociological rather than psychological, though both disciplines may be the basis for data collection in a practical application.

The starting point for many of the recent attempts to examine the impact of residential environments is recognition of, and occasional borrowing from, the seminal contributions of Goffman (1961) and Kleemeier (1961). Goffman's essays on 'the social situation of mental patients and other inmates' introduced the concept of the total institution, and subsequent discussions of environments have often focused on criteria of totality laid out by Goffman. Probably most forms of institution have at one time or another been the subject of investigations of such an orientation. Kleemeier, in contrast, was specifically interested in environments of the *elderly* and distinguished 'congregate', 'segregate', and 'institutional control' dimensions. This dimensionality has been adopted and adapted in a number of gerontological studies, with the contributions of Pincus (1968) and Kahana (1974) being perhaps the best known.

Other investigators have preferred to go back further for their theoretical bases, and particularly to the works of Lewin (1935) and

Murray (1938). Lewin asserted that behaviour was a function of the relationship between a person and his environment, and in subsequent studies concentrated on such climatic features as leadership atmosphere, social norms, and opportunities for new role acquisitions (Lewin, 1946, 1952). Murray also wrote of the relationship between person and environment, but emphasised the importance of an *optimal balance* between personal needs (whose strength characterises 'personality') and environmental press (the forces or stimuli of the environment). Expansion of this 'need-press' model by Stern, Stein and Bloom (1956) and Pace and Stern (1958) was later followed by the empirical applications of Moos, Lawton and others. As with the works of Goffman, Kleemeier and Lewin, we shall have more to say about Murray's theoretical contribution in our consideration of some of the more important theoretical perspectives on social climates for the elderly in section 5.2.

The next section of this chapter therefore takes a look at the social ecology model of Lawton and his associates. This model is based on Murray's need-press theory, emphasising the relationship between the elderly individual's level of competence ('a diverse collection of abilities residing within the individual') and the environmental press. This approach can be viewed as a special case of DeLong's (1974) theory of Coding Behaviour and is consistent with a large body of sociological research collectively known as Exchange Theory. We shall also examine those gerontological studies that have built, respectively, on the contributions of Goffman and Kleemeier. Principal among the former is Ruth Bennett's ten item scale of totality, but there are also very many other studies which have, either explicitly or implicitly, examined elements of totality and their relationship to aspects of well-being among the elderly. Kleemeier's dimensionality has most notably begotten Pincus's 'Homes for the Aged Description Questionnaire', which in turn partly inspired Kahana's congruence model of residential care. The fact that Eva Kahana focuses directly upon the degree of congruence between the elderly person's needs and the properties of his environment, and that she extensively references Barker's (1968) study of behaviour settings, illustrates the interrelatedness of these approaches and, to a limited degree, the artificiality of the distinction adopted here. We shall, however, persist with this trichotomy, in an attempt to impose a little order on what is a vast and various body of literature.

Section 5.3 pulls together these various theoretical perspectives by distinguishing and discussing a number of common themes, or dimensions, of the social environments of old people's homes and related residential settings. For example, writers focusing on aspects of totality, researchers applying the 'competence-press model', and investigators working in the Kleemeier tradition, have all emphasised the importance for quality of life of residents' privacy and the regime of the institution. These aspects of milieu therefore receive separate treatment in the third section, along with such other dimensions as the degree of stimulation afforded by the environment, individuality and environmental homogeneity, and communication and interaction.

5.2 Theoretical perspectives on social environment

5.2.1 Environmental totality and the elderly

There can be little doubt that Goffman's introduction and formalisation of the concept of *institutional totality* is one of the most important milestones in the development of institutional care and confinement. Whilst in many respects his essay, *Asylums*, represented a synthesis of views and propositions that had been recognised before, the fact that almost every subsequent treatise on the social aspects of residential living has extensively referenced his work stands witness to his impact.

Goffman (1961, section III) distinguished four characteristics which served to define an institution as total:

> First, all aspects of life are conducted in the same place and under the same single authority. Second, each phase of the member's daily activity is carried on in the immediate company of a large batch of others, all of whom are treated alike and required to do the same thing together. Third, all phases of the day's activities are tightly scheduled, with one activity leading at a prearranged time into the next, the whole sequence of activities being imposed from above by a system of explicit formal rulings and a body of officials. Finally, the various enforced activities are brought together into a single rational plan purportedly designed to fulfil the official aims of the institution.

Thus residential institutions are 'social hybrids, part residential community, part formal organisation . . . symbolised by the barrier to social intercourse with the outside'. Old people's homes fall into the first of five categories of institutions – for persons incapable and harmless.

Indicators and indices of environmental totality have been developed and applied to virtually all types of institution. For example, Wing and Brown (1970) developed a scale of ward restrictiveness for use in mental hospitals in Britain, and Kellam, Shmelzer and Berman (1966) proposed the concept of an 'adult status dimension' to assess the degree to which patients on psychiatric wards were 'allowed to maintain basic symbols of adulthood'. Both scales are closely linked to Goffman's characteristics of totality. Similarly, Apte's (1968) Hostel-Hospital Practice Profile and the social climate questionnnaire for approved schools and community homes developed by Heal, Sinclair and Troop (1973) have items closely allied to those of Goffman. Whilst there is possibly something to gain from a critical examination of these totality constructs in other fields, we here restrict our attention to those whose specific focus is the social environment of the aged person, and only deviate significantly from this path to discuss King and Raynes's (1968) Inmate Management Scale for children's homes. John Townsend and Ann Kimbell (1975) later adapted the Inmate Management Scale for use in a study of old people's homes in Cheshire.

The earliest development of Goffman's ideas in a gerontological direction came from Ruth Bennett (1963). In a series of papers, Bennett drew up and applied an Index of Totality based on ten criteria, each rated as high, medium or low in totality. These criteria are listed below, together with Bennett's descriptions of high and low totality in parentheses:

(a) the planned duration of residence (permanent *v*. temporary);
(b) the orientation of activities (towards the institution *v*. towards the community);
(c) pattern of recruitment (involuntary *v*. voluntary);
(d) the residential pattern (congregate living *v*. private quarters);
(e) the system of sanctions (standardized objective rewards and punishments vs. none);
(f) the scheduling of activities (group sequential activities *v*. individual choices);
(g) provisions made for disseminating normative information (formal provisions *v*. none);
(h) provisions made for allocation of staff time to observation of residents (provision for continual observation *v*. none);
(i) personal property of residents (most removed *v*. none removed); and
(j) decision-making about personal property (residents make no decisions *v*. all decisions).

Bennett's Totality Index has been applied in a number of different settings in the USA. In the original 1963 paper, the author describes certain aspects of the social structure of an institution for the aged in New York City which she had been studying for five years. This home received a rating in the middle to high range on the index. In a later study, Bennett and Nahemow (1965b) described how social adjustment criteria differed between the various types of institutional facility (geriatric ward of a mental hospital, nursing home, apartment residence of a home for the aged, institutional division of a home for the aged, and a public housing development), and how these differences reflect basic differences in the degree of totality. In institutions ranked high in totality (nursing homes and homes for the aged), adjustment criteria for residents were vague or non-existent. Socialisation, defined by Bennett and Nahemow (1965a) as the amount of information learned about the home, was better in settings of low totality, and normative knowledge was not a prerequisite for successful adustment in homes of low and high totality, but only for settings of medium totality. 'Only in the middle totality range is how well you do socially a clear reflection of what you know' (Bennett and Nahemow, 1972). Environmental totality by Bennett's criteria was found to vary considerably between nursing homes and high totality was related to the age of the institution and to the lack of gerontological training among staff (Bennett and Eisdorfer, 1975). Bennett's Totality Index thus differentiates well between residential settings which differ with regard to their basic philosophies of care and their resident populations. However, the gradations are insufficiently fine and the dimensions too broadly arranged for the index to be immediately useful in a study of British old people's homes. Most conventional homes would receive identical ratings on each of the first four criteria (at least), which would thus appear redundant, and the range of environments covered by the 'medium totality' label on most of the other criteria is far too wide to be sensitive to crucially important variations in residential practices and conventions.

Another Totality Index has been developed by Coe (1965), who contrasted the effects of three institutional environments of different degrees of totality. Higher totality was found to be related to more withdrawal and depersonalisation by residents themselves. The index of totality included concepts assessing the lack of privacy, rigidity of scheduling, limitations on access to personal property, and use of force by staff. Kahana and Coe (1969) built on this index in their study of conformity and deviance in a Jewish home for the aged. Where there were few formalised, clear, and unambiguous rules, the elderly were able to cope.

The most important study of totality in a British residential care setting was conducted by King, Raynes and Tizard (1971), using the scales developed by the first two authors a few years earlier. The King and Raynes (1968) operational measure of Inmate Management in children's homes has four dimensions of institutional variation:

(a) the rigidity of the routine (inflexibility of management practice — neither individual differences nor unique circumstances are taken into account);
(b) the block treatment of inmates (regimentation of inmates together as a group before, during, or after a specific activity);
(c) the depersonalisation of inmates (denials of opportunities for inmate privacy, self-expression, and personal possession and initiative); and

(d) the social distance between staff and inmates (separation of staff and inmate worlds, keeping their areas of accommodation apart, and limiting interactions between staff and inmates to functionally specific formal activities).

The scale has dimensions which can clearly be linked to some of the criteria of Bennett. However, the King and Raynes scale will be much more sensitive to subtle (though important) differences in social environment. It was applied in a study of three children's homes by King *et al.* (1971). Later the scale was adapted for studying old people's homes by Townsend and Kimbell (1975) who concentrated on three aspects of regime — structure of routine, depersonalisation, and social distance. With a sample of ten homes situated in the old county of Cheshire, they found no relationship between regime and dependency, but did find that confusion and the number of activities, and confusion and social distance between staff and residents, were positively associated, although they prefer to reserve judgment as to the direction of causation.

The totality scales of King and Raynes (1968) and Townsend and Kimbell (1975) have a number of drawbacks. In common with Bennett's index, the totality constructs fail to cover some of the dimensions of environment distinguished in other theoretical perspectives — for example, the segregate dimension in Kleemeier's schema (see section 5.2.2), the homogeniety of the environment in general, the frequency and nature of interaction, and so on. Later work by Norma Raynes uses the scale in conjunction with other dimensions of environment (Raynes, Pratt and Roses, 1979). The scale is also too general for a study specific to homes for the aged. King and Raynes deliberately kept their scale independent of the characteristics of the particular types of establishment studied, including the age of inmates. Furthermore, one of the items of the King and Raynes measure defined a home as institution-oriented (as opposed to child-oriented) when there was a sharp distinction between staff and inmate worlds; that is, greater social distance between staff and residents meant a greater degree of totality. This assumption contrasts sharply with the recommendation of Lipman and Slater (1977a) and Barrett (1976), among others, that staff and resident worlds should be kept apart as much as possible. Caring practices and principles are far too different to allow simple transmutation of the scale. Finally, and more fundamentally, the dimensions do not reflect personality theory. Indeed it seems that they are intended not to, since King and Raynes deliberately sought to avoid a reliance on any particular theory of child management (King and Raynes, 1968, p.43). Such scales were developed not for the measurement and explanation of output *per se*. They were intended as one item in an evaluation of differences in the quality of residential care based more on data on inputs and their use (such as staff ratios and staff deployment, information about staff role and staff performance, and management practices) than on outputs, the effects on the residents.

We discuss some of the more important aspects of totality – such as privacy, interpersonal interaction, and environmental constraint – in the next section of this chapter.

5.2.2 Congregation, segregation and institutional control

Another large body of research literature regarding the impact of a setting upon the life-style and well-being of its inhabitants was generated by Kleemeier's essay on 'The use and meaning of time in special settings' (Kleemeier, 1961). In that essay he distinguishes three 'descriptive dimensions of special settings' which serve to describe the environment-individual impact:

(i) *The Segregate-Nonsegregate Continuum*: 'the condition under which older persons may live exclusively among their age peers having little contact with other age groups'.

(ii) *The Institutional/Non-Institutional Continuum*: 'the varying degrees to which the individual must adjust his life to imposed rules, discipline, and the various means of social control used by staff'.

(iii) *The Congregate/Non-Congregate Continnum*: 'the closeness of individuals to each other and . . . the degree of privacy possible to attain in the settings'.

These Segregate, Institutional Control, and Congregate dimensions have been generalised in subsequent use. For example, the Segregate dimension was, in Kleemeier's initial statement, concerned solely with the age homogeneity or heterogeneity of the setting, but has since been expanded to include homogeneity of sex, health status, level of functioning, ethnic background and race, permanency and religion. Any social or individual characteristic, when prevalent among a group of persons concentrated in a single setting, which exerts an influence upon residents' well-being and behaviour should therefore be included within the Segregate Dimension. The Institutional Control Dimension will similarly cover all aspects of regime and constraint within the home, and particularly those totality characteristics stressed by Goffman, Bennett and others. The final dimension concerns the congregation of residents – their physical proximity and degree of enforced interaction, and the resultant degree of privacy afforded them.

The similarity of the approaches of Kleemeier and Goffman is fairly self-evident. Environments which are strongly homogeneous along salient dimensions, which permit little individual freedom of choice or movement, and which severely restrict privacy simply disregard most individual needs and preferences. 'Institutions which are high on the segregate, congregate, and institutional dimensions of Kleemeier's schema may ... be seen as having strong totalistic features in Goffman's sense' (Kahana, 1974, p.204).

There have been two major applications of Kleemeier's schema – the earlier work of Allen Pincus on the definition and measurement of the psychosocial milieu in homes for the aged (Pincus, 1968, 1968a; Pincus and Wood, 1970), and the general congruence model of Eva Kahana (1974). Pincus's 'Home for the Aged Description Questionnaire' (HDQ) is perhaps the more general tool for describing the institutional environment, but Kahana's systems of dimensions of congruence has the signal virtue of linking Kleemeier's contribution to the 'press model' of Lewin and Murray, and the subsequent ecological models of Moos and Lawton (see below).

Pincus (1968) defines the institutional environment as: 'The psychological milieu in which the residents live, as expressed through and/or generated by: (a) physical aspects of the setting ...; (b) rules, regulations, and programme ...; and (c) staff behaviour with residents' (ibid., p.207). These three generating dimensions do not, however, cover all salient aspects of the environment – neglecting, for example, the social and personal environments broadly defined, and the so-called 'supra-personal environment' (see below). The latter omission is all the more surprising in view of Pincus' desire to base his HDQ on Kleemeier's dimensionality, an important component of which is the homogeneity of residents with respect to age and such other salient characteristics as those listed above.

The second stage of Pincus's development of Kleemeier's perspective is to distinguish four dimensions of the institutional environment which will adequately and comprehensively describe the important aspects of each of the three generating characteristics (a), (b) and (c). These four dimensions are:

1 the public/private dimension (privacy);
2 the structured/unstructured dimension (regime and the degree of individual choice);
3 the resource rich/resource sparse dimension (stimulation and social interaction); and
4 the isolated/integrated dimension (communication and interaction outside the home).

The third and final stage is to cross-classify the generating factors (a) – (c) with the four descriptive dimensions (1) – (4) to obtain a twelve-celled framework to guide the measurement of the environmental climate. Some examples of environmental aspects for each of the cells are given in the following table, reproduced from Pincus (1968,

115

Table 5.1 The twelve cells of Pincus's 'Homes Description Questionnaire' (Taken from Pincus, 1968. p.208)

Aspects of the institutional setting	Dimensions of the institutional environment			
	Public/private	Structured/ unstructured	Resource sparce/ resource rich	Integrated/isolated
Physical plant	Proportion of single and double rooms; number of day rooms	Existence of signs displayed around the home reminding residents of rules and regulations	Availability of facilities where residents can cook a meal or prepare a snack; existence of a library	Distance from public transportation; distance from shopping area
Rules and regulations and programme	Existence of rules requiring residents to keep the doors to their rooms open at all times	Existence of rules regulating residents' bedtime; provisions for residents to help in planning activities	Existence of regular jobs around the home performed by residents	Extent of restrictions placed on visiting hours; frequency with which residents are taken on trips outside the home
Staff behaviour	Extent to which staff knock on doors before entering residents' rooms	Extent to which staff decide what programmes are to be watched on TV; extent to which staff expect strict obedience from residents	Extent to which staff encourage residents to participate in activities	Extent to which staff assist residents who need help in making phone calls or writing letters

(Reprinted by permission of *The Gerontologist*, 1835 K Street, NW, Suite 305, Washington, DC 20006; vol. 8, no. 3, 1968, p. 208.)

p.208). Items for each cell were gleaned from previous studies of old people's homes, and from the 72 item 'Characteristics of the Treatment Environment Scale' developed for mental hospitals by Jackson (1964).

The final version of Pincus's scale has 36 items, each in the form of a statement about life in the home. A 5-point scale is used for each statement, ranging from 'completely true' to 'completely false'. One of the basic assumptions of this approach is the multidimensionality of the institutional environment. The classification of aspects (1) – (4) above represents one possible arrangement; a second was examined by factor analysing responses from 263 staff questionnaires. At first, four factors were derived and found to conform reasonably well to the prior notion of public/private, structured/unstructured, resource rich/resource sparse, and isolated/integrated components. However, a more general analysis reported in Pincus and Wood (1970) allowed the extraction of five factors – a fifth (Personalisation) component, referring to the social distance between staff and residents, being added to the other four. Intercorrelation of dimension scores was fairly low, suggesting empirical independence.

The HDQ was found to give a picture of the residential environment not dissimilar to observations made by a researcher and project interviewers prior to administration of the questionnaire. Each questionnaire took no more than fifteen minutes to complete by staff members, and no difficulties were encountered by these respondents. In the second study, Pincus and Wood (1970) also administered the HDQ to 39 residents in one home and compared their responses and perceptions to those of the staff. Responses were significantly different on three of the five dimensions – the freedom (structured/unstructured), resources (rich/sparse), and the integration/isolation dimensions. Generally, staff saw the environment as providing more freedom and more resources for residents, but perceived residents as more isolated from the community than did the residents themselves. Second, the responses of skilled staff (nurses, technicians, office and administrative staff, and professionals) and unskilled staff (maintenance, domestic and kitchen staff) were compared. The only significant difference observed was on the structured/unstructured dimension – unskilled staff regarding the environment as offering less freedom. The authors can offer no convincing explanations for these differences.

The validity of the HDQ thus far is reasonable. It is based quite explicitly on the theoretical model of Robert Kleemeier and, apart from an inadequate coverage of the latter's Segregate dimension, appears to capture the essence of his approach. Within the 3 x 4 framework set out above it is possible to include most, but not all, of the dimensions of importance stressed by other writers. Of course, it would be possible to add, say, a supra-personal component to the vertical classification (see section 5.2.3(B) below) and a fifth category representing the Personalisation factor to the horizontal. As regards validity against the observations of researchers and professionals, the scale performs well, but the internal consistency of responses between staff and residents is less encouraging. Given the 'multiple realities' in an old people's home (Gubrium, 1974), such differences between staff and resident perceptions are to be expected and, indeed, are important data for an adequate production perspective on residential care. Finally, Pincus suggests the HDQ be validated against residents' behaviour, a suggestion taken up in a study by Reiter and Nuehring (1968) and cited by Pincus and Wood (1970). From this they concluded that:

> Except for the Resource dimension the subjective and behavioural measures with respect to the same dimension are significantly correlated. In addition the subjective measures with respect to the Freedom and Resource dimensions correlate significantly with the behavioural measure of Privacy.

Furthermore, subjective feelings about the environmental dimensions were better predictors of overall satisfaction with the home than was the residents' overt behaviour. These conclusions should, however, be taken as no more than tentative in view of the crude nature of the Reiter and Nuehring study.

In addition to Pincus's measurement of the institutional environment along the lines originally suggested by Kleemeier, there have been two *congruence* models of behaviour and affect which have used the Congregate, Segregate and Institutional Control dimensions. The earlier of the two, reported in the unpublished thesis of Mangum (1971), will be discussed in the section 5.2.3. The other Kleemeier-based congruence study was conducted by Kahana (1974).

Kahana focused directly on the degree of fit between the elderly person and the properties of his environment, positing a tension-reduction, but apparently not a tension-creation, model of human behaviour: 'The individual's profile of personal needs and preferences must always be considered in conjunction with the profile of the environment in evaluating residential settings' (ibid., p.203). The environment profile adopted by Kahana is precisely the classification of Kleemeier as described above. Each of the three aspects of environment are described, and individual resident preferences specified in order to establish the degree of congruence:

1 *Segregation* — homogeneity of residents, presence of routines, continuity or similarity of residential life as compared with community life.

2 *Congregation* – privacy, individuality of care and regime, availability of choices, pursuit of own interests.

3 *Institutional control* – control over resources, behaviour and personal possessions, tolerance of deviance, encouragement of dependence.

Four other dimensions of congruence are based on characteristics of the aged individual – particularly cognitive functioning and personality organisation – and 'the lack of congruence between environmental expectations and the needs and characteristics of the ageing individual may be especially difficult to cope with in these areas' (ibid., p.207). These four dimensions are:

4 *Structure* – ambiguity of expectations and roles, order and organisation.

5 *Stimulation activity* – availability, orientation and extent of stimuli from physical and social environments.

6 *Affect* – tolerance of 'affective expression' and emotion, amount of excitement and emotional stimulation.

7 *Impulse control* – immediate or postponed need gratification, tolerance of restlessness and wandering, importance of level-headedness.

For full details see Kahana, 1974, pp.209-10.)

This schema was applied in a study of three homes serving diverse populations – a traditional non-profit home for the aged, a professionally oriented home, and a proprietory nursing home mainly catering for fairly affluent residents. At least thirty residents in each home were interviewed about their personal life space, their preferences for segregation, congregation and so on, their morale (using Lawton's PGC morale scale) and their self-rated life satisfaction. In two of the three homes, a stepwise regression procedure indicated that congruence was an important and significant determinant of well-being. With samples of 43, 50 and 30 residents respectively, the congruence measures collectively explained 45, 29 and 83 per cent of the variation in scores on the PGC morale scale, and 51, 40 and 51 per cent of the variation in self-rated life satisfaction. Each of the subdimensions of the seven 'global' dimensions listed above was entered according to the usual criteria of a stepwise regression procedure. This unfortunately means that the excess of the number of residents over the number of subdimensions is relatively small and may serve to cast a little doubt upon the reliability of the empirical results. Five subdimensions emerged as important determinants of morale: privacy was among the best predictors of morale in all three homes, and motor-control, stimulation, continuity with the past, and change versus sameness were of considerable importance in two out of three homes.

It should be noted that in the third home, in which individual-environmental congruence was least important as a determinant of well-being, there were more options available to residents. 'This home had fewer total institutional features.' We shall find in the next subsection that this result lends support to the 'environmental docility hypothesis' of Lawton and Simon (1968).

5.2.3 Individual competence and environmental press

Henry Murray's (1938) treatise on personality was the first to recognise in a theoretical framework at least, the dual process of personal needs and environmental press. Murray argued that 'press' (forces, stimuli) acted in a way which either satisfied or frustrated personal needs, with the result that human behaviour could be most usefully studied by examining the nature of person-environment interaction. The strength of these needs characterises an individual's 'personality' and it was this side of the interactive process that received most of Murray's attention. His list of needs were *psychogenic* motivational tendencies which he distinguished from the 'viscerogenic' (biological and homeostatic) needs. No parallel development in the objective measurement of environmental press was forthcoming until the work of Stern, Stein and Bloom (1956). Defining a setting to include the social demands made upon individuals greatly improved the prediction of behaviour. Later, Pace and Stern (1958) looked at the 'perceived climate' of students at colleges and universities, and took the consensus of students' perceptions as a measure of environmental climate. This climate was demonstrated to exert a significant influence upon students' behaviour.

Further developments of the need-press model in the context of institutional care or containment have progressed in a number of directions. Of particular interest in this production model of the care of *elderly* persons are the social ecology models of Lawton and Moos, and the many empirical studies they have generated.

(A) Moos's social climate scale

We have already alluded to Moos's argument that there exists a 'prediction sound barrier' in the explanation of behaviour in various fields and his argument that a person's behaviour outside an institutional setting is unrelated to that inside. The more intensive, cohesive, and socially integrated the residential setting, the greater is its impact on behaviour likely to be: 'The press of the environment as the patient perceives it establishes the directions his behaviour should take if he is to find satisfaction and reward within the ward culture' (Moos and Houts, 1970, p.482). Thus, basing his work explicitly on that of Murray (1938) and Stern (1970) Moos was able to postulate a tightly-reasoned need-press model, and to develop scales for its testing – the Community-Oriented Programmes Environment Scale (COPES), its associated Ward Atmosphere Scale (WAS), and the more recent Sheltered Care Environment Scale (SCES) for the elderly.

Moos and his associates in Palo Alto, California, have only recently turned their attention to environments for the elderly after a number of years studying a wide variety of other institutional environments. Most of the earlier studies shared common dimensions, based in part on the theories of Murray and Stern, with a pool of questionnaire items collected after meticulous study of the respective environments. Ten dimensions were distinguished in these earlier studies:

(a) *Involvement* – of members in the day-to-day functioning of the environment.
(b) *Support* – are staff and residents supportive toward each other?
(c) *Spontaneity* – how much does the environment foster emotional expression?
(d) *Autonomy* – the emphasis on independence.
(e) *Practical orientation* – orientation towards future goals.
(f) *Personal problem orientation* – independence in personal problems.
(g) *Anger and aggression* – allowances for.
(h) *Order and organisation* – the importance of structure and organisation.
(i) *Programme clarity* – clarity of rules and procedures.
(j) *Staff control* – extent of staff control over residents.

These ten dimensions, which together constitute the COPES, form three clusters – relationship variables (dimensions a, b, c), programme variables (d, e, f, g) and system maintenance and administrative variables (h, i, j). The scales – with 100 true/false items covering the ten dimensions – were then used to ask both staff and inmates (patients, residents) about the usual patterns of behaviour. In this way Moos intended to ascertain the subjective perceptions that actually influence behaviour, obtaining data both for individuals and for the environment under the same dimensions. This allows better assessment of the congruence between the individual and his environment. Other scales based on the same items asked inmates and staff about the characteristics they would consider ideal, thus providing information about ideational quasi-inputs. Thus four sets of data are available for comparison in order to establish congruence: data from staff and from inmates about the environment as they perceived it; and data from staff and from inmates about how each would like the environment to be. Full details of the COPES instrument – its careful development and its application – are given by Moos (1972, 1974a, 1974b). Raynes *et al.*

(1979) have since developed this line of work in a related area of research (see chapter 4).

There is no evidence to suggest that either Moos or his associates in Palo Alto used the COPES instrument to assess environments for the *elderly*. Instead it was left to O'Donnell, Collins and Schuler (1978) to examine its usefulness in this context. These researchers administered the scale to '20 non-geriatric younger residents, 20 geriatric residents, and 20 nursing home staff' of a convalescent centre in Wisconsin. Using a slightly reworded version of COPES, O'Donnell and his associates compared the perceptions of the three groups of respondents along each of the ten dimensions. On the whole they found that older residents and staff held much more positive feelings about the environment – they placed 'more emphasis on relationships, and consistently perceived more involvement, support and spontaneity than the younger residents' (ibid., p.270). Unfortunately, the sample of residents and staff used for the study – and the limitation to a single nursing home – make it dangerous to generalise from their results and conclusions. Furthermore, Rudolf Moos has himself recently reentered the fray, developing a Sheltered Care Environment Scale (SCES) to evaluate sheltered care settings for the elderly (Moos, Gauvain, Lemke, Max and Mehren, 1979).

There are a number of similarities between the earlier COPES instrument and the later SCES instrument – although a few slight changes in nomenclature tend to disguise them. The three 'global clusters' of environmental dimensions used earlier are retained for this latest scale, although they are now called the Relationship, Personal Growth, and System Maintenance and System Change dimensions or clusters. The constituent subscales of the SCES are listed below, the first two assessing the Relationship dimension, the third and fourth the Personal Growth dimension, and the final three the System Maintenance and Change dimension:

(a) *Cohesion* – help, support and involvement of staff with residents and residents with each other.
(b) *Conflict* – extent of expression of anger and criticism by residents.
(c) *Independence* and self-sufficiency of residents in personal affairs, encouragement of responsibility and self-direction.
(d) *Self-exploration* – can residents openly discuss and express their feelings?
(e) *Organisation and order* – their importance in the home. How explicit are the rules and procedures?
(f) *Resident influence* – over rules and policies of the home; restriction of residents by staff through regulations.
(g) *Physical comfort* – privacy, pleasant decor provided by physical environment.

In their paper, Moos *et al.* (1979) describe the stages of development of their measuring instrument — how they narrowed a large pool of items selected from related previous research into a scale of 63 true/ false items. As a first step, overlapping items were eliminated, an approximate balance between positive (true) and negative (false) responses was sought, and pretesting was carried out. The items were all carefully worded so that they could be understood by typical residents of facilities for the elderly. The second stage was to select about a dozen items for each of 'twelve rationally-derived subscales'. These subscales were the seven listed above, plus staff support, expressiveness, expectations for functioning, clarity and innovation. The initial steps had reduced the item pool from a total of over 300 items to 140, and this number was further reduced to 63 following careful statistical analyses of the responses from over sixteen hundred residents and five hundred staff members of skilled nursing and nursing home facilities, residential homes, and federally-assisted apartment house facilities. These 63 items were equally divided among the seven subscales listed above (a through to g), the other five subscales initially distinguished being discarded because of their apparent empirical similarity and intercorrelation with the retained subscales.

How good a basis does the Sheltered Care Environment Scale provide for the measurement of the social environment of old people's homes? Its dimensionality is directly derived from the work of Murray and his intellectual inheritor Stern; and although Murray himself was basically a psychoanalytic theorist, his typology of needs drawn on by Moos has had a strong influence in other areas of study, particularly amongst the so-called 'consistency theorists'. A number of Murray needs appear to have the properties of stability and partial independence which are preconditions for their existence as entities. However, the Moos and Murray dimensions do not correspond exactly. Affiliation, the need to obtain close and warm interaction between people and avoid a sense of loneliness is of obvious relevance to life in old people's homes. However, Moos dropped Murray's Affiliation dimension from his earlier COPES instrument because its items were highly correlated with Involvement (Moos, 1974a), and it is not clear that this dimension is adequately reflected in the SCES instrument. Again the dimensions do not directly reflect the concepts of other personality theorists, for instance Rogers's positive regard and self-regard might well be reflected in subject responses to items on some of the dimensions. It should not be difficult to develop items about positive regard and self-regard in the perceived climate instrument. The same *prima facie* lack of direct coverage is evident in respect of some other important dimensions, such as Erikson's Integrity, Fromm's Full Functioning, and Maslow's Belongingness, for although some items are salient, no dimension either singly or in combination covers the concept adequately. There are no items directly focused on fullness of the subject's own life or his fear of death for instance.

These criticisms — that Moos's dimensions require adaptation because they omit some aspects of importance for old people's homes specifically mentioned in some other American approaches and clearly important in the British literature, and that the items are not directly salient to some personality characteristics of direct importance in old age — do nothing to undermine the potential value of his approach as part of a wider collection of data. His earlier work — with the COPES instrument and in non-gerontological settings — eschewed all multivariate modelling and ignored the dependence of his scale scores on other characteristics. As part of the welfare production model, however, the SCES instrument would appear as an extremely interesting intermediary — determined in part (and possibly to a large extent) by staff attitudes, experiences and ideologies, by residents' characteristics at the point of entry to the home, and by the physical environment, whilst at the same time being itself an important determinant of the well-being of residents. The three parallel forms of the SCES — the Real Form (staff and residents' perceptions of the current social environment), the Ideal Form (conceptions of an ideal home), and the Expectations Form (expectations of prospective staff and residents regarding the environment they are about to enter) — provide invaluable data for the description and understanding of residential care environments.

(B) Lawton's Social Ecology Model

Possibly the most important, and certainly the most impressive, of the social ecology models of ageing and the care of the aged is that of Lawton and his colleagues at the Philadelphia Geriatric Center. Lawton's earlier work led to the development of the so-called 'environmental docility hypothesis', whereby the proportion of behaviour attributable to environmental vis-à-vis personal characteristics increases as individual competence decreases (Lawton and Simon, 1968), later placed more squarely in the need (competence)-press models of the Murray genre (Lawton, 1970a, 1970b, 1970c), and culminating (in some sense) in a general social ecology theory of the ageing process (Lawton and Nahemow, 1973). In subsequent research, he and his colleagues have applied and tested the theory in a variety of settings for the elderly.

Lawton and Nahemow define the ecology of ageing as 'a system of continual adaptations in which both the organism and the environment change over time in a non-random manner; either environment or the organism is capable of initiating a cycle of action, or of responding'. Environments surround the perceiver, enfolding and all-embracing, constituting a system of human communication (DeLong, 1974) and always containing a surplus of information, some redundant, some contradictory, and some inadequate or ambiguous. Many aspects of the environment are determined or influenced by the organism, particularly those 'supra-personal dimensions', whilst the process of adaptation to these environmental press or messages is effected through a dual process of assimilation and accommodation. 'Man and environment exist in an inextricable and mutually-pervasive relationship . . . Neither is satisfactorily seen to be *a priori* independent of the other — the influences are intrinsically mutually directional. The man-environment relationship constitutes a mutual causal system' (DeLong, 1974, p.103). DeLong, in fact, has been instrumental in the development of a general theory of 'coding behaviour', asserting that it is through 'codes', whether genetically determined or socially learned, that the organism and its environment come to influence one another. It then follows as a corollary that dominance of one component in the interaction will lead to maladaptive behaviour, as in the Lawton model.

As we saw in chapter 3, as a person progresses through middle and old age, almost invariably his competence will decrease. Losses experienced during these years are cumulative and in most case irreversable. Physical, social, economic, vocational and sensory losses have important psychological consequences, in addition to those 'naturally occurring' deteriorations. For example, deteriorations in hearing and sight tend to screen environmental impact in one form or another, resulting in sensory deprivation. Other environmental stimuli are deliberately excluded to conserve available resources — by routinisation and a preference for simplicity, by compliance and disengagement. Reduced competence, therefore, is the occasion for retrenchment, the seeking of stability. However, as the person ages he becomes less able to discriminate among environmental cues and those that are received become increasingly important as their number decreases. Furthermore, his power resources which permit environmental mastery are steadily ebbing away — his health and solvency not least among them. The *environmental docility hypothesis* follows naturally: 'the less competent are more vulnerable — not vulnerable in terms of receptor sensitivity, but in terms of their behaviour being controlled by environmental, rather than interpersonal forces' (Lawton and Nahemow, 1973).

There are a number of studies which lend support to the environmental docility hypothesis. Lawton and Simon's (1968) original statement of the hypothesis was accompanied by supportive evidence, and Rosow's (1967) findings are consistent with such a statement. Lawton and Nahemow (1973) report the work presented in the Ph.D. thesis of Mangum (1971) who directly tested the congruence hypothesis in a sample of six housing projects. The adjustment of the elderly individual was hypothesised to be a function of the degree of consonance between the activity level of the individual and the activity-inducing properties of the housing setting, indexed as a composite of the three Kleemeier dimensions (see above). Contrary to expectation, Mangum found that the hypothesis was not generally borne out. However, he did find that environmental characteristics were more important than status and personality characteristics in the prediction of adjustment for lower socio-economic groups, but less important for higher socio-economic groups. If one takes socio-economic status as a determinant of competence, as it most certainly was in general in the population examined, this provides strong evidence in favour of the docility hypothesis. Gubrium (1970) similarly produced evidence to suggest that those aged persons with good health and solvency resources had greater behaviour flexibility, and Smith and Lipman (1972) concluded that the relationship between peer interaction and life satisfaction was statistically significant only for those residents defined as constrained (poor health and low monthly income). And finally, Lawton himself found supportive evidence in a recent study of the adaptation process in the relatively dependent elderly following intra-institutional re-location (Lawton, Patnaik and Kleban, 1976).

The environmental docility hypothesis led naturally to a full *transactional model* relating the ageing individual to his environment. Lawton and Nahemow (1973) distinguish the following components:

(a) *The degree of individual competence* — 'conceived as a diverse collection of abilities residing within the individual', and defined strictly in relation to external phenomena and tasks. Competence is task performance. Domains of competence are hierarchically arranged in order of increasing complexity of behaviour: *life maintenance* (e.g. breathing); *functional health, perception-cognition, physical self-maintenance* (grooming, eating); *instrumental self-maintenance* (employment, basic cooking, housekeeping); *effectance* (creativity, exploration, curiosity); and *social role* (love, leadership, contact, sensory contact) (Lawton, 1970c, 1972b; Golant and McCaslin, 1977).

(b) *Environmental press* — those forces in the environment that evoke a response when interacting with individual needs (Murray, 1938). The social ecology model is concerned only with what Murray called 'alpha press' — the objective aspects of environmental demand — and not with the subjective 'beta press'. Environmental press may be distinguished (and thence 'measured') in terms of the demands they place on residents and the reciprocity afforded, in terms of the stress they induce and the support they offer, in terms of their normative meanings, and so on. Furthermore, 'press are neutral in that their positive or negative quality is defined by the interacting individual, rather than residing intrinsically in the environment' (Lawton and Nahemow, 1973).

(c) *Adaptive behaviour* – the observed manifestation of individual competence within the social environment. For example, in an 'age homogeneous' environment, such as an old people's home, age-related norms will naturally develop and the range of adaptive behaviours will widen. What is and what is not adaptive is determined by social norms and other environmental characteristics and certain individual values, such as those based on self-actualisation.

(d) *Affective responses* – the inner aspect of the individual-environment transaction (corresponding to the outer manifestation of adaptive behaviour). Any internal emotional state influenced by the transaction – including, for example, the twelve domains of morale or life satisfaction described in section 2.2.3 above – are to be included.

(e) *Adaptation level* – the state of equilibrium between environmental press and individual competence, attained when the stimuli received by the individual 'are perceived as neither too strong or too weak'. Two processes characterise adaptation – the process of *assimilation* whereby the individual modifies or 're-codes' the environment in order to be able to take it in, and the process of *accommodation* in which the *individual's* characteristics are modified to meet the environment press (Helson, 1964; DeLong, 1974; Piaget and Inhelder, 1970).

These five elements provide the key to the ecological model of Lawton and Nahemow and are defined with sufficient generality as to include as special cases most other gerontological approaches to the environment-individual transaction. At any point in time an individual exhibits a specific level of competence in relation to a given set of environmental press. Clearly, both competence and press must be assessed along a number of dimensions. There will be a set of situations in which environmental stimuli will be 'just right' for a particular individual – he will be at his adaptation level. Presumably, more competent individuals will adapt to stronger press. When an individual is close to this adaptation level he will exhibit positive affect and adaptive behaviour. The range of press or stimuli that allow behaviour consistent with full adptation and positive affect will be wider for the more competent than the less competent – an immediate corollary of the environmental docility hypothesis. Frequently, and perhaps generally, however, environmental press will be either too strong or too weak. Certainly, as Lawton and Nahemow argue, there is no inherent reason for a state of equilibrium to remain indefinitely – individual competence changes, generally decreasing in elderly populations, and environmental press become less complex as role demands become fewer, as contemporaries die or move away, as the elderly person's economic status dwindles, and as environments themselves become more familiar.

At this point, it is illuminating to contrast the ecological model of

Lawton and Nahemow with certain other transactional models of ageing. Many writers have emphasised the desirability of matching individuals and environments in order to facilitate the satisfaction of needs. Kahana's (1974) congruence model focuses directly on the degree of fit between the elderly person and his environment, morale being higher in settings displaying greater congruence, and Schooler (1974) is principally concerned with matching the rates of change between the two components. The matching scheme proposed by Sherwood, Morris and Barnhart (1975) (using discriminant function analysis) similarly attempts to match an individual's needs with an appropriate level of service supports. What is implicit in these schema is that well-being is solely a result of need satisfaction or tension reduction. In contrast, it has been argued by many psychologists that tension reduction as an explanation of all behaviour is inadequate, and that it is imperative to recognise the part that tension creation, exploration, and the search for stimulation play in determining affect and behaviour (Berlyne, 1960; Calhoun, 1963; Fiske and Maddi, 1961; White, 1959). 'Under conditions of sensory, affective or cognitive boredom . . . people will create stress, problems, or conflict for themselves' (Lawton, 1970c, p.39). A preoccupation with tension reduction is also characteristic of residential care in Britain (PSSC, 1977, paragraph 1.16):

> The community has high expectations of public authorities, although these tend to be expressed only in reactions to those instances in which harm befalls people in care. As a result, a greater emphasis may be placed on the avoidance of risks than on the promotion of high standards of residential life, and may profoundly influence the context in which residential care is provided. In consequence, there is considerable tension between ensuring the safety yet promoting the freedom of people in care.

In Lawton's schema, the 'zone of maximal performance potential' is that area of the competence-press map in which the demands made by the environment are just noticeably greater than the accustomed level of performance of the aged individual. The need to create tensions is evident.

The final element of the ecology model is the set of 'interventive strategies' to enable an elderly person to move towards an adaptation level — either by changing the environmental press, or by influencing the individual's competence. Lawton and Nahemow distinguish four sets of manoeuvres, arranged in the following matrix (p. 129).

This matrix allows a classification of all extant personal social service policies and recommended interventions. For example, home improvement, rehousing and institutionalisation fall within the top left-hand cell, and of course the impact of the resource inputs discussed in chapter 4 can be included here. The top right-hand cell

The individual is:

A passive responder   *An active initiator*

The point of application is:

	A passive responder	An active initiator
The environment	Social and environmental engineering (e.g. institutionalisation)	Individual redesigns his environment (assimilation)
The individual	Rehabilitation, prosthesis	Self-therapy, growth (accommodation)

will include a diverse collection of manoeuvres. An elderly resident of an old people's home may leave her door open to signal that she is open to visitors — a move to compensate either for reduced competence, through immobility, or for reduced press, through fewer interactions or role demands. On the bottom line of the matrix we have the interventions which are aimed at the *individual*, rather then the environment. Passive response interventions will include the physical prostheses discussed by Kushlick — such as false teeth, glasses, walking frames, and so on, whilst active initiation by the individual can take the form of self-therapy or self-help. In general, of course, most forms of care use interventive strategies of all four varieties.[1]

Lawton's social ecology model stems from the same base as the model of Moos but differs from it in a number of respects. Moos's work has the advantage of having a fairly well validated and widely applied battery of congruence indicators which attempt to measure *directly* the differences between individual needs and environmental press or stimuli. The respondent, whether staff member or elderly resident, is asked to describe the 'real' and 'ideal' environments by agreeing or disagreeing with each of a number of statements. However, the length of Moos's SCES instrument, even after its reduction to 63 items, may present problems. The questionnaires may be too long and too complex for use with the institutionalised elderly in Britain, a large proportion of whom are very frail and/or confused. Lawton's model certainly has contextual validity and has carefully built on a vast body of supportive gerontological literature, but apparently still lacks a set of instruments and methodologies for its practical application. However, implicit in Lawton's writings and in some of the works he cites, is a methodological approach which is rather more relevant for an elderly sample. Instead of attempting to measure the dimensions of congruence or the degrees of environmental or individual dominance directly, he prefers to obtain separate indicators of press and competence. With separate indicators of press and competence, the implications of the dominance of one over the other would be assessed indirectly through the final set of empirical relationships characterising the welfare production model. It may, of course, be possible to measure press and competence separately but on the same dimensional basis, as Kahana (1974) has done (see section 5.2.2).

Furthermore, if by press we mean Murray's objective alpha press, then we need not attempt to quantify the elderly residents' perceived environmental climates. Opinion is divided on the efficacy of using residents' perceptions as indicators of the social milieu of a home for the elderly. Pincus moved from a concentration on purely *staff* perceptions in his 1968 study to a comparison of staff *and* residents' perceptions in a later study (Pincus and Wood, 1970). Some of the other practical approaches to environmental assessment discussed in this chapter have done likewise, and there is currently a trend among British commentators and researchers to take much more account of residents' perceptions and views. On the other hand, there is still considerable scepticism regarding the accuracy and usefulness of residents' responses to gerontologists' vast and various questionnaires. McClelland argued that self-description yields a schemata more than underlying motives; culturally appropriate images more than individual needs. It is well known that self-description is subject to response styles and in particular statements that are culturally acceptable are thought acceptable to the interviewer. Plank (1977) noted when reporting that only 10 per cent of residents of old people's homes in London stated that they disliked living there, that residents were more inhibited in the expression of criticism than residents of sheltered housing schemes. For whatever reasons, not only did a lower percentage of home residents express a dislike for their new place of residence, but also a lower percentage expressed both likes and dislikes. It is this unwillingness to criticise, whilst at the same time clearly not being warmly enthusiastic, that is evidence of nervousness, ambivalence and the unreliability of residents' perceptions.

(C) Some other transactional models

As well as the impressive social ecology models of Rudolf Moos and Powell Lawton, there have been some other approaches to the assessment of the caring environment which have adopted a transactional stance. Graney (1974), for instance, distinguishes between two types of variable which intervene between a person and his environment — the environmental characteristics which help to explain how external influences can come to specify the normative meaning of behaviour (such as the age, sex and health homogeneity of the environment), and the characteristics of the social selves which serve to define the meaning of the environment to the older person (in particular, his ability to cope with changes in physical and social milieux). Similar arguments can be found in Gubrium's socio-environmental theory of ageing (1972, pp.281-2):

the environment of action for the aged is two-sided and consequently built on the interrelationship of two contextual dimensions. The first of these is social, referring to the normative outcomes of social homogeneity, residential proximity, and local protectiveness. The second dimension will be referred to as the 'individual context' indicating those activity resources such as health, solvency and social support that influence behaviour flexibility.

Weinstock (1974, p.269) draws on the work of Lewin (1946) to support this theory of ageing:

Optimal adjustment or adaptation for any human being involves an integration of available inner resources within the social system surrounding the person. Social systems which make demands above and beyond the capacities of the individual produce stress and tip the balance in the 'failure' direction. Just as stressful, however, are those social settings which offer no expectations, no challenge, no opportunity for use of accumulated individual resources. A situation which has become too familiar, which offers no new roles, may result in adaptive failure as well.

Dowd (1975) and Paulig and McGee (1977) have adapted the exchange theory or power theory of Blau (1964) to the problems of ageing and adjustment. To exercise power to influence behaviour and affect one must possess sufficient 'power resources', defined as anything that is perceived as rewarding and which therefore renders one susceptible to social influence. Blau argued that there are four generalised power resources: money, approval, esteem and compliance. Money is 'inappropriate for repaying diffuse social obligations' and approval has little social value, so that the elderly person is generally reduced to the expression of esteem and compliance in order to engage in exchange/ transaction relationships. Esteem is 'less expensive' than compliance and is thus used first, but is unlikely to prove an adequate incentive for exchange in transactions of some duration. The aged are consequently left with only compliance resources: 'the relative power of the aged *vis-à-vis* their social environment is gradually diminished until all that remains of their power resources is the humble capacity to comply' (Dowd, 1975, p.587). Behaviour, that is, becomes maladaptive and affect decreases as the individual's own power resources are steadily eroded away. Paulig and McGee (1977) use a similar power theory perspective to analyse and explain observed 'patterns of male-female interaction at senior citizen centres'. Whilst the detailed findings of this study are not immediately relevant for the production model outlined in this book, it is clear that the exchange (transaction or power) perspective on ageing will usefully contribute to our understanding of the social environments of old people's homes and the situations of residents within them.

The theoretical models or perspectives on the social environments of old people's homes, and on environments for the elderly in general, that we have reviewed in this section have been taken almost *en masse* from the American literature. In contrast to this impressive body of well-argued theory and (generally) careful application, the state of the art in Britain looks very primitive. Students of the British personal social services, with very few exceptions, have been very reluctant to scratch the well-polished veneer of simple description and comparison. To all intents and purposes, there is no theoretical argument in the British literature on old people's homes. However, there are encouraging signs that a 'theoretical breakthrough' may be on the way. Recently, the social work press has published a few papers which attempt to distinguish alternative 'models', or more accurately, 'scenarios', of residential care in the British context. For example, David Harris (1977) describes seven models of care, Howard Harris (1977) compared (unfavourably) an old people's home and an hotel, Payne (1978) describes 'The Hollow' and 'The Beehive' as polar examples of residential environments – with a third scenario, 'Newvista', being added as a fairer and more realistic example by Prosser (1978), and Palfrey (1976) has distinguished the Clinical, Democratic and Charitable homes on the basis of visits to homes in Gwent. Whilst these alternative 'scenarios' provide only anecdotal evidence they may well be important stepping stones in the development of a theory of environments and environmental impacts in British old people's homes.

5.3 Some important dimensions of social environment

In this section of the chapter on social environments we briefly consider a number of the more important constituent dimensions of these environments. Most of the dimensions are well-integrated into the scales and assessment instruments that have been developed out of the theoretical perspectives presented in the previous section. For the present, therefore, we are concerned with pulling together some common themes and, of more pertinence, in reviewing briefly some of the empirical evidence apposite to each dimension of social milieu. We distinguish seven dimensions, which do not necessarily span the whole universe of social environment in residential settings for the elderly but which have attracted most attention from gerontologists. These dimensions are: Regime and Social Control (including independence and individuality); Motor Control; Privacy; Stimulation and Participation; Communication and Interaction; Homogeneity; and Continuity.

5.3.1 Regime, social control and independence[2]

The dimension of environment that most readily springs to mind and which has attracted much attention in gerontological studies is regime or social control. It is rare to find a survey of the elderly, and of their position in society, that does not examine their real and perceived independence. Certainly regime plays an important role in the theories of Goffman, Kleemeier and Murray and virtually all the scales and instruments based on their models include regime or social control items — the rigidity of the routine dimension of King and Raynes (1968), the scheduling of activities and sanction system of Bennett (1963), the rules, regulations and programme of Pincus (1968), Kahana's (1974) institutional control items, and the organisation subscale of Moos *et al.* (1979).

The Social Work Service of the DHSS, looking at a sample of old people's homes, distinguished four kinds of social control (Utting, 1977, p.17):

(i) control 'derived from the perceived responsibilities of communal living, including the responsibility to protect residents' (including restrictions on smoking habits and drug administration);

(ii) control 'apparently required for efficient management in the light of staffing levels and qualifications' (routinising the day to fit into the staff rota);

(iii) control required to protect staff 'in view of their assumed accountability for things that might go wrong' (avoiding risks); and

(iv) control apparently 'without a rational purpose in the operational context' (lack of consultation over menus, enforced dependence).

As Utting remarks, there may be some purpose to the first three, but the fourth is without justification. Using an alternative classification of controls — into behavioural, cognitive, and decisional — Averill (1973) has also demonstrated how social controls can be both purposeful and purposeless. The recent Personal Social Services Council report, *Residential Care Reviewed* (1977, p.52) provides a most succinct statement of the organisational meaning and 'justification' of routine:

Is the timing of the day's routine and hours of going to bed based on what staff consider appropriate for residents, what residents desire, what a small number of residents want, what is necessary in order to fit a certain number of activities into the day, what is administratively convenient, or the hours when staff are available?

The report then goes on to list a set of 'questions for staff' – questions that usefully serve to describe the most important characteristics and aspects of institutional regime in British old people's homes today.

The weight of empirical evidence would suggest that resident self-determination and personal control is necessary for, or at least strongly associated with, general well-being and survival among the elderly. Removal or loss of personal control is associated with depression, physical decline, a false sense of helplessness, early death (Gresham, 1976; Schulz, 1976; Seligman, 1975; Streib, 1971), with lower morale and life satisfaction, and with poorer adjustment (Chang, 1977; Fawcett *et al.*, 1976; Felton and Kahana, 1974; Wolk and Telleen, 1976). Regime and social control often take the form of 'infantilisation' of residents through enforced dependency and patronising statements, thus initiating or contributing towards negative self-attitudes among residents. Incongruity between expectations about residential regime and the realities of life in the home will be confusing as well as debilitating (Chang, 1977). Expectations of a routinised environment can be so strong as to induce residents to introduce elements of regimentation even when the management deliberately tries to avoid it (Dorset County Council Social Services Department, 1977).

Closely related to the concept of regime is the extent to which the environment allows residents to retain their *independence* and *individuality*, and to exercise their *rights*. Independence is a state of self-reliance, whether economic, physical, mental or social, and is associated with at least one of three behavioural states – autonomy, environmental mastery or internal control (Atchley, 1977, chapter 11; Golant and McCaslin, 1977). Economic independence is generally denied the resident of the old people's home, whilst physical independence depends crucially on the individual's mobility and the physical prostheses provided by the home. Mental independence requires 'an alert mind that can exercise knowledge, experience, and skills to solve problems posed by the social and physical environment' (Atchley, 1977, p.197), and social independence means having the power to demand one's rights.

5.3.2 Motor control

Eva Kahana's study of the impact of environmental characteristics and incongruities on the lives of 123 residents of three American nursing homes found that motor control was one of five important predictors of morale in two of the homes (Kahana, 1974). Motor control –

covering the environmental tolerance of motor expression, restlessness and wandering, and the residents' corresponding degree of 'psychomotor inhibition' — is usually discussed and compared with social and psycho-pharmacological control, and in many regards the three are indistinguishable (Maxwell, Bader and Watson, 1972). In chapter 4 above we discussed the impact of design on life in an old people's home, and certainly poor design can substantially constrain the movements of physically frail residents. Snyder *et al.* (1978) tackle the motor control dimension from the perspective of the resident, studying 'wanderers' in an American nursing facility. Wanderers were found to be better oriented in time and place, to respond more appropriately to conversation, and to have more 'psychosocial needs'. Wandering behaviour fell into three categories — searching behaviour, often for something unattainable; industrious, seemingly inexhaustible driving to remain busy; and aimless behaviour — and was found to have a number of causes, most of them rooted in the wanderer's previous lifestyle. This led Snyder and her associates to argue that (ibid., p.276):

> neither pharmacological nor physical restraints are 'cures' for wandering. . . . In any event physical control and drugging should not be used as the first and only response to wandering, since both approaches complicate and obscure the causes and consequent approaches to wandering.

Nevertheless, physical bullying probably remains a weapon of importance in old people's homes. Carelessness can be a form of punishment. 'Accidents' may often not be reported. Moreover, it is easy subtly to induce fear among old people nervous about their physical capacities. There is some evidence that resource inputs may influence the security of an old person's environment. Bennett *et al.* (1968) showed a negative association between the number of fractures and staffing levels.

5.3.3 Privacy

What degree of privacy is afforded the individual resident by the social environmental characteristics of the home? This question, in many guises, is common to most sociological studies of residential homes and attempts to tap a most important feature of the caring and living milieu. Privacy takes a number of meanings in a number of different settings, and Pastalan's (1968) four-fold classification has done much to clarify them and to relate them to their respective expected individual feelings. First we have the conventional, lay, definition of privacy as *solitude* — separation from the group. Solitude is related to feelings of autonomy. Second one can distinguish privacy as *intimacy*, where the individual is part of a small, closely-knit group, with concomitant feelings of emotional release. A third type of privacy is *freedom from identification and surveillance* in public places – anonymity – related to self-evaluation, and a fourth is *reserve*, the erection of psychological barriers against unwanted intrusion, which is related to feelings of limited and protected communication.

Armed with this dimensionality it is possible, as Pastalan illustrates, to investigate the factors affecting privacy – behaviour forms, situational contexts, antecedent factors, and organismic factors. In the typical British old people's home, sharing of bedrooms is not uncommon. This can cause many problems and give rise to unnecessary frictions. One resident, quoted in the Personal Social Services Council report, *Residential Care Reviewed* (1977), put it simply (ibid., p.53):

> My opinion is that single rooms should be available for each resident if that is what they want. The choice of a single or shared room should be up to the individual. Some people prefer privacy and some like company, but the choice should be theirs.

With such enforced room-sharing, the opportunities for solitude are considerably reduced. However, co-operative staff behaviour and a resident's determination can together allow the resident a certain amount of intimacy, freedom and reserve. Thus, for example, staff can avoid entering a resident's room without knocking and can ensure they seek permission before showing visitors around the home; the warden or matron can allow residents to have locking cupboards; the resident can be given privacy in the bath and toilet. In other words, in Pastalan's terminology, the resident should be free from surveillance and intervention.[3] We may quote the PSSC again (ibid., pp.53-4):

> A great deal of lip-service is paid to the idea of privacy, but there is alarming neglect of it. It is surprising how often staff will claim that they always knock on residents' doors and yet immediately afterwards walk into a room without knocking or with so perfunctory a knock as to be meaningless. ... A private area to which he may withdraw, and a private, lockable place for his possessions are the basic right of every resident. He may wish to share but he should do so by choice, not by necessity.

Regarding the resident's available set of strategies to obtain privacy in the face of adverse design characteristics and staff behaviour, the studies of Ittleston, Proshansky and Rivlin (1970) and of Weiss (1977) are most informative. Ittleston *et al.* emphasised the potential for functional privacy – a situation in which one has the widest range of personal choice – in rooms of different sizes on a psychiatric ward. They found that large, multiple-occupancy rooms provoke patient withdrawal – 'there are functional equivalents of privacy which do not necessarily involve physical separation' (ibid., p.269). Schwartz and Proppe (1969, 1970) likewise argue that where the environment does

not provide opportunities for privacy, residents take it by not interacting with one another. The study by Weiss (1977) focused on intimacy, arguing (and finding supportive evidence) that a minimum or
threshold level of intimacy can act as a buffer to the stresses accompanying the ageing process.

A lack of privacy, in whatever sense, can have many and serious
repercussions, some of which we can easily recognise from the dimensionality of Pastalan. Certainly, behaviour will often be forced towards
a more primitive level of response — constant physical proximity
without relief leading to a search for social distance manifested in a
refusal to talk or interact with near neighbours (Schwartz, 1975).
Privacy is frequently seen as an important intermediary between
environmental press and individual competence, behaviour, and affect.
For example, Aloia (1973) found privacy contributed directly to a
sense of effectiveness, mastery, and hence self-regard, so that privacy
functioned as a catalyst in the attainment of transactional competence.
Kahana (1974) found privacy to be significantly predictive of residents'
well-being for 'the erosion of their privacy probably strikes at the very
roots of their identity, independence, and dignity' (Howard Harris,
1977, p.13). As Lipman and Slater (1977a) state: 'Access to privacy . . .
can be regarded as a buffer between the pressures met in everyday
social intercourse and people's abilities to manage them' (ibid., p.149).

In some respects, the obverse of privacy is interaction and communication. We return to these aspects of social environment in section
5.3.5.

5.3.4 Stimulus and participation

Environmental stimulation is at the very core of the need-press models
of Murray, Moos and Lawton. The individual resident's need for a
degree of stimulation congruent with his level of competence is a
common thread running through the various arguments of these theorists. Similarly, stimulation has been the principal focus of the various
research studies of physical prostheses to foster engagement and well-
being. The importance of activities and stimulation is also well recognised in the British policy literature, (for example, see PSSC, 1977,
p.56) although the reality of care may be rather different (Jenkins et
al., 1977, p.429):

> Admission to an old people's home . . . reduces the need to engage
> in many practical activities of daily living; all too often it also fails
> to provide the chance to engage in them at all, or in alternative
> recreational activities. . . . Low levels of observed activity may be
> as much a function of very limited opportunities to engage in
> activities as of the characteristics or disabilities of residents.

We discussed the importance and variety of activity amenities in Section 4.2 (j) above and therefore keep our present comments fairly brief. McClannahan's (1973a) series of experiments in social engineering within a home for the aged is one of the more interesting of recent examinations of activity *generation*, and the work of Kushlick and his associates in Wessex with various physical and social prostheses for the elderly and mentally handicapped is perhaps the most thorough (see, for example, Kushlick and Blunden, 1974; and Jenkins *et al.*, 1977). Running parallel is the vast body of literature on the so-called Activity and Disengagement Theories of ageing which examine the association between the level of engagement with the environment and subsequent morale and affect (see chapter 2 above and also Knapp, 1977b). Few studies, however, have been directed towards the social construction and meaning of activities in residential homes and their effects upon the elderly population. It is generally agreed that activities should be readily available to, but not forced upon, all residents within the home regardless of physical or mental status. There should perhaps be a slight bias in orientation toward the more intellectually impaired persons whose options for improvement or maintenance of quality of life are rather more limited than the intellectually intact residents (Miller and Barry, 1976). If these activities can additionally be of specific therapeutic value, be resident-initiated and/or managed, or involve residents in day-to-day running of the home, so much the better.

One source of stimulation and participation often suggested comes from the provision of residential and day care services jointly under the same roof. Day visitors to the home, particularly those elderly visitors with similar disabilities and dependencies as the residents, may help residents maintain links with the community, may help break down some of the stereotyped views and fantasies about residential care held by the non-resident elderly (DHSS, 1976c, p.40), and may provide much-needed stimulation to residents. This 'stimulation' may be either direct, through the establishment or maintenance of friendships, or indirect as a result of the establishment of new activities and leisure pursuits. Integration of day care clients and residents in common activities within and outside the home may also help to dispel those feelings of resentment by residents that often accompanies the 'intrusion' of day care clients (National Corporation for the Care of Old People, 1976).

5.3.5 Communication and interaction

We have already touched on the communication and interaction characteristics of residential environments in our discussions of privacy, of stimulation and participation, and of social control. In these brief paragraphs we focus on the nature and frequency of staff-resident, resident-resident, and resident-community interactions.

One of the major problems facing elderly people living in the community is loneliness and it is often this factor which precipitates entry into residential care (East Sussex County Council Social Services Department, 1975; Wager, 1972). A fairly crude instrument devised by Tobin and Lieberman (1976) to examine the elderly person's perception of others as resources successfully differentiated between those on the waiting list for residential care and those coping adequately in the community. Admission into a residential home should hopefully provide opportunities for more and better interpersonal interaction and communication.

Staff-resident interactions generally reflect and determine the regime and social controls of the caring environment. Fairhurst (1978) has examined staff-resident *talk* in a geriatric hospital in Manchester. Talk, she argues, is a resource, and an examination of staff-resident verbal interaction provides a good indication of the meanings of work held by staff and their attitudes towards the elderly residents. Fairhurst suggests that there are four types of talk by staff to residents: time-out talk, ceremonial talk, superlative talk, and persuasive talk.

(a) *Time-out talk* is regarded by staff as an alternative to their 'real' duties — 'talk with patients was "time-out" from the pressing exigency of getting through their work. Once work had been "finished" time could be spent "talking to" patients' (ibid., p.4). Such conversation often took the form of joking, fun and sexual innuendo.

(b) *Ceremonial talk* is the most common of verbal interchanges, serving to punctuate and order interaction. Ceremonial talk is task-oriented ('it's time to get up') and is used to ensure the smooth execution of tasks.

(c) *Superlative talk* — such as 'jolly good' and 'wonderful' — has no meaning and is possibly used only to reduce stigma and as 'a mechanism for adapting to failure'. Unwarranted praise and congratulation is particularly showered on the senile demented.

(d) *Persuasive talk* is based on the claim by staff that they know best — both medically and socially — and is used to get residents to take unwanted medications and participate in activities.

Residents' reactions to these various types of talk will clearly differ, and Fairhurst concludes that it is by no means clear that policies to allow staff to spend more time talking with residents will necessarily improve the standard or character of this talk.

Romaniuk, Hoyer and Romaniuk (1977) focusing on the *patronising statements* of staff in a New York nursing home, suggested six categories:

139

    (i) *Suggestion and instructions* — uninvited prompts in residents' conversations which remove the opportunity for the residents to demonstrate their competence and self-sufficiency.

   (ii) *Requests for an explanation or clarification* — unsolicited requests on behalf of residents, preventing residents from requesting information independently.

  (iii) *Summaries and restatements* — again, as with (ii), the staff member assumes the resident doesn't understand some information and so summarises, restates and simplifies it.

  (iv) *Comments and evaluation* — unsolicited interjections in residents' conversations, either to explain or compliment, which prevent residents' expression of feelings and receipt of 'normal' feedback.

   (v) *Leading questions* — implying that the resident hadn't thought out a problem properly or completely, whilst the staff member had.

  (vi) *Answering another's question and providing explanations* — uninvited answers and statements to residents' questions to other residents, assuming incompetence and incapability.

In all cases, staff members assume that residents are not competent enough to answer, comment or comprehend, and in interjecting prevent residents from demonstrating their competence. Negative attitudes among residential home staff, as conveyed through such patronising statements, will undoubtedly lower the residents' own self-attitudes and distort their self-perceptions. Commentators on residential care frequently stress the need for staff to chat with residents, to be helpful, considerate and understanding, and yet chat or talk which is predominantly patronising or predominantly of the kind discussed by Fairhurst will clearly be damaging. Perhaps it is such a predominance of 'negative talk' that explains Plank's (1977) finding that residents felt they had less social contact than other groups. Residents clearly did not classify many of their contacts with staff and other residents as 'seeing someone to talk to'.

In chapter 4 above, we discussed the small body of research literature that has addressed the problem of determining the nature of environmental characteristics which facilitate or hinder peer interactions. Slater (1968) found that the level of adjustment of residents in a British home, measured on a four item self-image index and a four item self-rated health index, was related to both the number of friends in the home and the number of visitors. Elias (1977) reached a similar conclusion in her study of 73 aged widows living in senior citizen housing, finding that social adjustment (as measured on the Cavan scale) was related to regular contact with close friends, neighbours and was associated with ageing group consciousness (group memberships and peer-identification). Adaptation to social stress among the aged has also been found to be better among those with a confidant (Lowenthal and Haven, 1968; and see the review by Bennett, 1970, p.103). On the other hand, Smith and Lipman (1972) concluded that peer interaction was only related to life satisfaction for unconstrained residents (good health and high income), a finding that lends support to Lawton's environmental docility hypothesis. This may explain why some residents feel unable to establish close friendships with staff and other residents within the socially constrained environment of the typical old people's home. Feelings of isolation among rational residents may be further exacerbated by the presence of too high a proportion of confused residents. The character of life in the home, and the quality of life of residents, will also be influenced to some extent by the frequency and nature of links with the surrounding community. Visitors to the home, whether friends and relatives of the residents, or professional and voluntary workers, will be important in this respect (see section 4.1 above). Of equal or greater importance is the need for residents to be involved in community activities, even if this only means an occasional visit to the shops or a local pub.

5.3.6 Homogeneity

Implicit in Goffman's discussion of institutional totality and in the press models of Murray and Stern was the assumption that a total institution strives for a 'homogeneous environmental stimulus field', implying lack of variety, and hence lack of environmental stimuli (Lawton, 1970c). In the gerontological context most attention has focused, not on homogeneity of the environment as a whole, but on homogeneity of the supra-personal environment: How similar or dissimilar are residents with regard to such characteristics as age, sex, confusion, health, religion, race and so on? What degree of segregation is practised or observed in the home, and what are the implications for residents' morale, behaviour, and general well-being?

Supra-personal homogeneity is an amalgam of two features — social similarity (Segregation) and proximity (Congregation). Integration and interaction are fostered by both social similarity and proximity, although residential propinquity is necessary, but not sufficient, for friendship establishment (Bultena, 1968).

The most widely studied of the supra-personal dimensions is age. Rosow (1967), Bultena and Marshall (1969) and Gubrium (1970) all found that age-concentration stimulated peer interaction and morale. However, the last two of these papers both stress the mediating influence of such factors as education, self-rated health, and solvency on the concentration-well-being association. Those individuals with greater flexibility, as determined by their income and health, were affected less by environmental variations. More recently, Bultena (1974) found evidence to support his hypothesis 'that planned retirement communities facilitate the adaptation of aged migrants to the retirement role', a finding which could not be explained away through differences in age, solvency, education and occupational status, and health.

Physical separation of the aged and infirm from younger members of society protects them from role expectations based on the work ethic, whereby personal importance is directly related to productive capacity. Age-concentration instead allows roles, norms and value systems more appropriate to retirement, senescence and, perhaps, disengagement to develop, and facilitates the qualification and specification of social participation norms, which in turn intervene between social interaction and well-being (Bultena, 1974; Bultena and Wood, 1969; Graney, 1974; Gubrium, 1972; Messer, 1967; Rose, 1965). Messer (1967), for example, found that the relationship between activity and morale pertained only in age-integrated environments. In age-segregated housing developments, the age-specific normative system freed the elderly 'from a compulsion toward continued activity and from feelings of inadequacy associated with inactivity' (Lawton, 1970c, p.39). For a subculture of ageing to emerge, the environment must be age-concentrated, proximate, and exhibit relative continuity as such. Such a subculture will differ substantially from society at large in the activities and roles that are expected, sanctioned or labelled as deviant. Only those individuals with strong power resources will be able to cope with an age-heterogeneous environment (Gubrium, 1972).

However, evidence of a lack of association, or of a negative association, has also been forthcoming. Kahana and Kahana (1970) randomly assigned elderly admissions to a state hospital to age-integrated and age-segregated wards and found that those on the integrated ward were superior on measures of cognitive and social functioning after three weeks. McClannahan (1973a) and Teaff et al. (1978) argued that age-*heterogeneity* fostered social interaction, life satisfaction and independence, and Rubenstein and Rubenstein (1972) illustrated the beneficial effects on the elderly of visits by young people, particularly when they were prepared to sit and listen. Thus, some age-integration appears beneficial.

Segregation by sex, within age-segregated environments, is a similarly contentious subject although there is little hard empirical evidence to call upon to resolve the issue, although Bennett and Eisdorfer (1975) cite evidence to suggest that the higher death rate of males following relocation into sexually-integrated environments is indicative of the deleterious effects of integration. Contrariwise, Silverstone and Wynter (1975) found that sexual integration of previously single sex floors in a geriatric institution, after some initial resistance, resulted in a higher affect level and more socially desirable behaviour on the part of the residents. The most recently opened purpose-built homes for the elderly cater for both men and women, but this generally does not stop spatial segregation by sex, either by staff or the residents themselves (Lipman and Slater, 1975). A letter recently published in *Social Work Today* best illustrates this voluntary segregation (Wilson, 1977, p.9):

> We have four lounges at this home . . . no doubt you will be shocked to hear that three are occupied by ladies and one is the men's lounge. I can just hear you screaming 'segregation'. We don't segregate them . . . they segregate themselves. The men prefer it that way. They can break wind to their hearts content, smoke their grim pipes and swear in good old fashioned 1914-18 style and offend no-one.

Apart from these investigations of age- and sex-homogeneity and concentration of the suprapersonal environments of the elderly, a few other residents' characteristics have been distinguished as important and discussed in the gerontological literature. Meacher (1972) argued for integration of the confused and rational elderly in residential care, but Lipman and Slater (1975) found that rational residents *chose* to segregate in sitting spaces. Rational residents frequently prefer to sit in their own rooms rather than share a lounge with the confused and incontinent, although they generally tolerate the company of the physically handicapped. Where the confused are not segregated, *all* residents may be deprived of physical freedom and social autonomy (Snyder *et al.*, 1978). Integration of the confused and rational, and of the frail and active will, however, increase the opportunities for enhancement of competence (Graney, 1974; Schoenberg, Carr, Peretz and Kutscher, 1972). Other dimensions of interest include 'isolates', permanency, religious, and ethnic and racial homogeneity (Bennett and Eisdorfer, 1975; Graney, 1974; Nahemow and Bennett, 1968).

Segregation, therefore, promotes the establishment of friendships and hence raises morale. Secondly, environments characterised by homogeneity along certain suprapersonal dimensions 'can facilitate the emergence of social norms among the aged which are better suited to the realities of their status in society than are the role expectations promulgated in [heterogeneous] settings' (Bultena, 1974, p.74).

5.3.7 Continuity

The continuity of the physical and social environments of elderly people, and indeed the continuity of every aspect of their life-styles, has long been regarded as an important determinant of behaviour, well-being and survival. The sources of discontinuity are many and various, but in the context of residential care it is particularly the experience of relocation to and between residential homes that most concerns us. This, too, has been one of the most popular topics of gerontological research, particularly since Carp's (1966) study of elderly persons moving into apartment dwellings. Tobin and Lieberman (1976) are among a number of researchers who have suggested that it is the act and experience of *moving into* an institution which accounts for many of the noxious effects often attributed to *living within* an institution.

Schulz and Brenner (1977) argue that, because relocation is generally a stressful experience, its impact can be lessened by increasing both the controllability and predictability of the relocation. *Controllability* refers to the voluntary/involuntary nature of the move, whilst *predictability* 'is inversely related to the severity of the environmental change . . . and directly related to the amount of preparation given individuals before the move' (ibid., p.324). This simple theoretical framework is similar in many respects to that of Tobin and Lieberman (1976, p.20):

> Effects in this framework are thus seen as a function of the difference between the two environments. The larger the difference between the new and old environment − with expectations (anticipated losses) being equal − the greater the possibility that the elderly person will need to develop adaptive responses often beyond his capacity. In this light, the effect of an institution can be viewed less as a product of its quality or characteristics than of the degree to which it forces the person to make new or overtaxing adaptive responses.

Furthermore, because the ageing individual's adaptive capacity or competence is deteriorating steadily, the chances of his coping with the new environment will be lessened, and the chances of demoralisation increased.

The effects of relocation were initially measured in terms of survival rates and morbidity levels alone, but later studies have extended the list of impact dimensions to include most salient psychological and psychosocial factors. Using one or more of these impact criteria, the empirical studies of relocation largely support the theoretical propositions of Schulz and Brenner, and of Tobin and Lieberman. Voluntary relocation is less harmful than involuntary relocation, suitable preparation neutralises many of the deleterious effects, and 'similar' environments are less harmful than 'dissimilar' environments (see Schulz and Brenner, 1977, for a review).

Attempts to lessen the severity of relocation from a home environment to an institutional one in the British context at least, have largely followed these recommendations. Although voluntary entry into an old people's home will be increasingly rare during a period in which potential residents are both more numerous, more frail, and more confused, it is still possible for administrators, social workers and relatives to prepare the potential resident more thoroughly and to lessen the extent of the environmental change by personalising the new resident's room in the home. The Department of Health and Social Security has long encouraged authorities to allow old people to bring into homes small pieces of furniture and other links with their past. The practice of building furniture into the structure of the homes greatly limits the feasibility of doing so.[4] Evaluation of a new home in Dorset bears this out (Dorset County Council Social Services Department, 1977, paragraph 7.12):

> The extent to which residents can keep their own possessions once they have been admitted to residential care is of course limited by the space available. Unfortunately the design of the bedrooms does not leave much scope for personalisation by different arrangements of furniture or introduction of residents' own large items of furniture. Call-bells and sink units are situated so that in each room there is only one sensible position for the bed.

Sherman and Newman (1977) provide empirical verification of the importance of cherished personal possessions — the lack of a cherished possession was found to be associated with lower scores on Neugarten's Life Satisfaction Index.

The nub of the Tobin and Lieberman thesis is that behaviour, affect and general well-being within the old people's home are the product of both the characteristics of the institution itself and the experience of relocation. These two authors have, to the best of our knowledge, conducted the only study that has attempted to weigh up the relative effects of environmental discontinuity and environmental characteristics *per se*. This study is, in fact, a conglomeration of a number of studies co-ordinated by these two authors at the University of Chicago. Although Tobin and Lieberman had difficulty disentangling the effects of environmental discontinuity from those of institutional life, the data from a sample of 100 persons studied over a period of four years suggested that discontinuity had a critical impact, especially on well-being one year after admission to the home (Tobin and Lieberman, 1976, p.219):

> Those who manifested the extreme outcomes of a marked deterioration or death were more likely to have lived transitionally in nursing homes, to be more passive and to exhibit physical deterioration, as well as emotional reactions, shortly after admission. These findings taken together suggest that the move itself is taxing.

Inputs and the production process

Three additional studies by Lieberman (1974) support this conclusion. Individuals most likely to suffer adversely as a result of environmental discontinuity are more passive, less able to mobilise psychological coping resources, and more physically debilitated.

5.4 Conclusion

This discussion of the social environment has been long and, at times, tortuous. It is clear that the study of environmental language and coding, of therapeutic settings and institutional totality, of individual needs and environmental press, is vast and various. From this conglomeration of research will hopefully come a co-ordinated theory with associated instrumentation. Environmental characteristics and the corresponding individual needs should be studied preferably in conjunction, the dimensionality of the former incorporating those climatic aspects stressed by, for example, Kleemeier, Goffman, Moos, Pincus, Kahana and Lawton, and the dimensionality of the latter incorporating those areas of competence which we will discuss in the next chapter.

Chapter 6

Personal characteristics and experiences

In chapter 4 we discussed the main resource inputs of the production of welfare model, and then moved on, in chapter 5, to consider the place of the social environment in the causal structure. In this chapter our attention is focused on other, personal, influences on individual well-being — personality differences and habitual style of life, the importance of events immediately prior to admission, individual characteristics at the point of entry, and the process of adjustment to the institution. Of these, the first two are historical factors. Pre-admission effects are distinguishable from those relatively stable characteristics that contribute to the description of the degree of disjunction between institutional life and previous career.

6.1 Resident personality

In the second section of chapter 2, we discussed certain personality theories in order to glean from them a conceptualisation and dimensionality of output. In this section we are, in contrast, concerned with those traits of a resident's personality which predict well-being among the elderly. Much has been said in chapter 5 about those needs and preferences which are reflections of a resident's personality, and the manner in which they combine with environmental characteristics to determine behaviour and well-being through an ecological congruence model of human behaviour. We do not repeat the discussion here but instead report the results of a most interesting and, to our knowledge, unique study of personality predictors of well-being of the elderly which has come to our attention.[1] The study was carried out by Barbara Turner (1969) and submitted as a Doctoral thesis to the University of Chicago. The substantive results of the study are also reported in Turner, Tobin and Lieberman (1972) and Tobin and Lieberman (1976).

The basic assumption of Turner's study is that (Turner *et al.*, 1972, p.61):

> those aged with pre-institutional personality traits that are congruent with the specific demands of the relocation environment will experience a minimum of distress due to relocation. Such congruent personality traits may facilitate adaptation because the impact of relocation is lessened when there is a fit between traits and specific adaptive demands of the environment. In this approach the unit of analysis becomes the person-environment relationship in which situational demands determine the predictive power of personality traits.

Personality traits were assessed for a sample of 85 elderly persons on the waiting list for a home, three to twelve months prior to admission. Adaptation to institutional life was assessed approximately twelve months after admission (23 of the sample of 85 were not assessed at this second stage because of poor health, morbidity, or refusal).

Nine personality traits were distinguished, drawing upon earlier literature on institutional living (Goffman, 1961; Martin, 1955; Sommer and Osmond, 1960; Townsend, 1962) and a detailed study of 37 'old-timers' who had successfully adapted to this sample of homes (Lieberman, Brock and Tobin, 1968). Each of these traits was assumed to relate to successful institutional adaptation, and was measured on a five-point scale, independent of the other eight. These traits were: activity-passivity; aggression; narcissistic body image; authoritarian; status drive; distrust of others; non-empathy; extrapunitive; and non-intrapunitive.[2] It was assumed that high positive scores on each of these dimensions indicated a greater degree of congruence with the institutional setting, an assumption justified by the results of an assessment of a subsample of the successfully adjusted 'old-timers'. The nine congruence traits were submitted to a principal components analysis, and four factors emerged, named as: punitive-authoritarian, aggressiveness, non-reflective, and unfriendly. For the purposes of predicting adaptation and adjustment, however, a single total congruence score was used. This score was found to be independent of cognitive functioning and feelings of dominance, but related to denial of impending institutionalisation (those with higher congruence tend to deny less), and a measure of mental health (higher congruence associated with more psychopathology). Individuals revealing higher congruence between personality traits and institutional setting also had *lower* feelings of well-being, more anxiety, better quality of interpersonal relations, and described themselves as less loving. This variety of associations implies a complex adaptation process. In general, however, a person who has such personality traits as those distinguished above (Turner *et al.*, 1972, pp.67-8):

may not experience the initial impact of severe environmental stressors, whereas the aged person without such traits may react adversely to initial impact and, because of physical fragility, show consequent morbidity or die. The congruent traits identified as predictive for the present relocation environment suggest that a vigorous, if not hostile-narcissistic, pre-admission style is related to intactness one year after institutionalisation.

6.2 Experiences prior to admission to the home[3]

In view of the difficulties and expense in following a sizeable sample of elderly persons through the various stages of application or referral, waiting list, entry, and adjustment to a residential home, it is not surprising that there have been few studies of the effects of pre-admission characteristics and experiences upon the well-being of the elderly once they have entered and adjusted to the home. Apart from Morris's (1974, 1975) argument that reaction to an institution occurs *prior* to admission, there being a differential response along the institutional path depending upon the needs of the individual,[4] and the longitudinal studies by the Gerontological Centre in Nijmegen (for brief details, see Coleman, 1976), and by Maas and Kuypers (1974) in California, the only major studies that have come to our notice are those reported by Bennett and Nahemow (1965b), Spasoff *et al.* (1978), and Tobin and Lieberman (1976).

Tobin, Lieberman and their colleagues at the University of Chicago at Illinois seek to explain the deleterious influences frequently attributable to institutional life *per se*, by taking account of four factors: biases in effect caused by selection policies (residents are necessarily more incapacitated than the community-resident elderly), pre-admission effects, environmental discontinuity, and institutional life itself. They see no *a priori* reason to relegate any of these factors to being merely incidental perturbations of the institutional path, but instead examine each one fully. Pre-admission effects are of two kinds — major events in the resident's life history, and factors experienced in the process of becoming a resident (admission and waiting). The first of these appears to have received little attention. Maas and Kuypers (1974) emphasise the importance of the 'life review' in their report of a forty-year longitudinal study of adult life-styles and personality (Maas and Kuypers, 1974, p.215):

for those small proportions in our study whose personalities and life styles seem problematic, it is not merely old age that has ushered in the dissatisfactions and the suffering. In early adulthood these men and women were in various ways at odds with others and themselves or too constricted in their involvements. Old age merely continues for them what earlier years have launched.

This longitudinal study is very useful for its conceptual framework for the description of life-styles. Maas and Kuypers distinguish a dozen *arenas* of life-style (home and visiting, work and leisure, marriage, and so on) as well as four *dimensions* of life-style (interaction, involvement, satisfaction and perception of change). This framework is of some interest for the possible prediction of who it is that enters institutions, their environmental needs in them, and their general well-being. The second aspect argues that the individual whose needs are met 'through an institutional solution may be so changed by the forces set in motion in the process that he or she comes to approximate institutionalised elderly in his or her psychology before entering the institutional environment' (Tobin and Lieberman, 1976, p.17).

Stage 1 　The first step in the process of becoming a resident is the application by, or on behalf of, the elderly person for a place in a residential home. The elderly person's attitude to institutional care at the time of the application may well not be at all conducive to the success of the residential intervention. Elderly people often hold negative views about all forms of personal social service care, and particularly about residential care, and thus may attach negative meanings to otherwise unimportant role losses. They may envisage their independence to be severely curtailed in the home whilst they are anyway currently housebound and dependent upon the daily visit of the home help for many tasks (Kleemeier, 1961; Montgomery, 1965; Shanas, 1961). For the large number of residents admitted in an emergency there can be no time for preparation on the part of the resident. Emergency admissions are often unavoidable but, as the Personal Social Services Council (1977) recommend, they should only be short-term and essential.

Following the application for a residential home place there then follows, for all non-emergency cases, a waiting period before admission during which time the prospective resident must be 'prepared' for the move and for the new mode of living. Responsibility for preparation should be shared by the community-based social worker, friends, neighbours and relatives, and residential home staff. The type of preparation necessary will obviously vary from individual to individual, but it is a common fact that inadequate preparation can be an important reason for the subsequent failure of institutional care to achieve its aims and objectives. The essential characteristics and components of preparation have recently been thoroughly discussed by, for example, Brearley (1977, pp.56-7), the British Association of Social Workers (1977, p.11), the Personal Social Services Council (1977, p.23) and Pope (1978). As Pope argues, the period of waiting is the

Field
s.w.

150

period during which the elderly person comes 'to terms with feelings of rejection from family, neighbours and community' and begins (1978, p.12):

> to anticipate exactly what this new life in an old people's home will comprise. Whether it is anticipated with eagerness, fear or indifference will leave its mark at the moment of admission for it is then that the expectations and ideas that have been built up possibly over many months face the test of reality.

It is argued that those elderly who receive preparation for the move, particularly by visiting the home to meet the matron and view the situation at periods before admission, will experience less anticipated loss and perceived loss after the move and thus adjust more favourably to the home (Dominic, Greenblatt and Stotsky, 1968 and 1968a; Stotsky, 1967). The admission period in fact can be divided into two (Pope, 1978): the *preparation phase*, lasting from the time of application to the time of notification that a place is available, and the *separation phase*, lasting from notification of an available place to the moment of admission. Each phase has its own constituent elements and activities for social services staff and residents' significant others, and the experience of each can have an important impact on the subsequent welfare of residents.

Two important empirical studies of the impact of the pre-admission experiences on the welfare (generally defined) of the elderly resident can be found in the American literature. The research of Bennett and Nahemow (1965b) was concerned solely with the impact on adjustment of social isolation experienced prior to entry to the home. Social adjustment was assumed to comprise three processes: integration (the number of group activities engaged in), conformity (behaviour conforming with social norms extant in the home) and evaluation (of various aspects of home life). A measure of *socialisation* to the home was obtained measuring the amount of information about the home learned by the new resident ('the ability to perceive group affairs in accordance with the perception of the majority'). These indicators of adjustment and socialisation were examined in relation to two indicators of isolation prior to admission. One index, the Adulthood Isolation Index, was concerned with eight major roles during the elderly person's entire life-span: organisational membership, contact with children, contact with siblings, contact with relatives, contact with friends, relationships with parents, spouse and work associates, throughout the entire lifespan. The reliability of this index was reasonable, each item scoring 0, 1 or 2 and aggregated. The other index, the Pre-entry Isolation Index, was concerned with only the first five of these statuses and only for the year immediately prior to investigation. Scores on both isolation indices were related only to the integration component of the adjust-

151

ment concept, and also suggested that isolation prior to entry hindered socialisation within the home (see section 6.4 below).

The study carried out at the University of Chicago generally confirmed these results (Tobin and Lieberman, 1976, p.218):

> The psychological portrait of the institutionalised older person who enters one of the better long-term care institutions is sketched in before the person actually enters and lives in the institutional environment. The psychological effects of institutionalisation are less attributable to institutional life than to reactions to the waiting period preceding admission. The effects are particularly attributed to the loss meaning of separation imparted to the process and to the experience of being abandoned that reflects both separation and the dread of the impending event. Our findings suggest that reactions or effects occur in response to meanings of loss and anticipated loss and not to the events that precipitated admission.

They thus conclude their study with the assertion that: 'The gray portrait, which has been attributed to actually living in an institutional environment, can thus be understood as the end stage of a process that begins well before entering and living in these facilities' (ibid., p.21).

6.3 Individual characteristics at the point of entry

Indicators of output measure change in the state of welfare over time due to the impact of the institution. Arguably the initial states of a resident can affect this change considerably, although the evidence is ambiguous and difficult to evaluate because of statistical inadequacies and the inevitably large errors of measurement. Individual characteristics at the point of entry will often reflect the very reasons for admission to residential care — poor physical health or functioning, loneliness, depression, or anxiety about independent living for example — and certainly will in part be influenced by the amount of preparation afforded the resident before admission. A number of characteristics have been identified or suggested as important determinants of the subsequent well-being of the resident, and are thus included as quasi-inputs in our production of welfare model.

6.3.1 Resident attitudes

Firstly, as we discussed in section 5.3.7 above, the attitudes of the newly admitted resident will be crucially important in determining the outcomes of institutional care. An elderly person admitted involuntarily will be expected to fare less well than a person voluntarily entering the home. Schulz and Brenner (1977, p.325-7) review a number of studies which collectively support this hypothesis. Although these two authors set out a number of methodological inadequacies in some of the studies covered by their review, they nevertheless conclude that 'the remaining studies taken together are compelling in the consistency of their results and in their support of the proposed model' (p.327). In other words, voluntary entrants to institutions fare better than involuntary entrants. A recent Canadian study provides further support. Spasoff *et al.* (1978) studied just over 300 applicants for 'chronic care' in Ontario and found that (ibid., pp.284-5):

> those with a more favourable attitude toward the move at the initial interview [either before or soon after admission] more often expressed satisfaction at the follow-up [approximately one month after admission], although even of those with an initially negative attitude three-quarters were not satisfied.[5]

Spasoff and his colleagues themselves have some doubts about the validity of these findings, however (p.286), and a further complication arises from the fact that the elderly subjects were sometimes interviewed after admission, by which time the impact of admission and the environment of the home itself will almost certainly have had some effect.

6.3.2 Well-being on admission

Secondly, there is evidence about the impact of psychological well-being and adjustment at the time of entry into the home. Morris (1974, 1975) studied a group of elderly applicants to a 'long-term care facility', some of whom were admitted during the five-year study period, and others not. Morris found that those in greatest need by clinical criteria tended to have the lowest scores on the Life Progression component of the PGC morale scale (see section 2.2.7 above) but had, on average, increased their scores during the subsequent year. This was the only group in his sample of 269 to have increased their score. On average, this group also showed a slight, but not significant, increase in scores on other components. The judgment of need was carried out by a research clinician and would have been based on much more than the PGC scales but could nevertheless have been pervasively biased – the subjects could have been interviewed, and data collected for subsequent scaling, at an unrepresentative stage when the errors of measurement would have been consistently in one direction. No doubt the research clinician would have discounted this to a degree. More serious, however, it appears that Morris failed to take account of the death or hospitalisation of subjects. The more usual effect to appear from the literature is that psychological ill-being or lack of adjustment has a negative effect on subsequent psychological well-being and outcomes generally. Such results apply to indicators of depression, failures in developmental task adjustment, low psychological well-being and other criteria (Smith and Lipman, 1972; Wolk and Telleen, 1976; Lieberman, 1965). Much depends upon the quality of the environment in the home. Oberleder (1962, p.31) concluded that

> The ability of the adjusted residents to live so effectively and think so youthfully in an environment which is possibly unpalatable to them suggests among other facts, of course, the mechanism of denial referred to in the Butler and Perlin study (1957). It is possible that the old age person who is able to deny reality — in this case, the reality of segregation and institutionalisation — and at the same time is able to engage in compensatory, even escape-type activity, may perhaps possess the most effective combination of traits for adjustment in a home for the aged.

Again it seems that Turner (1969) concluded that being aggressive, distrustful and hostile towards others can help in the adjustment process. However, Turner also found that those who had coped well in this in the past could cope well with institutionalisation.

The developmental task adjustment scale of Wolk and Kurtz (1975) has fourteen items covering a number of developmental tasks: adjustment to decreasing physical strength and health, to the increased susceptibility to illness and hence to invalidity, to retirement and reduced income, to forcibly redefined goals and orientations, to death of one's spouse and loneliness, to an explicit affiliation with the age group, and generally and finally to an admission that one is old. Some of these items are clearly related to the output of homes and could thus be appropriate quasi-inputs. Similarly, Sherwood and Nadelson (1972) found that the non-clinically derived, sociological theory of relative deprivation proved to be a better predictor of 'despair' in an aged population applying for long-term care than was Erikson's clinically derived developmental theory. Aspects of relative deprivation — the greater the perceived differences between current circumstances and more favourable circumstances of peers in one's reference group the greater the feelings of deprivation leading to despair, low morale and misery — might therefore with advantage be included in scales measuring quasi-inputs as well as in scales measuring outputs.

6.3.3 Health status on admission

Physical health and capacity for self-care are also known to have an influence on subsequent well-being. For instance, Morris (1975) found that those who perceived that their health had improved over a twelve-month period had also improved in morale. This however, is not an

154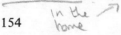

unambiguous result — the mood component in self-perceived health is substantial and again there is the possibility of a regression effect. Indeed, that it is likely to be a regression effect seems compatible with one of the results of Bull and Aucoin (1975); that among those with very poor health an improvement in health appears to have a substantial effect on satisfaction and adjustment while improvements beyond this level appear to have little effect. Much the same arguments apply if one controls for those items of incapacity for self-care in the residential home context. This is the most relevant single health indicator since, *de facto*, the residential home is a long term care facility, a semi-permanent surrogate home.

6.3.4 Mental status on admission

The literature also demonstrates the relevance of mental impairment. Organic brain damage has been shown to predispose towards increased morbidity and mortality at relocation because the senile psychotic cannot prepare for change and lacks adaptive responses. The senile psychotic person, although not sufficiently in contact to understand advance explanations of a move, is nevertheless sufficiently alert to recognise and respond to familiar environmental cues. The removal of these cues and their replacement with unfamiliar environmental stimuli results in cognitive dissonance and disturbance which is greater the less the aged individual possesses the adaptive capacity to cope, because of the loss of the capacity for recent memory.

6.4 The stages of admission, adjustment and institutionalisation

The reactions of residents depend not only on the type of quasi-input factor discussed above; they are also qualitatively different at the different stages of adjustment. The social work literature differentiates three stages of the adjustment process — that of decision and preparation, that of impact, and that of settling in. The importance of an adequate preparation for life in an old people's home was discussed in the second section of this chapter. In this section we look at the second and third stages — the impact of admission and the period of 'settling in', this latter stage itself often having two components — adjustment[6] and institutionalisation. Adjustment need not necessarily mean the apathy, withdrawal or submissiveness that has been called 'institutionalisation', but the vulnerability of residents in their first few days in the home and the apparent hostility of many residential environments frequently render the two indistinguishable.

The impact stage, as Yawney and Slover (1973) call it, extends from the moment of entry until the elderly resident masters the new institutional environment or, as often happens, until the environment

see p 150

155

masters the resident (institutionalisation). The admission process is thus crucially important in determining virtually every aspect of the resident's future life in the home. Pope (1978) discusses three aspects of admission that make it so important.

(a) First, there is 'the impact that the actual admission appears to have upon the people concerned' (ibid., p.12). The enormous changes that the new resident undergoes come at a time of vulnerability, when 'psychic and physical energy are diminished and when long established modes of life are only reluctantly changed' (BASW, 1977, p.11). The so-called 'relocation literature' reviewed by Yawney and Slover (1973) and Schulz and Brenner (1977) has addressed the problem of *who* survives this initial impact stage (see below). Generally, the greater the control over, or preparation for, the admission and the less marked the difference between the old and new environments, the greater the likelihood of survival.

(b) Pope's second aspect 'is to be found in the admission practices and the implications that these may have for the subsequent life of the residents. . . Practical everyday necessities for the smooth running of a home . . . take on a symbolic significance that extends deeply into the lives of those who experience them' (Pope, 1977, p.13). The new resident must be received with kindness and reassurance and must be allowed to retain his or her rights to humanity, autonomy, lucidity, and fidelity (Fried, 1974). The invasion of personal privacy by staff and other residents is probably one of the most common characteristics of admission and one of the most damaging.

(c) Third, 'whilst an admission may represent the ending of one phase of life it is also the beginning of another. Thus it provides the opportunity to reassess and on occasion revitalise the life of the elderly person to give a greater satisfaction or security to life than was hitherto the case' (Pope, 1978, p. 13).

During the impact stage most elderly residents will experience grief, helplessness, anger, and depression (Yawney and Slover, 1973). Parkes (1972b) discusses how shock and numbness give way to anxiety and distress, and then to reorganisation and redirection of feelings. Much higher mortality and morbidity rates have been observed during the impact stage (Aldrich, 1964; Lieberman, 1961; Pope, 1977, 1978; Yawney and Slover, 1973), although researchers have not always used the same time-scale in their studies. It is also clear that many residents have an unrealistically favourable view of the home during the early part of the impact stage.

The length of the impact stage has been operationally defined as the period 'from the end of the first day until the new resident looks on the home as "home"' (Pope, 1978, p. 14) or, alternatively, as the time it takes to lift the newly admitted aged person from his initial feelings of dissonance and disorientation to a mastering of the new environment (Yawney and Slover, 1973) or submission to that environment. Yawney and Slover argue that it takes between one-and-a-half and six months for the resident to adjust, Ruth Bennett (1963) estimated that it took at least two months for the loss of self to dawn upon new entrants, and Rodstein, Savitsky and Starkman (1976) estimated that over three-quarters of new residents had overcome any problems of adjustment within six months of admission. Contrariwise, Spasoff *et al.* (1978) felt that 'by one month after admission most of the subjects had made a fairly satisfactory adjustment to institutional life' (ibid., p. 286). Of course, these studies have all been conducted in the North American context where both the characteristics presented by residents at the point of entry and the environments of the homes may well be different from those typical of the British old people's home.

Bennett and Nahemow (1965a, 1965b, 1972) have analysed the process that leads to adjustment. They argue that socialisation, the process of learning the norms and mores of the home, is a prerequisite for, but distinct from, adjustment. Adjustment has three components: integration (participation in activities, the membership of informal groups, and friendships — including the conversational integration emphasised by Meacher), evaluation (the development of opinions regarding specific aspects of life in the home), and conformity (behaviour enacted in accordance with social norms). Socialisation, conceptualised as an intervening mechanism between experience prior to entry and subsequent adjustment, was found to be a predictor of adjustment after one, two, and six months of residence, indicating the importance of rapid social learning. Learning was not fully complete, however, sometimes until two years had elapsed. Furthermore, the probability that socialisation will lead to integration, evaluation, and conformity clearly depends upon the degree of anabolism of the social environment.

A similar period of adjustment was assumed by Jackson (1974) in his study of the relationship between residence, education, socialisation, and cognitive task performance with a sample of residents from a 'private rest home' for the aged. In order to increase the reliability of the responses to the various tests and questionnaires he only sampled individuals who had resided in the home for longer than the six-week 'orientation period'. He found, incidentally, that duration of institutional residence as negatively related to cognitive task performance.

Spasoff *et al.* (1978) report a longitudinal study of a sample of elderly residents in Ontario long-term care institutions (chronic hospitals, nursing homes, homes for the aged, and foster homes supervised by homes for the aged). Interviews were conducted before or immediately after admission, after approximately one month in the institution, and after one year in the institution. The changes in resident well-being and activity were observed by the researchers

157

using both objective indicators and the subjective assessments of residents, their relatives, and staff. These changes paint a fairly clear picture of the processes of adjustment to long-term care, although the variety of caring environments studied and the variety of characteristics presented by the elderly at the point of admission will render these processes untypical of those to be found in homes for the aged alone. Furthermore, Spasoff and his colleagues point out the shortage of nursing homes in the Ontario area, so that new entrants may be rather more needy than will typically be the case. Anyway, differences between Canadian and British policies, and hence differences in the inputs and quasi-inputs entering the production of welfare process at each and every level, will mean that the phasing of adjustment in British old people's homes may differ somewhat.

Just over 300 elderly persons applied for admission to a long-term care institution during the intake year of the study (June 1973 – June 1974), two-thirds of whom were interviewed either before or soon after admission. Exactly one-half of the original applicants had entered an institution by the end of the second year of data collection. The second interview was conducted approximately one month after admission, by which time 15 of the 151 new entrants had since left care – 14 had died and 1 had been discharged. Of the remaining residents, just over a third could not be interviewed because 'The subject's condition precluded participation in a meaningful interview' (Spasoff *et al.*, 1978, p. 282). For these residents, interviews were conducted with a close relative. Interview data from residents and from relatives was combined for the purposes of the report where the authors felt this did not represent a serious misrepresentation. After one month in the institutions, Spasoff and his colleagues observed that:

- – 'The proportion of subjects who sat for hours on end doing nothing was almost identical to that at the initial interviews, before admission' (p. 283).
- More residents had become less involved in social and recreational activities than had become more involved, a pattern apparently established before admission.
- Self-perceived health had improved for 43 per cent of residents, and remained unchanged for 30 per cent, but dependency in the activities of daily living had generally increased, presumably because of the greater availability of help.
- The psychological status of most residents had improved.

These findings led them to conclude that most of the elderly had 'satisfactorily adjusted to institutional life' after one month in the home.

One year after admission to the institution, 38 of the 151 original entrants (25 per cent) had died, and 9 had been discharged, and one year follow-up interviews were obtained for 95 of the remaining 104 residents (54 interviews with residents themselves, the remainder with relatives). Observed changes between one month and one year after admission included:

- There were no significant changes in visiting by relatives and friends, in the use of the telephone, in concern over the lack of privacy, or in the enjoyment of the company of other residents. Significantly more residents reported having close friends in the institution.
- Activity rates were somewhat lower after a year in the institution than after a month. Half the residents listed their major activity as 'sitting or lying around or doing nothing at all' (ibid., p. 288), as compared with 41 per cent after one month.
- Self-perceived health had now improved for only 27 per cent of residents, and remained unchanged for 36 per cent. A third of the residents had developed new health problems since admission, most of them new physical problems. Dependency had changed very little.
- Psychological state for all residents together had changed very little, with improvement more frequent than deterioration.
- Satisfaction with care remained generally high, but there had nevertheless been a drop in satisfaction with the physical and emotional aspects of care.

Adjustment to the home may not always be successful. Residents who survive the impact of admission may display the characteristics of apathy, withdrawal, uninterest, resignation and submissiveness (Bates, 1976, pp. 26-30). Such institutionalisation or 'institutional neurosis' (Barton, 1966) develops from initial feelings of incompetence at the point of entry, feelings which are reinforced by the dominance, restrictiveness, impersonality and 'totality' of the home environment (Kutner, 1969).

The development of institutionalisation, like the process of adjustment, takes place in a series of stages, each of which varies in symptomatology. The following table, from Yawney and Slover (1973), gives one account of the dangers during the period of adjustment for a resident who is suggestible, lacking in confidence and generally feeling 'incompetent'. He then develops doubts about his physical and mental conditions (induced by the expectations of staff and others) in turn leading to the acceptance of a passive role and diminished interest in personal care. Identification of the self with others in the institution then results, itself leading to psychosocial degradation and with it the progressive loss of personal skills and actual (rather than felt) competence. Of course, in a situation where adjustment would be made to an environment that can yield only a low level of life satisfaction, an unwillingness or inability to adjust can actually in some circumstances contribute to life satisfaction. We have quoted above some results of Oberleder and Turner which are compatible with this view.

Table 6.1 Stages in the development of institutionalisation

Developmental stage	Symptoms	Prognosis
Stage of uncertainty	Loss of identity	Readily reversible
Deprived of cultural and social reinforcement	Looks for success and adaptation: hyper-suggestible	
Doubts about physical and mental condition	Questioning: faltering	
Feels relieved of responsibility because he is receiving message: 'something is wrong with you'	Less interest in personal care: resents being treated as incompetent	Therapy is increasingly difficult
Compliant but still feels more competent than other residents		
Loss of contact with family and friends	Fewer letters and visits; socially awkward	
Identifies self with others in institution	Complete psychosocial degradation	Not readily reversible

(Copyright 1973, National Association of Social Workers. Inc. Reprinted with permission from Yawney and Slover in *Social Work*, vol. 18, no. 3, 1973 p. 93.)

We therefore conclude that not only will the pattern and rate of reaction of residents differ greatly (for reasons that will be clear from the argument of various parts of this and other chapters), but also that the symptomatology will vary between stages in the experience of institutional life and also with the anabolic characteristics of the social environment. It does not seem to us that ground work research on the description of adaptation processes of individual residents to life in different kinds of homes has been carried out with the extensiveness and rigour which allow one to make firm judgments about the importance of the various 'individual quasi-inputs' discussed in this chapter and their impact on resident welfare. As this book has demonstrated, the production of welfare process in old people's homes is both broadly-based and complex. To disentangle reliably the influences of the resource inputs of the environment, of residents' characteristics at the point of entry, and of experiences in the process of becoming a resident will thus require a very carefully designed empirical study. The use of a change measure of individual well-being to reflect a major part of the output of an old people's home complicates the model yet further, for it will be dangerous to place undue reliance on indicators of residents' well-being obtained at, or shortly after, the point of entry.

Part four

Conclusion

Chapter 7

Concluding discussion

The aim of this book has been to describe and evaluate concepts, theories that embody them and associated measurement tools. For this, we have needed a framework, partly in order to organise our account, and partly to provide criteria about what issues must be mentioned and what can be omitted. The framework we have chosen is the economist's — the production relations approach which focuses on the analysis of the relationships between resources and outputs. The framework has certainly proved valuable. The application of the framework has allowed us to see more clearly than would otherwise have been possible a most striking characteristic of the literature — the failure of any of it to take a sufficiently general view of causal processes in the production of welfare in old people's homes. The literature we have reviewed draws on very disparate sources. Some of the literature was so closely focused that in reading it it is often difficult to see the wood for the trees. Certainly, none of the literature systematically asks all the questions posed by the production relations approach.

7.1 Applying the production relations approach

The book separately analysed outputs and inputs.

7.1.1 Outputs

The introductory chapter was mainly concerned with output as a general concept. Outputs, we argued, consist of welfare consequences of different combinations of resources in long-term care facilities for the elderly, outcomes sufficiently advanced in the process of producing welfare to be valued in their own right. In principle we would not include less global outcomes of care because their presence would probably have consequences which would not be valued for themselves;

165

though in practice we might be forced to do so because there appeared to be no reliable method of measuring these consequences.

We must take separate account of a large number of such outcomes. One reason is that residential homes are sufficiently closed communities to cause nearly all aspects of the quality of life to be influenced by varying resource constellations. A second is that variations in inputs have consequences that vary between kinds of outcome. Such relationships are sufficiently diverse for it to be sensible not to attempt to indicate the numerous and various outcomes by a single or even a relatively few measures. It would be equally sensible to measure outcomes of a variety of degrees of generality. The literature reviewed in Part three has discovered many quite specific effects — specific effects which cumulate to influence more general aspects of the quality of life. For this reason, Part two did not contain a lengthy discussion of how to value outcomes so as to aggregate them into a single measure, although a few arguments about such evaluative processes were presented. However, a description of welfare consequences has only a limited meaning in the absence of evaluatory information. For instance, knowledge about consequences for the capacity for self-care assessed in terms of household maintenance activities is of limited use for assessing programmes unless we either postulate that people value the capacity to undertake activities fairly equally, or we have some information about people's evaluation of the importance of such activities to them.

How then should we select a dimensionality of outcomes? Certainly account should be taken of organisational goals, latent as well as manifest. However, to rely on the latent and manifest goals of actors would be dangerous when these aims are considered explicitly by them only infrequently. It will be remembered that, in one of its more persuasive documents, the Personal Social Services Council lamented the absence of 'a philosophy of residential care'. An analysis of latent and manifest goals is one valuable basis, but certainly such an analysis would need to be supplemented by drawing on the whole of the international social welfare paradigm. The existence of this paradigm allows the researcher to draw on a larger international literature. This contains theoretical argument about what consequences are likely to be important as well as the nature of the causal processes. It also describes and evaluates instruments for collecting data to apply the theoretical concepts. The paradigm allows the research worker to use a far broader intellectual base than would otherwise be possible: not just the British and American social work literature and the American gerontological literature, but also the work of the personality theorists and of others that together make the intellectual bases for argument that much more explicit.

International comparisons have much to contribute to extending the range of our imagination about the variety of types of care. This is so of American as well as European provision. In the American system, the nearest equivalent to our residential homes are 'health related facilities' which are not intended to provide much personal care. However, nursing homes, which do provide some personal care, are relatively more important than in the UK. There is therefore an overlap in the clienteles of British old people's homes and American nursing homes. Among the most important ways in which they differ from British homes is their scale, many having more than 400 beds. Being large, they are able to employ a wide range of specialised para-professional personnel and provide a wide range of facilities. Indeed, they are required to do so by state licensing authorities in such states as New York. Facilities can include a shop, restaurant, coffee lounges and recreational facilities. In some states, there is the requirement that no bedroom should accommodate more than three persons; and most residents are accommodated in single or double-bedded rooms. In the better homes, all floors have telephones for patients and private tele-vision sets. Residents' councils are often active and seem not to be inhibited from fighting battles with the management. All homes in New York must employ a dietician. Every resident has to have a planned programme of activities and the record of them is open to state inspec-tion. All homes are required to employ activities staff and post a pro-gramme of activities on a bulletin board.

Far from being dissatisfied with the large scale of their homes, the trend in New York is to take further advantage of potential economies of scale by increasing the size of facilities. Clearly the level of inputs is more generous than is the case in Britain. Whereas the whole philoso-phy of care in the American model directly reflects an awareness of economies of scale, the models of provision in the UK reflect an as-sumed relationship between scale and the dangers of institutionalism. No doubt the Americans have developed their philosophy through a history in which large institutions have generated scandals in voluntary and private homes and in which the response was the development of state regulation to achieve the same standards of services in *all* institu-tions as were available in the *best* voluntary and private ones. In Britain, the best institutions at the time of the Nuffield Survey, when the post-war policy was being thought out, were small, voluntary homes. When the state came to replace the workhouse, it modelled its provision on these small homes. Bevan's argument focused on the able-bodied and stressed privacy, independence and autonomy. In doing so, he neglected the effect on these residents of sources of stimulation in the environment of the home. It was not understood that the creation of a stimulating environment for the physically and mentally infirm that were increasingly to dominate admissions to residential care would require specialised resources. (For the early history of post-war policy see Davies (1968, pp. 64-72) and Sumner and Smith (1969).) Now, the problem for Britain is to provide these facilities that are most worthwhile given the scale of homes and their inherited facilities.

There are three main beneficiaries from the welfare outcomes of variations between residential homes: individual residents, their significant others, and society in general. It is most important to study the effect of variations on the first. In our review of American approaches to measuring the psychological well-being of residents we distinguished between the *quality of life*, of which such well-being is a component, and the *quality of care*. The latter has received far more — in comparison, rather too much — attention in the British literature. The two would be synonymous only if the best environments for some are the best for all. This is an invalid assumption, as became clearer to readers of later chapters. It is the fit between the environment and the individual that must be the focus of attention. It was the unacceptability of the assumption of a common ameliorative environment for all that caused both the 'disengagement' and 'activity' theories of ageing to seem naive, and to focus attention instead on the implications of typologies or patterns of ageing. Though related to the arguments of personality theory, the approach does not postulate rigid and unchanging intra-psychic characteristics. Clearly, however, the practical importance of the argument that different types of environment are 'best' for different people depends on such continuities. The evidence suggests that such continuities are important.

Our analysis of the measurement of engaged activity, as currently undertaken, led us to conclude that it can make a valuable contribution to the measurement of outcome where no more direct measures of well-being could be sufficiently valid and reliable. Also it is valuable as one quasi-input among others in studying the processes of producing welfare. However, it takes too little account of the congruence argument to be a valid and reliable measure of final output in studies seeking to understand the relationships between inputs and outputs for persons of varying dispositions.

We have therefore focused more on the direct study of morale and life satisfaction. We discussed in detail some of the more important life satisfaction ratings and indices (LSR and LSI), the Affect Balance Scale (ABS), and the Philadelphia Geriatric Center (PGC) scale. First their content was examined in relation to the writings of the personality theorists, so as to form an impression of their degree of content, concurrent, and construct validities, test-retest reliability, and the stability of the dimensions yielded in factor analysis. None of the scales seemed to be for all purposes superior to the others. All indices and their dimensions are interrelated. Compared with others there is clearly a trade-off to be made between the opportunity cost (in other data foregone) in using LSR and the greater validity and reliability of the data to be obtained. Some scales were directed at more general populations, others at populations near or above the margins of need for institutionalisation. But all those reviewed were sufficiently valid and reliable to be usable.

This essay has not discussed in great detail outcomes enjoyed principally by residents though not central to their overall psychological well-being. Indeed, only two among a vast number of effects distinguished in the literature — mortality and (more briefly) morbidity — were at all extensively discussed. One reason is the very pervasiveness in the studies of such factors. The study of their interrelationship is worthy of a monograph in its own right. Second, many of them are intermediate and not final outputs. Third, it is what the citizen (or his representative) values which can legitimately count as output. It is the citizen who pays, and is therefore the consumer. Benefits to residents (or significant others) can be legitimately counted only because they contribute a satisfaction to citizens that exceeds their costs. Some conclusions that at first sight may seem paradoxical follow from the fact that it is the citizen who is the consumer. If citizens' representatives derive subjective benefits from Picasso reproductions on the walls of their old people's homes while residents are impervious to their magic, the psychological satisfaction of the representatives can legitimately be counted as output as long as the councillor does not form his satisfaction from thinking that residents are in fact enjoying them. Again, if citizens' representatives consider some amenity as a prerequisite for the civilised life of those in their care but residents leave it unvalued and unused, it may be legitimately counted — again, as long as the councillor does not consider it to be a prerequisite only because residents do. If an increment of standards of care adds to the satisfaction of representatives though not to that of residents, it may be separately counted. But legitimacy is one thing; making the best judgment about the use of resources is another. It is this distinction between wise and legitimate judgment that resolves our paradoxes. We should put great weight on residents' psychological well-being and little weight on factors that warm the hearts of councillors but are little valued by residents because such factors are — mainly because of simple misjudgment — often where resources are most likely to be wasted. Indeed some features of standards often seem to yield absurdly little for their high resource cost. An example is the overkill in fire prevention in well-designed buildings with minimal fire risk. What is of practical interest about some of these features is the cost which small improvements in safety impose in diminution of welfare of other kinds both indirectly, by reducing the resources available for more welfare-producing expenditure, and directly. A letter to *The Times* from a school headmaster described wittily the nil effect of fire doors on the zero probability of injury through fire and the large number of broken limbs caused directly by them. Again, satisfaction from services should not in all cases be counted separately; since in some it is already to some extent reflected in salary payments received, and it is important not to count the same effect twice. If the consequences for residents are already counted, it is only those other consequences that contribute to citizens' satisfaction that need be included — or indeed *can* be included if we are to avoid double counting.

We did not devote much space to outputs enjoyed mainly by significant others. One reason is that studies of production relations in old people's homes examine the influence of varying combinations of resources on outcomes. In such studies the implicit comparison groups are persons in other residential homes 'similar' at the point of admission or at the time of the decision to admit, and not similar persons not resident in long-term facilities. This is a partial admission of the complexity of the knowledge-building task. There is a pressing need to compare the consequences of alternative resource patterns which combine short 'one-off' or periodic stays in homes with long-term stays. (To restrict the argument to long-term care may be necessary, but it is certainly not desirable.) Of course, there can be great differences in the consequences for significant others of residents being situated in one environment rather than another; but not nearly as great as the difference between being a long-term resident and receiving most packages combining residential and other care. Again, only to the degree that they are valued by citizens should they be included; and if significant others value them because residents do, it would be double counting to include them also as benefits to significant others.

Important though such considerations are, they hardly form a major conclusion. One such conclusion is that many of the most impressive classifications and measurements of welfare are closely interrelated. Several instruments and classifications seem to be both reasonably reliable and valid, and reliable and valid to a similar degree. In practice, therefore, the choice between them need not depend on their intrinsic qualities. Several supplementary conclusions follow. We can no longer take refuge in assuming that measures of the quality of *care* are sufficient indicators of the quality of *life*. We must use more direct indicators of outcomes. The scholarly experience of the Americans described in chapter 2 should aid sensible choice given the purpose in hand. Secondly, it follows from the interrelatedness of scales and the dimensions they yield that we can shift the focus of the issue about the measurement of this kind of output. Questions of the form 'What is the best dimensionality of outputs?' and 'How best can they be measured?' need not be viewed separately from the processes of production themselves. Since these kinds of output are interrelated, we can as sensibly start from a classification of resource and non-resource inputs, and so from a set of policy choices in the deploy-

Table 7.1 Outputs from the process of production of welfare: description and operationalisation

(A) General well-being of residents

(i) *Psychological well-being*

Description: life satisfaction or morale, with constituent or separate dimensions of happiness, mood, self-concept, intra-psychic and psychophysiological symptoms, self-rated health, attitude, loneliness, etc.

Operationalisation: well over 100 different scales available. Most popular scales are the *Life Satisfaction Index*, with dimensions of zest, resolution, goal congruence, self-concept, mood, contentment and achievement (see section 2.2.5); the *Affect Balance Scale*, with dimensions of positive affect, negative affect and long-term satisfaction (see section 2.2.6); and the *PGC Morale Scale*, with dimensions of tranquility or agitation, satisfaction with life progression or attitude towards ageing and lonely dissatisfaction (see section 2.2.7). Very widely applied in gerontological research in North America; very limited application in UK and elsewhere. Reliability and validity in UK not yet rigorously examined.

(ii) *Engagement*

Description: engaged activity is 'interacting with materials or people in a manner likely to maintain or develop skills and abilities'.

Operationalisation: measures of engaged activity developed by Wessex team under Kushlick and the 'Living Environments Group' of Kansas University (see section 2.1). Limited application in both North America and UK.

(iii) *Benefits not related to psychological well-being*

Description: Principally mortality, morbidity (physical, mental and sensory), and certain other dimensions. These are benefits valued in their own right but which may not make a major contribution to psychological well-being. Nurture (nutrition, cleanliness, warmth) may also be included.

Operationalisation: Large number of scaling techniques and scales currently in use. For reviews see Wright; Challis; Lieberman and other references in section 3.1.

(B) Narrower sources of resident satisfaction

Residents' significant others

Description: Residents' significant others are major beneficiaries from residential provision – through relief from strain and tension (intolerance, overcrowding, aggravation of illness, tension from inadequacy); psychological well-being (altruism, etc.).

Operationalisation: Isaacs, Livingstone and Neville, 1972; Davies and Duncan, 1975; and see section 3.2.

ment of the more controllable of them. Again, we can just as well use as our baseline a set of ideas about the welfare producing processes themselves as we can a particular conceptualisation of outputs and the indicators developed to measure it. Using the literature on the inter-relation of outputs, we can be eclectic in the way we ensure coverage of important outputs and allow their description as dimensions to be substantially empirically determined in the analysis of the relation-ships of inputs and outcomes. Only conceptually are inputs and outputs divisible in the study of the production of welfare. Table 7.1. illustrates the breadth of choice faced by researchers into the production of wel-fare in old people's homes by summarising the types of output dimen-sions most thoroughly explored in Part II.

7.1.2 Inputs and the production process

The plan of the book has separated resource inputs from non-resource and quasi-inputs. This plan was chosen because it makes it easier to follow streams of literature by doing so, not because resource and other inputs work independently of one another. As has frequently become evident from the argument, resource inputs are often enabling factors which have an effect quite different in magnitude when accompanied by non-resource and quasi-inputs. If they have a significance as a group, it is more because they tend in general to be more controllable by the organisation. But even this generalisation does not universally hold. There are many slips between the cup of intention and the lip of achievement even in implementing planned provisions of some of the more important physical resources. However, there can be no denying that in general, quantities of physical resources and design features of homes are more controllable than, say, the practices and attitudes of care staff, or the characteristics that highest priority residents bring with them to the residential context and the stages that immediately preceded it.

Following the fundamental distinction in economics between current and capital resources, we deal separately with manpower services and imputed flows of services from the physical structure of homes. In chapter 4, we organised our discussion of manpower inputs around the types of manpower, their numbers, and the nature and quality of all services rendered. Dealing with *types* of manpower we discussed theoretical arguments about the manpower input financed from sources other than the manpower budget of the home itself. But the literature testing the general impact of such peripatetic manpower services as those supplied by skilled nurses, physiotherapists and oc-cupational therapists is surprisingly sparse, case studies excepted. The 'marginal productivity' for different kinds of output of such inputs are most important to assess since the importance attached to them is one of the major ways in which the American model of long-term care differs from our own. The Americans go as far as to require a minimal standard of a variety of types of such input defined by state regulation. Of course, many of them, particularly the 'therapists' of various kinds, dieticians and the larger nursing input, reflect the medical model whose application to the American intermediate care facility is so criticised by writers from that country. But it also reflects a feature not much stressed by American writers, probably because it seems too obvious to mention. The American model is one in which the best facilities are in competition for consumers and thus seek to sell their services by offering — or at least appearing to offer — a wide range of services that those shopping on behalf of potential consumers believe will contribute to the quality of their lives as well as to the quality of their care. Until we know more about the consequences for quality of life of the different kinds of input for residents with different characteristics, we shall be unable to learn properly from the American experience. Transplanting ideas from one system to another is fraught with difficulties — particularly difficulties of understanding exactly what the consequences of the application of resources will be. Production relations research is useful precisely because it sharpens the perceptions of cause and consequence which must be at least implicit in cross-national emulation. However, the potential of cross-national emulation is only one aspect of the problem. Emulations of the practices in some areas by social services managers and others is even more directly important. An example is the increased use of nursing staff in homes, sometimes funded by joint financing arrangements.

Of course, the central focus of analysis should remain the impact upon output of the staff on the manpower establishment of homes themselves. 'Hit and run' staff tend to have their effect indirectly rather than directly, so that the impact is often — indeed in some cases generally — weak though pervasive.

A discussion of the numbers of the main types of staff suggests some further conclusions. First, both econometric modelling from large surveys and the analysis of descriptive data from small numbers of homes imply that there is rather less substitution between four main types of staff than might be expected from casual observation or from some depth studies. Of course, the principal studies may underestimate the actual degree of substitution of one form of staff for another. Imber (1977) may do so because her study is based on job descriptions provided by matrons. Almost certainly, these are likely to be biased: to be partly statements of intent and not entirely descriptions about tasks generally performed. Often it is at crisis points that staff substitution has its most powerful effect on the welfare of residents. Such crisis points can be enormously important for welfare though quantitatively a small proportion of the total time. Therefore, even if matrons' statements are unbiased accounts of how, in general, time is used they may understate the true importance for welfare of substitution in the performance of tasks. Therefore Imber's results must be viewed with caution. One must look for different types of reasons for the low degree of substitution found in earlier work by one of the authors (Knapp, 1979). As the study makes clear a very probable source of bias is the weakness of the indicators. The crudity of the measures of manpower input unweighted by the timing of that input are bound to attenuate relationships. Again, the data source did not permit measurement of the quality of life even in the crudest terms. We must therefore conclude that the literature has not yet produced reasonable estimates of the degree of substitution of forms of manpower in the production of welfare.

And of course, even if it had done so, we must make clear that *what is* is not necessarily to be identified with *what ought to be*. There are several places in the book where it is implicit in the argument that rigid role specification during staff-resident interactions has evil effects, but few places where a rigid role specification between the primary manpower groups can have beneficial effects. We should as a matter of policy be working towards the diminution of rigidity of those specifications. In this, we would be swimming against a powerful tide in many social services departments. One reason for swimming hard is that in many such departments it is necessary to do so in order to retain that degree of flexibility that now exists. To lose it could disastrously impair the ability of the residential home to cope with clients who cannot be cared for in any other way in the short term. Such a role may not be desirable. It should never dominate. But in many areas it remains an inescapable function of residential homes. The changing balance between demands and resources may make it so in more authorities.

The literature allows a second conclusion. Partly because of the apparently low degree of substitution, types of staff are easily predictable from the characteristics of residents and of the home itself. The numbers of care staff are surprisingly predictable from information about the dependency distribution of clients. Though there is evidence that it is the very few most dependent clients who consume a high proportion of care time, variations between homes in the numbers of staff are sensitive to the broader distribution of clients by incapacity. The number of care staff is also responsive to home characteristics. The causes of relationships are not necessarily as straightforward as they may seem. For instance, one might have expected that new homes would have more generous staffing than old ones because the staffing requirements of the new homes would be deliberately fought out in the context of the social environment it would be hoped to create in them, and their staffing would be negotiated *ad hoc*. However, one's expectation would be false. Other findings help to fill gaps in the jigsaw. The greater the range of functions undertaken, the higher this ratio of staff to residents. The range of functions undertaken (particularly the presence of day care clients), a distribution of residents heavily weighted with the more frail, and the design features that predict the ratio, have one thing in common; they all increase the work-load of staff. What the results show, therefore, is that there is some responsiveness of staff-resident ratios to work-load.

As might be expected, numbers of domestic staff are more sensitive to differences in the design features of the home than are numbers of care staff; though the number of domestic staff also is responsive to the work-load generated by the presence of day care facilities. The British work so far completed is a little more elaborate than any American studies of the same *genre*. However, the one American team which has explored similar questions — that at the Battelle Centre, Seattle — comes out with much the same picture (see McCaffree *et al.*, 1977; Battelle Health Care Study Centre, 1977).

Third, there is some evidence that the influence of the staff-resident ratio is felt indirectly. For instance, Linn found that the effects of staff-resident ratios were felt in the quality of care, and Curry and Ratliff argued that they affected milieu by influencing the amount of time that staff and residents could spend in personal contact. In this country Neill *et al.* show how care staff want more time to be able to talk with residents. However, not all the results discussed in chapter 4 were compatible. For instance, it is not clear whether the staff-resident ratio itself, that is, the *physical* resource, is the chicken or the egg. It is possible that a consciousness of the need for generous staff ratios among higher management might be associated with a commitment that influences the selection of staff and the management of day-to-day affairs which in turn encourages a personalised approach to the care of residents.

Much of the literature tends to be inexplicit about causal processes in the way it handles ideas and evidence about the impact of the quality of staffing. Some studies treat as equivalent inputs and quasi-inputs of very differing degrees of causal priority in the production of welfare. The main task is to explain variations in the quality of staff contacts with residents. There have been important developments in the arguments about this. Two examples may be quoted from chapter 4. One is about the influence of the formal organisation of homes and their organisational milieu: Raynes and others have shown that organisations might well make a distinctive contribution to the explanation of the nature of client/resident contact. In the study of American homes for the mentally handicapped, Raynes *et al.* (1979) developed an argument showing the impact of organisational dimensions whose theoretical importance and measurement has been developed by the Aston group — in particular, they suggest the importance of centralisa-

175

tion, formalisation, specialisation and (not an Aston factor) communication. The results provide support for some, though not all, of the predictions from the argument; the effects working directly through staff morale and indirectly through morale by way of turnover. Again, Raynes's pioneering study shows that characteristics of different levels of the organisation seem to influence aspects of the quality of care: the characteristics at the highest levels influencing the factors whose influence is most pervasive, like the resource framework. The argument might well be applied to British old people's homes. Though smaller and more separate from the residential sections of their authorities than Raynes's 'homes' are from their institutional management, some have themselves management structures with geographically defined sections which define the span of control of one manager. Variations between the authorities in the style of higher management are certainly great.

It is true that contingency theory argues that variations in formal organisation and style are themselves responses to environmental features, as is the degree to which members are concerned to avoid politically costly scandals, or the acuteness of executive concern to safeguard their autonomy. Some of these responses are functional. Therefore, it may well be that the most effective method of tackling organisational features may be indirect; for instance, by means of an almost invisible attempt by chief officers over a long period of time to educate new committee members into accepting organisational features which seem to reduce executive accountability. However, we should not make too much of such caveats. Relationships in contingency theory are as weak, indirect and complex as in most other areas of social science. More important are context-specific factors – the personality of crucial decision-makers for instance. However, there can now be no excuse for ignoring the consequences of formal organisation at various levels for the nature of resident/staff contact.

A conclusion of this book may well be that those causal processes about which expert, non-academic, opinions are most strongly held are not necessarily those that have been most researched. This is so for the literature examining the influence of such characteristics of the personnel as their training, education and experience, and that on the provision of expert support staff and their attitudes to residents. Although views about the effects of such factors are certainly strongly held by policy-makers and those with more direct experience, they tend not to be based on formal research evidence. Therefore, although they are in the vague terms in which they are stated no less convincing, the absence of formal research to describe relationships and define issues more precisely makes our choice of strategies to secure improvements a hit and miss business. For example, we lack precise evidence about how many persons are affected by misjudgments about personal care strategies that follow from lacunae among home managers and others in specific areas of knowledge like current best practice in the management of residents with varying symptoms of mental disorder. We have no precise evidence about what consequences follow for the quality of life and use (or rather misuse) of care resources. Again, is it because of professional self-selection of those with some personality traits that there seems to be a tendency for homes headed by former nurses to neglect residents' psychosocial needs? If that is even partly true the policy of training new appointees might be most successful if it were to be accompanied by the screening of candidates using psychological tests (Baltz and Turner, 1977, show some success at this). We are not here to question the relatively greater effect of current social environment, attitudes and behaviour than long standing personality characteristics. Rather we are arguing that for those areas able to attract a range of candidates for posts in homes, such screening is an inexpensive complement of a programme of training. Research of two types is needed: research that more clearly distinguishes causal factors which are manipulable by policy intervention, as well as research which directly contributes to the development of such tools as screening devices and educational kits. However, such narrowly focused research is very dependent on general production relations knowledge. It certainly makes little sense to examine exhaustively the twigs unless we have a reasonable map of the wood.

It is with a diminished sense of frustration with the gap between policy argument and research-based knowledge that we view the literature on the relationship between flows from capital and outputs. Our disappointment was less not (mainly) because our expectations were lower. In fact, the literature is relatively strong; and it is an area where British research is second to none. It has quantified the relationship between capital costs per place and the number of places in the home: a set of relationships that is by no means of trivial importance to those needing to be able to predict this relationship in order to issue guidelines to authorities on capital costs per place. It has also shown the ways in which the larger homes tend to have characteristics that tend to make them more institutional in character. But it has achieved something more important: it has replaced a simplistic set of half-truths by one grounded in evidence and approaching nearer an understanding of the complex reality. In both the USA and in England the patterns of variation in the design features of homes are extremely complex, as work by Knapp and Schooler show. Neither has succeeded in finding a simple dimensionality that has much theoretical meaning. Even the direction of the influence on residents' well-being of some of the dimensions of variations in design derived using such techniques as factor analysis are open to question. So the literature on the effects of the capital inputs on the well-being of residents contains some studies which use evidence to develop a sophisticated normative argument, and others which describe the consequences of design features for well-being in a small number of circumstances. But even in this relatively well developed field our understanding of causality is patchy, and so is the degree of precision with which we can anchor policy recommendations in established causal relationships.

One of the ways in which it has replaced simplistic notions by a more complex view of reality is the treatment of scale. The research has clearly shown that scale itself is not the most important of the causal factors reflecting capital, but it *is* a variable that is associated with other characteristics of the capital stock which are of more fundamental causal importance. Certainly scale as measured by the number of places in the institution (or the living unit) would seem to be no more than one among a large number of factors of importance. It should continue to be a central variable only in the most general statistical analysis, where its ready availability allows the collection of large data sets for the estimation of broad but useful relationships.

The goal of the designers of homes is to enable a form of domesticity that maximises a resident's ability to exercise a degree of independence necessary for psychosocial well-being. The literature summarised in chapter 4 goes some way to making this fuzzy platitude rather more concrete, and discusses several ways of achieving the goal. The literature also distinguishes features that have undesirable effects. However, it is not only space that precluded an analysis of that key issue for the design of homes – the balance that might be appropriately struck between competing goals for residents with different characteristics. The complexity of the processes is formidable – and all the more so because home design is probably more important for enabling certain kinds of staff behaviour than for its direct effects on the quality of life. It is legitimate to complain that the direct and indirect effects have not been clearly distinguished in very useful contributions to the literature.

The research on the impact of capital stock has made real progress. But perhaps the best developed stream of literature is the sociological approach to the analysis of the impact of social environment on the quality of life. Much of it is built on the concept of institutional totality. Goffman's work is too well known to need summarising in this book, far less in this concluding chapter. (The indicators of the dimensions of institutional totality he described have been discussed in some detail in chapter 5.) Though developed initially for research in other types of institution, these indicators have also been used for old people's homes. For instance, John Townsend and Ann Kimbell used the Inmate Management Scale developed for children's homes by King and Raynes in their study of old people's homes in Cheshire. However, as early as 1963 Ruth Bennett had developed and used an index of totality specifically for long-term care facilities for the aged. Despite its development for a more similar setting, its calibration would in our view be insufficiently fine to be of much use for the comparative study of old people's homes. King and Raynes' scale more sensitively and subtly describes differences in the environment. For instance, it worked well in differentiating between homes in Cheshire.

However, the generality that is an advantage in developing a theory of the production of welfare for all institutions is a disadvantage if our focus is narrower, and our objective is to produce a more sophisticated causal argument of practical use to policy-making for one kind of institution. The Inmate Management Scale, it will be remembered, was quite deliberately made as independent as possible of the type of homes. It has other problems. The scale is based on predictions from theoretical argument that are by no means uncontroversial. For instance, to King and Raynes, greater social distance between staff and residents implies greater totality, whereas almost the opposite is so to Lipman and Slater. Moreover, this scale, like the Bennett scale and others, does not cover some important dimensions of environment.

Some of these are better covered by Kleemeier. Kleemeier published at much the same time as Goffman. His approach was similar but more general. In essence it concentrated on three continua: Segregation; Institutionalisation; and Congregation. In a most imaginative study Pincus elaborated Kleemeier's approach empirically. He developed his 38-item Homes Description Questionnaire and subsequently showed that the criterion validity of the instrument is reasonable, as is the correlation between subjective assumptions and behaviour. However, although it is better able to comprehend various perspectives, we argued in chapter 5 that some other components could well be added. Kahana developed out of Kleemeier's work a congruence argument and thus linked Kleemeier's dimensions of environmental variation with dimensions of variation between individual residents. Kahana's empirical work, although too small in scale to be convincing in every detail, forces us to take into account the need to make central to our theory of production of welfare in old people's homes, the fit between the person and his environment. This is accomplished by showing that doing so adds greatly to the explanatory power of evidence. However, the mainstream development of the argument that it is *congruence* that is important rather than environmental and personal characteristics viewed separately, flowed from a different source — Murray's pre-war argument about personal needs and environmental press. This so-called 'need-press' model has been applied to a wide range of settings. One of the most highly developed variants of the approach is that described by Moos. Behaviour, he argues, is very responsive to the environmental press, and the more cohesive and socially integrated the setting the greater its impact. Moos and his associates have developed scales for a variety of settings including long-term care facilities for the aged. Their scales are applied both to residents and staff, and describe the perception of the environment as it is, how the subject would like it to be, and how the subject expects it to become. Although eminently clear in its theoretical basis, Moos's scales omit some important dimensions stressed by the personality theorists; and so could with advantage be further developed. But there is no denying that it is potentially a very important device for measuring intermediate inputs and outcomes in the production of welfare.

Parallel with the work of Moos has been that of Lawton and Nahemow. Their work on long-term care facilities for the elderly is certainly the most impressive of its type. Central to their work is the 'environmental docility hypothesis': the less competent an individual, the more his or her behaviour is controlled by the environment. They present a transactional model which we described in detail in chapter 5. The model explores the interrelationships between the degree of individual performance, environmental press, adaptive behaviour, affective response to the environment, and the level of adaptation to it. The argument embodies the insight that the individual approaches an acceptable or 'equilibrium' combination of environmental press and individual competence in circumstances in which the stimuli or press are neither too strong nor too weak. This acceptable position is achieved when the individual subjectively adjusts to the environment and also modifies his own characteristics and behaviour. Tensions should be just slightly greater than those to which the aged residents are accustomed, argue Lawton and Nahemow (as do, for instance, Maddi and McClelland). The model is supported by a large amount of gerontological evidence. It has also the advantage that it sidesteps tricky problems in the collection and handling of evidence. In particular, it depends far less than that of Moos on a collection of a large quantity of data on the subjective responses of elderly residents themselves, and separates the collection of data about environmental press and competence, and the other focal concepts. It does not even require them to be forced into the same dimensionality. But unfortunately, its instrumentation is not yet well-developed. But although this is the crowning theoretical achievement of the literature on the role of social environment in old people's homes, there are essential components missing. One of them is a dimensionality of social environment common to the literature. We attempted to make a contribution towards providing this in the closing pages of chapter 5, and also to delineate the particular ways in which they contribute to welfare.[1]

Since we soon concluded that 'fit', the congruence between individual characteristics and dimensions of the environment, is central to understanding the processes of determination of the quality of life, a whole chapter was devoted to discuss dimensions of personal variation just as a whole chapter was devoted to discussing social environment. Arguments of a variety of kinds were reviewed. One set related to the influence of personality characteristics. Some notable progress has been made. Turner, for instance, succeeded in both predicting the adjustment of residents to long-term care facilities using such data, and also providing a dimensionality of personality that makes theoretical sense. However, Turner's work was not linked to variations in environments between homes. Recently, increasing stress has been laid on the causal importance of experiences prior to admission, particularly in the work of Morris and of Tobin and Lieberman. Although personality and processes of development of the whole life-span are no doubt causally prior to many of the factors discussed by them, it is difficult to collect reliable data on the former over short periods of time. If valid, the arguments of these writers lead to an inescapable conclusion: we may well have overstated the importance of the effect of home factors on the well-being of residents compared with others. The same is less so about the effects of factors operating at the time of entry — such factors as the attitude of residents to admission or mental impairment.

The chapter structure of this essay has kept separate resource and other inputs, and among other inputs social environmental factors and residents' characteristics appear. In this way we have been able to describe more coherently than would otherwise be possible those streams of literature that have often competed with one another but that have each been seen in this essay to contribute important insights into the nature of causal processes. However, it would be wrong to conclude from this that we see such factors to be causally independent. Indeed, if the opposite is the case we have argued that congruence between environment and personality needs must be central to a theory whose focus is variations between homes. Similarly we would argue that resources operate in conjunction with non-resource factors. Often they just enable other factors to work. Sometimes they are themselves created by non-resource factors.[2] Only in the most broad-brush models can resources be regarded as causally prior to other factors. But what so much of the literature seems to have missed is the obverse of this: that we cannot develop a satisfactory theory of impact of residents' characteristics or environment unless we take into account the very complex patterns of variations in resources any more than we can develop a satisfying theory of the impact of environment without taking into account that different environments are best for different types of resident. We return to the central theoretical proposition of this book. The idea of fit between residents who differ greatly in their needs and environments, which also often vary greatly within as well as between homes, must be accepted as a central feature — possibly *the* central feature — of the theory of production of welfare in residential

Table 7.2 Inputs into the process of production of welfare: description and operationalisation

(A) Flows from capital		
(i) Home characteristics		Description: original function; ownership; overall home layout (institutional, communal or family layout); and size (places and building scale.) Operationalisation: most surveys and censuses of homes cover these characteristics. See section 4.2.1, (a), (b) and (c).
(ii) Facilities and resources		Description: basic resident facilities (number and siting of bathrooms, showers, WCs, social rooms); sitting and dining rooms (number and size, layout, rigidity of design); and general resources (minibus, kitchenettes, sunshades, library, access). Operationalisation: surveys of Townsend and Residential Census for evidence; commentaries of Barrett and Lawton for recommendations. See section 4.2.1 (f) (g) (h) (i) and (k).
(iii) Spatial dimensionality		Description: siting of home in relation to local amenities, activities and transport; internal scale (distances between rooms, availability of locomotive prostheses); spatial proximity of residents and staff; and sharing of rooms (including provision for couples). Operationalisation: see (ii) and section 4.2.1 (d) (e) (f) and (o).
(iv) Micro-design		Description: condition of the home (state of repair) and micro-design features (e.g. bedroom layout, position of light switches, taps, bells).
(B) Consumables		Description: minor capital items (furniture and fittings, equipment, physical prostheses); clothing, books and entertainments; provisions, fuel, light and cleaning. Operationalisation: see sections 4.2.1 (j), 4.3 and 5.3.7.
(C) Manpower resources		Description: staff classification (domestic, care, supervisory, office; part- and full-time; resident and non-resident); numbers of staff (hours, effective ratios, interactions, functions); staff turnover and continuity; help from other residents. Operationalisation: see Townsend; DHSS Residential Census; Imber; and Knapp for evidence; and see sections 4.1.1 and 4.1.2.
(D) Non-resource manpower		Description: staff training (qualifications, in-service training, specialist skills); staff experience (social work and residential experience, general background); personal characteristics (age, sex, marital status, ethnicity); staff perceptions (attitudes, opinions, goal perceptions, objectives); staff morale (including support). Operationalisation: see DHSS Residential Census; PSSC; Williams and see section 4.1.3.2.
(E) Formal organisation		Description: unit scale (institutional, communal or family groupings); autonomy of home and living units; organisational and environmental diversity. Operationalisation: Barrett; Lipman and Slater; Tizard, Sinclair and Clarke; PSSC; and see section 4.1.3.1.

Table 7.2 (cont'd).

(F) Characteristics of clients as a group.	Description: homogeneity of the supra-personal environment (similarity of residents with regard to age, sex, health, religion, race) segregation (social similarity) and congregation (proximity). Operationalisation: see Bultena; Gubrium; Lawton for examples; and see section 5.3.6.
(G) External manpower	Description: trained personnel (health and personal social services visitors, therapists); and others (voluntary visitors, significant others). Operationalisation: see section 4.1.1.
(H) Social environment (i) Regime, social control and independence	Description: rigidity of routine, scheduling of activities, sanction system, rules, regulations, programme, institutional control; independence, individuality and rights. Emphasised in all theoretical models. Operationalisation: nearly every study of social environment includes an examination of regime and control. See virtually all studies in section 5.3.1 and particularly Utting and PSSC.
(ii) Motor control	Description: environmental tolerance of motor expression, restlessness and wandering, and residents' corresponding 'psychomotor inhibition'; social and psycho-pharmacological control. Operationalisation: see Snyder et al. and see section 5.3.2.
(iii) Privacy	Description: solitude (separation from the group); intimacy (part of small, close-knit group); freedom from identification and surveillance (anonymity); and reserve (erection of psychological barriers against unwanted intrusion). Operationalisation: see Pastalan and see sections 4.2.1 (I) and 5.3.3.
(iv) Stimulus and participation	Description: activities and stimulation — at the very core of the need-press models of Murray, Moos and Lawton. Operationalisation: Wessex group led by Kushlick, Kansas University group, and see section 5.3.4.
(v) Communication and interaction	Description: nature and frequency of staff-resident, resident-resident, and resident-community interaction; loneliness. Operationalisation: Fairhurst's study of talk, Romaniuk's study of patronising statements, and see section 5.3.5.
(vi) Homogeneity	Description: homogeneity of general environment and supra-personal environment. See (F) above. Operationalisation: see (F) above and section 5.3.6.
(vii) Continuity	Description: continuity of physical and social environments, and all other aspects of life-style. Operationalisation: see Tobin and Lieberman; Schulz and Brenner; and see section 5.3.7.

Table 7.2 (cont'd).

(J) Individual characteristics

(i) Residents' personality

Description: personality traits such as activity-passivity, aggression, narcissism, authoritarianism, status drive, distrust, non-empathy, extrapunitive and intrapunitive natures.
Operationalisation: see Turner and section 6.1.

(ii) Pre-admission experiences

Description: major events in resident's life history and experiences during process of becoming a resident (admission and waiting).
Operationalisation: see Tobin and Lieberman; and see section 6.2.

(iii) Characteristics at point of admission

Description: psychological well-being, adjustment, attitudes, health and dependency.
Operationalisation: see Morris and see section 6.3.

(iv) Post-admission characteristics

Description: processes of institutionalisation and adjustment, decision and preparation, impact and settling in.
Operationalisation: Yawney and Slover; Morris; and see section 6.4.

homes, and possibly the theory of production of welfare in social care generally (Davies, 1979). Social environment and resident characteristics must not be viewed apart from one another.

We were able to present a summary selection of the most important of the dimensions and indicators of psychological well-being of residents and other outputs in Table 7.1. In Table 7.2 we organise around our central theoretical conclusion a similar summary of the inputs. Figure 7.1. links these together by schematically summarising, and in the process, simplifying, the production of welfare model. Presented here, we hope that it will prove to the reader a useful point of reference to some of the important sections of the essay.

7.2 The production relations approach and understanding the causes of welfare

In the introduction, we argued that the production relations approach focuses attention on some fundamental issues that would otherwise be easily neglected. It forces us to look at the whole range of major inputs; a variety of non-resource factors, current resources, and resources locked up in capital releasing flows of direct influence on welfare or creating circumstances in which other inputs are likely to affect them. It asks questions about the consequences of each input for each output — about the 'productivity' of inputs. It asks questions about how far inputs can compensate for one another — how far different combinations of input can produce similar output consequences. It asks questions about the efficiency of response of organisations to the possibilities created by their environments — about getting the most output from the given combination of inputs or using the most efficient combination of inputs to produce outputs in the light of input prices and constraints on their supply. These are coherent and standard questions; though we must not pretend that each has not got a whole host of alternative forms; and complex analyses are necessary in order to find answers which are not so oversimplified that they distort reality too much to provide a reliable basis for practical action.

It is with such questions as these in mind — in essence, a few simple standard questions — that we approached the literature. But although we were quite clear from the beginning what the questions have been, we do not feel that the literature had yielded coherent answers to even the simplest forms of the questions. Is this because the questions of the productions relations approach are of too little concern to have been a major focus of research in the vast literature we have read in writing this book? A moment's reflection will assure the reader that this is not so. These questions are amongst the must crucial for policy planning and administration. They are the questions for which we must

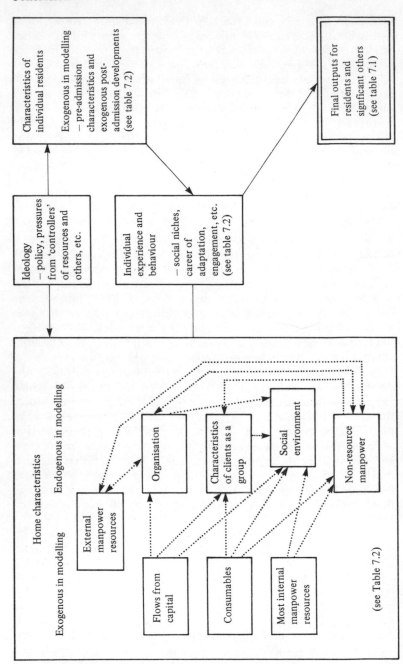

Figure 7.1 The production of welfare model

have reasonably credible answers before we can hope to answer other more finely grained questions about policy and practice. The reason why we have not been able to present straight answers to our standard questions is that the literature has grown up without such an overarching approach. The streams of literature are for the most part too partial and idiosyncratic to make the connections necessary for the questions to be answered. Without a meta-theory such as that provided by the production relations approach, coherence in the asking and answering of questions is unattainable.

But nevertheless, the reader may ask whether the difficulties in the way of applying the production relations approach are not so great as to be almost insurmountable? The subjective data from scales measuring psychological well-being have a substantial but certainly not a high degree of reliability and validity. Are not their reliability coefficients too low for analysis of a useful degree of precision? Is not the expense of supplementing such data with others involving direct judgment of experienced and trained observers too great to be faced? We have argued that research should separately measure a wide range of outputs, and that such outputs are interdependent. Therefore there may well be complex interactive production relations of a kind which economists call 'joint supply'. Joint supply, taken with many inputs and outputs, and inputs of varying but often uncertain causal priority, must suggest models that are highly complex. Because the models are complex, are there not great dangers of mis-specifying them and so making false deductions from the data? Surely the evidence of the literature is far from being sufficiently full to provide the insight based on independent evidence necessary to avoid such mis-specification in all important respects? Surely the modelling analysis of such complex forms requires not just the usual mix of systematic procedures and 'gut judgments' always needed in exploratory modelling, but also the handling of technical devices that are on the horizon of the subject?

The answer to all of these must be in the affirmative. However, three countervailing points must be made. No doubt the first full study will make many mistakes; but little progress would be made unless we undertake it because of the interdependence of questions one with another. This interdependence is one of the basic lessons of our review. Second, such a study must be country-specific. Concepts, causal arguments and measurement tools can generally be drawn from literature based on a variety of cultures and institutions, but the institutional context of each country is too specific to avoid empirical research in each setting, even though credible studies of production relations must border on 'big social science'. This is particularly so for old people's homes which are themselves very different from their nearest equivalents in the USA. Third, the application of the production relations approach has had a clear success in such other fields as universities, schools and hospitals. (In some ways, the measurement problems have always been vast. The data available for analysis has never been ideal. The validity and reliability of the outputs of universities are less acceptable than those of the outputs of old people's homes.) The researchers have generally complained that their studies have run up against technical statistical difficulties at the theoretical horizon of econometrics; and have often had to hurry the crucial analysis stage, so modelling with less thoroughness and imagination than the data deserved. Yet is has proved possible to provide credible answers to questions of theoretical importance, and so to provide a framework in which narrow investigations can take place, and also to provide valuable data, ideas and argument for the policy-maker and service manager.

7.3 The production relations approach and policy

Although there is never a logical inevitability about the connection between causal argument and policy recommendation, the production relations approach goes far to providing the data needed for policy-making. As we illustrated in the introduction to this essay, the successful application of the production relations approach contributes a basis for estimating the quantitative consequences of policy change. It shows the likely consequences for outputs of variations in each important form of resource; the amount of one type of resource that is necessary to compensate for another type in the production of very much the same mix of outcomes; and other information necessary for planning of a type outlined in the introduction. It provides equally useful data for short-term management.

These are general contributions that the approach can make. There are also specific contemporary issues which can be handled only with the help of knowledge of production relations. Space does not allow us to deal with the more obvious of these. Instead, this chapter takes up only one; creating a policy framework in which the best use can be made of local authority, voluntary and private homes while safeguarding the interests of residents.

7.3.1 Inter-sectoral co-ordination

Most British policy-making and analysis has almost totally ignored the issues that arise because we not only have local authority but also private and voluntary homes, probably because it was assumed that the sectors were diminishing in importance with the beneficent and inevitable growth of local authority provision. However, the reduction of capital expenditure on old people's homes to a level far lower than would be necessary to keep pace with increasing need must force us to think again about the policy implications of the existence of the three sectors.

Indeed, both the private and voluntary sectors are important in relation to local authority provision. The number of elderly persons supported by local authorities in independent homes (excluding chartered institutions) grew substantially during the 1960s and early 1970s. By the spring of 1976 the DHSS statistics suggest that there were 82 per cent more old people supported by local authorities in such homes than there were in 1959 and 31 per cent more than there were in 1969. By 1976 there were some 21,000 aged residents in registered private homes and 24,000 aged residents in voluntary homes. However, the growth in local authority support exceeded the overall growth in the number of residents; the 31 per cent increase in numbers of persons in independent homes supported by local authorities was exactly double the increase in the total number of residents in voluntary and private homes.

No firm data are available which would allow a precise forecast of numbers in the future. Consider some of the factors affecting the demand for places in private and voluntary homes. First, standard charges to residents have been rising fast, though less quickly than gross unit costs. The rates of increase have been lower in private or voluntary homes, so far as can be judged from the charges they have made to local authorities. The evidence is circumstantial only, but worth quoting. Whereas it has been estimated that net unit costs in local authority homes were £900 per resident (at 1975/6 prices) in the financial year 1970/1 and rose by three-fifths by 1975/6, net unit costs of residents supported by the authority in other homes rose from the lower level of £795 and by less than 15 per cent. So, in 1975/6, net unit costs to an authority averaged £905 per resident in independent homes and £1465 in the local authority's own homes. Thus, over the period, the relative prices to authorities of the two types of home had changed substantially. It is true that some — perhaps much more than a quarter — of the greater increase in the unit costs in local authority homes was due to improved staff-resident ratios and so rising standards. However, it would be surprising if authorities with a constrained budget and an increasingly heavy pressure of demand were not to respond to this increasing price differential. Certainly, some are doing so far more consciously now than they were five years ago. Others anyway believe that it would be unwise to have a system which relied exclusively on local authority provision. Indeed, some chairmen of social services committees go so far as to believe that local authorities cannot compete for value for money with some private and voluntary providers.

Second, private demand may be increasing. Only a small proportion of the elderly are in homes, so that demand can be sensitive to

Conclusion

trends important for minorities only. Despite the reluctance of authorities to put up standard charges in line with gross unit costs, the gap between the increase in unit costs in the two sectors has grown enough to make it likely that standard charges in local authority homes increased faster than standard charges in the private and voluntary sectors. Unfortunately (and surprisingly) we do not have precise data on trends in standard charges. (In this and some other respects our data is inferior to that available for the USA.) Meanwhile, increasing proportions of the population at risk have been becoming eligible for occupational pensions, albeit usually small amounts of money. More important, entrants to homes have increasingly been coming from a cohort who have owned houses whose value was substantial enough to use to buy substantial annuities. A higher proportion of demand, therefore, would have come from people who would have to pay standard charges in local authority homes and who would be able to afford, at least at first, to meet the charges in private and voluntary homes when their assets were put with the state pension, savings, and subsidies from children. In time, this has often made inevitable more support from public funds. During the period, inflation increasingly eroded the value of savings and annuities of residents in private and voluntary homes at the same time as it increased the unit costs, and therefore the charges. As a result, local authorities found themselves increasingly having to pay the charges on behalf of residents who had formerly paid their own. The voluntary homes themselves were often unable to put up their charges because the sources of charitable finance were becoming less profitable.

It would appear that demand may well have increased and for several reasons may well continue to increase in the future. Indeed it may rise faster. Whereas in the mid-1970s, increasing numbers of new places in local authority homes were becoming available, capital expenditure levels are now much lower than would be necessary to increase the supply of places in line with increasing numbers in need, thus making it more difficult to obtain a place in a local authority home and diverting demand towards the private and voluntary sectors.

So much for the demand factors. There is little evidence about the *supply* of places in the private and voluntary sectors. On the one hand, there has been increasing emphasis on adapting homes to meet fire regulations since the fire in Nottinghamshire in December 1974, and particularly since the report of the inquiry on it was published a year later.[3] Again, some local authorities are expecting the same staffing norms from the private and voluntary homes in which they support residents as in their own. For instance, authorities like Dorset require night staff to be available in all homes irrespective of the frailty of the residents of the homes. Yet others expect voluntary organisations to pay their staff at much the same rate as local authorities. Other factors than general inflation are affecting the supply costs of homes. Particularly important in the north-west, the number of persons in religious orders has been declining, a factor important not only in influencing the number of places provided by voluntary organisations but also for its effect on the cost per place. Also, the supply of places is likely to be affected by the diminishing flow of funds to charities. Again, among voluntary organisations there appears to be increasing emphasis on the provision of forms of care which are not quite residential in nature; for instance, housing association provisions, or organisations which provide combinations of shelter with domestic support in new ways, as is the case with the Abbeyfield Trust.

Such factors have adversely affected the supply of voluntary places more than the supply in private homes. Indeed, there are some factors that might cause *expansion* in number of private places. Between 1970 and 1973, and again since 1976, residential property has more than kept pace with inflation. Moreover, it is clear that private business can make at least a reasonable rate of return on capital as well as on proprietor's time in old people's homes. It is therefore at least possible that during the later part of the period, businesses have been entering this market as a form of investment in real estate. There is at least some anecdotal evidence of property companies buying large buildings like convents for use as old people's homes. Some directors of social services in the nine south coast counties talk about the affluence (indeed opulence) of some owners of chains of homes. (The largest operator in one English district is known to have extended his operations to the USA.) As has been demonstrated in the USA, it can be profitable for a company or private person making large profits in other sectors to 'tax farm' − to buy homes raising a loan with tax relief to do so. But in Britain, losses are unlikely. Any loss can be offset against profits elsewhere. After covering salaries a firm could be left with what would look like a modest rate of return on the capital invested. However, taking into account the gearing created by having a mortgage, the rate of return in relation to the money actually invested by a company or person ('the rate of return on equity') could be high after mortgage loans have been serviced and operating costs have been met. The rise in property values increases the potential for raising mortgages and so increasing the degree of gearing.

Of course, there is no real evidence that in Britain the commercialisation of the private old people's home has gone far by American standards. Our position seems not unlike that of the American nursing home sector in the late 1950s. Certainly private old people's homes in Britain tend to be too small to reap economies of scale that large profit-maximising operators would seek − though that might merely be a reflection of the relative prices of different kinds of property. But like the Americans, we lack official data about the structure of ownership of private sector homes, and the systems by which they are financed. One could well have a substantial share of the market and a substantial proportion of those residents supported by the local authorities in homes belonging to firms with a keen eye on rates of return on equity and the minimisation of costs.

Of course, this is not to suggest that private provision is necessarily bad provision. Local authority executives who have the closest contact with the private sector argue that it is enormously variable, and that some private homes do provide much better value for money than their local authority counterparts. Tom Hopkins, who has followed closely the analogous provision of private children's homes, is by no means condemnatory, although these homes give rise to problems similar to those raised by private old people's homes – negligible spending on staff training and state supervision, for instance (Hopkins, 1979a).

We may suggest conclusions in this discussion of trends in demand and supply of homes. First, overall demand for residential care is likely to increase because of the high rate of increase in the population of the age and sex groups likely to yield priority cases and the low rate of improvement in the relative effectiveness of domiciliary support services as a real alternative for residential care in most authorities. Second, the low rate of capital expenditure on local authority homes will divert demand to the private and voluntary sectors. Third, residents in private and voluntary homes are being increasingly supported from state funds.

Fourth, on the supply side the voluntary sector may be less well placed than the private sector. Voluntary organisations are facing increasing unit costs and diminishing sources of income. Whereas local authorities are prepared to pay a reasonable rate of return on capital as part of the charges made by private homes, the rules agreed between local authority associations and the voluntary sector do not allow voluntary organisations to earn a rate of return or indeed recoup depreciation allowances. It is partly for this reason that voluntary organisations are using their money for other purposes. In contrast, the provision of residential care might seem attractive to private providers, even to big commercial enterprises. Not only is the demand strong and underwritten by public authorities but also control over standards is weak in most authorities, and the instruments of control of standards are only indirect. Furthermore, the long-term boom in capital values can allow a high rate of capital appreciation on the original equity stake which can more than compensate for a modest rate of profit on the capital.

Indeed, the situation is uncomfortably like the American position in the early 1960s. At that time most American homes were owned by their managers. However, with increasing support for residents through Medicare and Medicaid and an increasing demand for places arising for demographic reasons, the demand for nursing home care increased rapidly. Both demand and supply were inelastic. The result was higher prices and a higher rate of profit; and as a consequence the attraction of large-scale commercial capital into what became an industry in which sources of finance, ownership and control became increasingly separated, in which owners put pressure on managers to keep down standards as cost-minimisation was sought; and in which what mattered as much as the rate of profit was the rate of capital appreciation. We must take care that we do not allow the American history to repeat itself here.

In the next section we discuss ways in which we can use production relations knowledge to control and co-ordinate the sectors more effectively than the Americans achieved despite their massively increased involvement in regulation since the late 1960s.

7.3.2. Towards a policy

The main aims of policy must be to ensure that both public and private consumers are ensured adequate standards and good value for money; and secondly, that residents should be guaranteed full civil rights and freedom from financial exploitation. The principle that the aged resident of a home requires protection, irrespective of the sector in which he resides, was acknowledged in the National Assistance Act of 1948. In many authorities registration is now applied to all institutions in which two or more old people are living as boarders. But the emphasis on obtaining the best value for money in ensuring at least adequate standards demands a more positive policy: one with carrots as well as sticks. The changed balance between the growth of need and local authority capital expenditure on homes forces us to look to the private and voluntary sectors as an important source of growth and flexibility. Although in Britain the two have behaved differently in the past, the experience in the USA shows that in circumstances in which there are opportunities for large and growing profits from existing and new provision, the vulpine commercial ends of the one, can be ruthlessly pursued in the sheep's clothing of the other, making necessary the application of the same vigilance in both sectors. More positively, both can enhance the variety of our provision, providing an element present for the more fortunate American consumer, but not part of the British tradition − a choice for residents, their relatives and those who help to place them. It need hardly be said that this choice would be increasingly demanded by new generations of potential residents who will be far more assertive than past entrants to homes have been. Both can help to provide for such special needs as homes for ethnic groups and persons to whom the provision of special facilities would add greatly to the quality of their lives.

Conclusion

Developing a policy which acknowledges that the voluntary and private sectors will grow, and probably grow far faster than local authority provision, demands a new conception of what roles the social services department should take most seriously. It demands that the social services department should primarily see itself as the political agency that sets objectives, formulates priorities, acts as entrepreneur in identifying needs and stimulating others to meet them, and performs the role of advisor as well as monitor of provision; and only secondarily, in its traditional function as direct provider. It is a conception of local government which has attracted increasing sympathy among the theoreticians of local government since the Maud report on management. Some attempts have been made to work it out. For instance, one of the authors has already elaborated the implications of such a role in another area of social welfare (Davies, 1978).

First we must review the current situation. It can hardly be claimed to adequately acknowledge the importance of the independent sectors.

(i) Most voluntary and private homes are rarely visited, certainly in most cases not as often as once every two years. Inspections are cursory and unsystematic in their coverage, and not made by teams of persons representing the range of disciplines and skills necessary for evaluating inputs and outcomes of a wide variety of kinds. (They are nothing like, for instance, the systematic inspections of schools by teams of Her Majesty's Inspectors or indeed the teams being developed by American federal agencies.)

(ii) When the inspections or casual observations by local authority personnel suggest that home care is unsatisfactory, there do not exist controls finely tuned to the problems diagnosed. It is easier to operate on fire hazards than on other forms of design feature which affect physical discomfort or safety. Nothing short of de-registration — with the most embarrassing consequence of having to find places elsewhere for residents thus made homeless — can be used as a threat to provide an incentive to improve non-resource inputs. On a rising market, a refusal to refer potential customers to homes is hardly a major threat. Of course, if new building is under consideration, the authority has some control through planning and building regulations, but these are often administered by an authority different from that responsible for monitoring standards in general, and certainly by a department with different objectives.

(iii) The financial treatment of the three sectors is riddled with anomalies. Local authorities pay charges to the private sector without scrutiny of their accounts. The accounts are not standardised — indeed they are often rudimentary — and are not subject to rigorous audit. The accounts of voluntary homes are also not standard in form. However, the local authority in which the home lies negotiates with it a charge which the local authority associations recommend that all authorities should pay. The criteria for negotiating the charge specify that the payment should not make allowance for certain items, including the depreciation of capital and a rate of return on it. In contrast, the local authority accounts for old people's homes are to a considerable degree standard in form. However, local authority home accounts do not cover all the costs in providing the residential service. For instance, the cost of relief and peripatetic staff and central administration are chargeable to other accounts. Again, local authority accounts do not make estimates of depreciation allowances at replacement cost, although the local authority accounts include their annual allowance for the amortisation of loan charges. Again, local authority accounts allow nothing for the imputed rental value of land though they do include actual rent payments.

So, the accounting practices differ greatly between sectors and within two of them. The accounts of homes in none of the sectors are such as to allow the treatment of the homes as 'cost centres', agencies whose accounts reflect all the costs generated by their activities. The charging rules are most favourable to the private sector and penalise the voluntary sector in relation to the private sector. Not even local authority accounting provides the financial information necessary to make judgments about what constitutes the best value for money in the area. The local authority administrator likewise has only the most casual knowledge of standards outside the local authority sector. He is also provided with no incentives to make use of the three sectors in such a way as to obtain the best value for money — behaviour that in our new situation will increasingly contribute to an important degree to the quality of lives of residents.

What policy developments could help achieve a better system? Space does not allow us here to develop an elaborate argument, since the subject is being discussed at all only to illustrate the importance of production relations studies. In particular, we can do no more than mention the energy shown by American policy-makers in developing devices to secure citizens' rights for residents as well as freedom from financial exploitation; the need for demonstration projects to assess the value of ombudsmen; the need to open homes to the community by encouraging the voluntary adoption of residents by people who are able to fight for their rights; and the need for codes or rules to which long-term facilities must adhere.

To these and a large number of other American devices may be added one whose influence might be great in the small British private sector. There are now possibly fewer than 2,000 private residential homes and just over one thousand private nursing homes housing mainly old people. It would be feasible to follow up samples of persons some time after they had entered homes, and assess their well-being with the aid of a multi-disciplinary team. The assessment would include the financial consequences of the policy of the home. This would be possible only if standard information on all persons admitted to the homes were collected prior to entry, and if there existed a system of sanctions for owners, managers and staff. For this reason, it would be necessary to register the ownership of homes, and licence and register the principal administrators. American federal regulations demand that homes should have boards of governors with responsibility for administering rules and regulations, for appointing principal staff, and for providing an assurance of compliance with home regulations. The licensed administrators would have the responsibility of defining the objectives of the home, communicating them to staff, co-ordinating activities and bearing responsibility for the welfare of individual residents, including the development of policies for the care of individual patients and the maintenance of records describing the implementation of policies. Old people should be supported by the authority only in registered homes.

Controlling standards while getting the best value for money is a more complex subject. The central principle of a policy of control would put the three sectors on a par with respect to important features of their financial relations with government. It would make a major contribution towards achieving this if the following could be accomplished:

(i) Accounts should be standardised and audited. Part of the objective would be to reflect the full range of costs – resource costs as well as cash flow – incurred in providing services to residents. This is a formidable task, not only because many private homes are small and their accounting is unsophisticated, but also because, particularly in the voluntary and local authority sectors, it is difficult to differentiate costs incurred for different kinds of output in facilities providing services additional to residential care. However, we could create a powerful incentive to standardise the accounts and have them audited as would be necessary to avoid gross abuses, the opportunities for which have been shown by American practice. Retrospective adjustment of payments would be negotiated on the basis of the accounts. (We are not proposing that the actual costs incurred by a home should be the principal basis for fixing an agreed charge with authorities for that home.)

(ii) An allowance should be made in all these sets of accounts for a notional rate of return on capital at a rate of profit sufficient to attract the level of private investment needed in that local authority area. This is because it is these sectors on which we shall in many areas depend for expanding facilities. The notional rate of profit might have to differ substantially between areas.

The basis for fixing (imputed) rents on land values would differ according to whether it was an existing facility or a facility that had not yet been designed according to operation that was a consideration. For *existing* facilities there should be an allowance for the following factors:

(A) Depreciation at replacement costs. American experience shows that careful treatment is necessary. (Replacement cost depreciation allows the accumulation of a fund which would allow the replacement of the assets at current prices.) Such depreciation allows the quick accumulation of large funds which can be transferred elsewhere if uncontrolled. This is a danger that is particularly great if there is subsidisation of loans for the building of homes — subsidisation that is valuable for small private providers and for voluntary organisations. Shulman and Galanter (1976) suggest that only if the state itself acquired the assets of nursing homes, could American abuses be avoided. Perhaps this may not be necessary. For instance, part or all of the depreciation allowance could be paid into a public trustee accumulation fund whose dispersement could be negotiated by agreed criteria.

(B) An allowance for the rent of land.

(C) Other current costs. These would be paid prospectively on the basis of statistical estimates. The statistical estimates would be based on costs and production function research in which these other recurrent costs would be predicted from:

    (i) the capital features of the home (whose importance in determining what current resources are necessary is shown by Knapp, 1979);

    (ii) the number and the characteristics of residents (whose effects on operating cost variation has been shown by Davies and Knapp, 1978; Knapp, 1978a and others);

    (iii) the local price level for care and domestic manpower; and

    (iv) some main output dimensions.

It is for the derivation of these estimates that cost and production relations studies would be essential.

The actual rate paid would be at a level at which the most efficient would achieve a higher rate of profit. The relatively inefficient would be penalised and those providing a higher standard than was regarded as requisite would be expected to finance that additionally high standard from other sources of funds. The local administrators would have to select their probabilities of penalising inefficiency, supporting standards higher than those applied elsewhere, and/or providing high

profits to the efficient; in effect balancing them against the
need to expand supply to a greater or lesser degree. Again,
they could choose the degree of incentive to give providers to
get them to conform. No doubt different local authorities
would choose different solutions. Ro and Auster (1969) present
a formula by which rate-setting authorities can choose the degree of incentive to efficiency, and the desired standard of cost
efficiency at any point in relation to the average that seemed
to it sensible given the relative need of the area for capacity.
Of course, as Hixson and Worthington (1977) point out, the
predictions must be outside the immediate control of providers.

The methods suggested are not quite those recommended or evaluated by American economists developing schemes for the 'incentive
reimbursement' of hospitals.[4] Such American writing invariably concentrated on total costs, not merely current costs. Our reason for making
separate allowance for the rate of profit for land costs and depreciation
is that the inheritance of capital is highly variable. The value of the land
on which a facility is situated is even more variable, and the needs of
areas to attract more investment funds from the private sectors and
therefore the needs for profit incentive also differ. However our proposals for new facilities not yet constructed are much more similar to
those developed in the American literature. Our scheme would provide
an incentive to suppliers to choose efficient designs. For new facilities
the rate would be fixed in the light of production relations knowledge
for total costs including depreciation at replacement cost. However,
separate account should be taken of the imputed rental value of land
and again a part share of the estimated replacement cost depreciation
should be withheld and maintained in the public trustee accumulation
fund.

Computation of the estimates would demand a substantial cost and
production function study covering homes for the three sectors. The
theory of the production of welfare is such that there should be two
basic units of analysis – the home and the resident within it. The
Long-Term Care Facility Improvement Study conducted by the US
Department of Health, Education and Welfare (Public Health Service,
Officer of Nursing Home Affairs) in 1975 provides what in many ways
could be a model for the design of the procedures for collecting data,
though because of the vagueness of its theoretical premises, it would be
necessary to collect slightly different data. It would also be necessary
to do so for residents at two points in time. It is our hope that this
essay has made it more feasible to attempt such a production relations
study.

It is American experience that fixing charges prospectively is acceptable both to the bodies paying charges and to the providers. To the

latter it offers a firm commitment from a contracting agency before contemplated expenditures are made. To the former, it is attractive since to withhold altogether charges retrospectively proves in general impracticable in the context of continuing negotiation. However, what would be important would be the negotiation of precise criteria for retrospective adjustment of rates. In Britain, unlike America, authorities would be able to negotiate a basis for charge-fixing that is favourable to them. There is still time to establish criteria that will encourage greater effectiveness, to obtain from private operators a substantial level of provision without paying excessively for it.

Although it is important for securing the best value for money in residential care, fixing appropriate charging structures is in itself insufficient for the control of standards. The Americans have done more to develop inspection techniques than we have. There can be no denying the necessity for them. We must learn more about such American methods and experience of inspection and other techniques of control.

However, an extension of the survey discussed in relation to the maintenance of citizens' rights and the prevention of financial exploitation could add enormously to the power of the system to secure good standards. The Americans are increasingly disenchanted with attempts to control inputs alone. We conclude on the basis of the earlier chapters of this book that a survey should capture data mainly about outputs of varying subjectivity, generality, and finality in the production of welfare. Some should be based on residents' statements, others on assessment of skilled and trained observers of residents and their environments. Some should be highly general, like the indicators of psychological well-being discussed in chapter 2, and others should be highly specific like indicators of satisfaction with food, warmth and privacy. For some residents and some inputs it would be necessary to measure factors early in the production of welfare because outputs produced from them are in themselves too difficult to measure with any reliability. It follows also from the argument of the book that such a survey would additionally need: (a) data about residents collected prior to their entry using standardised instruments such as have been developed in the USA and Britain; and (b) some data on the characteristics of residents and other factors necessary to assess the congruence between the needs of the individual and his social environment.

These then are essential features of a new policy built around the production relations knowledge and which recognises the importance of the independent sectors of provision. There would of necessity be peripheral elements of the policy, designed, for instance, to meet training and administrative costs in a cost-effective way, to provide specialised design services to independent providers, and to provide local information to potential residents and those who refer them. Again, our treatment of charging is merely a brief and superficial outline. We would hope to develop the arguments sketched out here in a later work.

What seems to us to be vital now is to launch a system that provides basically the right incentives and to get it established before the private sector becomes large and politically powerful. Otherwise we shall not just have some contextual similarities with the USA but the same basic political problem. It is a problem that is pervasive in the governmental control of the private sector. It is that the power of established political interests in the independent sector with a continuing and major stake in manipulating the political process in its own interest would quite overwhelm the assertion of the public interest, since the guardians of the public interest provide political support only conditionally and intermittently (Wilson, 1974, pp. 135-68).

The Life Satisfaction Rating Scale of Neugarten, Havighurst and Tobin

(A) Zest versus apathy

5 Speaks of several activities and relationships with enthusiasm. Feels that 'now' is the best time of life. Loves to do things, even sitting at home. Takes up new activities; makes new friends readily, seeks self-improvement. Shows zest in several areas of life.

4 Shows zest, but it is limited to one or two special interests, or limited to certain periods of time. May show disappointment or anger when things go wrong, if they keep him from active enjoyment of life. Plans ahead, even though in small time units.

3 Has a bland approach to life. Does not seem to get much pleasure out of the things he does. Seeks relaxation and a limited degree of involvement. May be quite detached (aloof) from many activities, things or people.

2 Thinks life is monotonous for the most part. May complain of fatigue. Feels bored with many things. If active, finds little meaning or enjoyment in the activity.

1 Lives on the basis of routine. Doesn't think anything worth doing.

(B) Resolution and fortitude

5 Try and try again attitude. Bloody but unbowed. Fights back; withstanding, not giving up. Active personal responsibility — take the bad and the good and make the most of it. Wouldn't change the past.

4 Can take life as it comes. 'I have no complaint on the way life has treated me'. Assumes responsibility readily. 'If you look

for the good side of life, you'll find it.' Does not mind talking about difficulties in life, but does not dwell on them either. 'You have to give up some things.'

3 Says, 'I've had my ups and downs; sometimes on top, sometimes on the bottom.' Shows a trace of extrapunitiveness or intrapunitiveness concerning his difficulties in life.

2 Feels he hasn't done better because he hasn't gotten the breaks. Feels great difference in life now as compared to age 45; the change has been for the worse. 'I've worked hard but never got anywhere.'

1 Talks of hard knocks which he has not mastered (extrapunitive). Feels helpless. Blames self a great deal (intrapunitive). Overwhelmed by life.

(C) Congruence between desired and achieved goals

5 Feels he has accomplished what he wanted to do. He has achieved or is achieving his own personal goals.

4 Regrets somewhat the chances missed during life. 'Maybe I could have made more of certain opportunities.' Nevertheless, feels he has been fairly successful in accomplishing what he wanted to do in life.

3 Has a fifty-fifty record of opportunities taken and opportunities missed. Would have done some things differently, if he had his life to live over. Might have gotten more education.

2 Has regrets about major opportunities missed but feels good about accomplishment in one area (may be his avocation).

1 Feels he has missed most opportunities in life.

(D) Self-concept

5 Feels at his best. 'I do better work now than ever before.' 'There was never any better time.' Thinks of self as wise, mellow; physically able or attractive; feels important to others. Feels he has the right to indulge himself.

4 Feels more fortunate than the average. Is sure that he can meet the exigencies of life. 'When I retire, I'll just substitute other activities.' Compensates well for any difficulty of health. Feels worthy of being indulged. 'Things I want to do, I can do, but I'll not overexert myself.' Feels in control of self in relation to the situation.

3 Sees self as competent in at least one area, e.g. work; but has doubts about self in other areas. Acknowledges loss of youthful vigor, but accepts it in a realistic way. Feels relatively unimportant, but doesn't mind. Feels he takes, but also gives. Senses a general, but not extreme, loss of status as he grows older. Reports health better than average.

2 Feels that other people look down on him. Tends to speak disparagingly of older people. Is defensive about what the years are doing to him.

1 Feels old. Feels in the way, or worthless. Makes self-disparaging remarks. 'I'm endured by others.'

(E) Mood tone

5 'This is the best time of my life.' Is nearly always cheerful, optimistic. Cheerfulness may seem unrealistic to an observer, but shows no sign of 'putting up a bold front'.

4 Gets pleasure out of life, knows it and shows it. There is enough restraint to seem appropriate to a younger person. Usually feels positive affect. Optimistic.

3 Seems to move along on an even temperamental keel. Any depressions are neutralized by positive mood swings. Generally neutral-to-positive affect. May show some irritability.

2 Wants things quiet and peaceful. General neutral-to-negative affect. Some depression.

1 Pessimistic, complaining, bitter. Complains of being lonely. Feels 'blue' a good deal of the time. May get angry when in contact with people.

The use of Bradburn's Affect Balance Scale with the elderly in residential care

Sheila Peace,[1] John Hall[2] and Graham Hamblin.[2]

Experience of our current study offers much conflicting evidence regarding the validity of using Bradburn's Affect Balance Scale (ABS) with elderly respondents in residential care. The scale was included as a measure of life satisfaction in a recent questionnaire designed to investigate the feasibility of applying to the residents of old people's homes survey measures of the quality of life developed on general population samples (Peace, Hall and Hamblin, 1979).

Our sample of 155 respondents in care differs widely from those used by both Moriwaki (1974) and Graney (1975), both of whom were concerned with relatively small samples of elderly respondents living in the community (27 and 46 respondents respectively). Our work is therefore, to our knowledge, the first to use this scale with a sample of residents in care. Because of this, respondents differ from those in other studies not only in age-structure, being far older,[3] but also in health, suffering from far greater degrees of physical and mental frailty. For these reasons our work with the ABS can be considered in two respects, first, in terms of its practical application with an elderly sample, and second in terms of the results obtained.

(A) Practical application

The problems of administering a scale of this nature to a very elderly sample lie mainly in comprehension. It is, frankly, a difficult scale to administer and requires a great deal of time, as well as patience and skill on the part of the interviewer. The elderly are not as used to survey techniques as younger age-groups, and declining auditory and visual health only serve to make matters worse.

In our study we employed a system of interviewer coding, developed by Cannell, Lawson and Hauser (1975) for problems encountered with the actual questions asked. This coding frame allowed us to judge each

question in terms of a number of factors, including respondent understanding, willingness to give information, problems with precodes and
clarity of question. The results of this coding exercise were illuminating. The most commonly used code referred to the number of times
the respondent asked for the question to be repeated or explained. In
this case 40 per cent of all such instances concerned the ABS, no other
question eliciting anything like this level of confusion among respondents. However, it was not just the elderly who found the scale
difficult. Another code referred to how difficult or easy the *interviewer* found it to administer each question. Once again 25 per cent
of all such instances involved the ABS.

Why is there such apparent difficulty in administering and inter-
preting the ABS with this particular client group? The main problem
lies in the specificity of the measures used in relation to the environment in which the majority of the institutionalised elderly find themselves. It is a sad reflection on residential care for the elderly that
items such as 'bored', 'depressed or very unhappy' and 'very lonely
or remote from people', have immediate meaning and yet others, such
as 'pleased about having accomplished something' or 'on top of the
world' have none. We could therefore conclude that elderly residents
in care are more likely to relate to negative than to positive affect
items, as a reflection of their circumstances. However, the problem also
lies in the fact that the positive affect items relate to current degree
of involvement, instead of long-term satisfaction and contentment.
They are concepts which appear to be outside their immediate experience. Other factors therefore need to be considered, and the work of
Beiser (1974) exemplifies one step in this direction.

We would accordingly suggest that, although responses to this scale
can be obtained from elderly respondents in care, it will, in most
cases, prove a time-consuming and difficult exercise, owing to the basic
characteristics of the elderly, and the nature of some of the questions.
Thus although it was possible for our interviwers to spend extra time on
certain questions, the fact that ours was a feasibility study means that
our findings must nevertheless allow for some degree of distortion within the data. The problems of relying on survey self-reports in this type
of research are therefore magnified with a very elderly sample.

With these reservations in mind, our findings nevertheless offer
some comparison with conclusions reached in earlier studies. It should
be remembered, however, that all the studies using this scale with the
elderly have been conducted in the USA, and with non-institutionalised
samples. These facts alone may well account for differences in the data.

(B) Results

(i) General characteristics

The ABS is based on a model which assumes the existence of two independent dimensions: a positive affect scale (PAS) and a negative affect scale (NAS). (See section 3.7 above.) In our own study this duodimensionality of the scale is still apparent. Both the PAS and the NAS correlate highly with the overall ABS (correlation coefficients of 0.74 and -0.78 respectively, both significant at the 0.001 level), indicating that the scale is made up of two independent dimensions and the low correlation between the PAS and NAS (-0.17, not significant) lends further support for the independence of the subscales.

It would appear therefore that the scale has some degree of construct validity, and can be taken as an indicator of overall psychological well-being. Moriwaki (1974) compared the ABS scores of two elderly groups and found that he could discriminate between them. They consisted of a 'normal church group' (n = 19), and a 'psychiatric outpatient group' (n = 8). The mean score of 8.27 for the 'normal' group was significantly higher than the 'psychiatric' group mean of 4.25. In comparison the mean score for our sample was 5.01, which compares with a mean score of 6.41 for a cross-sample of the British population.[4] We hesitate to compare our data with that of Moriwaki, feeling that his samples are not only extremely small, but also that his 'normal church group' is not really representative of the general population. There is no significant difference in mean ABS scores for all age-groups in our sample, and the range of scores is also low, with standard deviations of approximately 2.4 for all groups (Table B.1).

Table B.1 Comparison of ABS scores between studies

		Mean	Standard Deviation
Moriwaki (1974)	Psychiatric outpatient group	4.25	
	Normal church group	8.27	
Quality of life data general pop. 1975 (Hall, 1976)		6.41	
Quality of life data residents in care 1978		5.01	2.47
	Residents in care 54-74 years	5.5	2.39
	Residents in care 74-85 years	4.8	2.54
	Residents in care 85 plus years	4.9	2.43

The subjective well-being of this sample of elderly residents in care is significantly lower than that of a group of elderly respondents in the community. Analysis of ABS scores for those respondents aged 60 years or over in the 1975 Quality of Life Survey, undertaken by the SSRC's Survey Unit shows a distinct difference between the two groups (chi-square = 22.83, significant at the 0.01 level) for both mean scores and frequency distributions. Elderly residents in care are therefore more likely to report lower subjective well-being, having higher scores on the NAS (Table B.2).

Table B.2 Distribution of responses on Index of Affect Balance

	Index of Affect Balance (Positive minus negative range -5 to +5)				
	-3 or less	−2 or −1	0	+1 or +2	+3 or more
Urban elderly 1975 (% of sample)	7	14	17	38	24
Elderly in care 1978 (% of sample)	19	23	17	24	17

Both Moriwaki (1974) and Graney (1975) have looked at the relation between the ABS and a number of other independent criteria.

(ii) Well-being and activity

Graney found a direct relation between social activity and happiness. He looked at three areas of activity (media use, interpersonal interaction and activities in voluntary associations) and concluded that involvement in some form of activity, however passive, has a beneficial effect on the well-being of the elderly, thus supporting the activity theory of ageing. However, Graney's sample is relatively small (n = 46) and consists of females, all capable of living alone in the community and therefore likely to be more active than a sample of residents in care. Nevertheless, our work offers some tentative support for these claims. Part of our questionnaire asked whether respondents took part in a number of indoor and outdoor activities. (See Table B.3 below.) Scores were obtained to give a crude overall measure of activity rates, as well as of both indoor and outdoor pursuits. However, the distribution for outdoor activities is heavily skewed, and therefore affects the overall activity score. Even so, indoor activities (items related to Graney's 'media use') correlated positively with the ABS, and overall activity with the PAS (Table B.3). Graney also found differences between age-groups and a similar relationship difference appears in our data. It must be noted however that individual items of activity show little correlation with the ABS and therefore our data offer only partial evidence of a relationship between activity and morale.

Table B.3 Relationships between activity scores and ABS[1]

Graney (1975)		Quality of life data (1978)	
Total sample		Total sample	
Listen to radio	0.19 (0.05,41)	Indoor	0.33 (0.001,155)
Visiting neigh-	0.28 (0.01,40)	activities[2]	
bours		Overall	0.37 (0.001,155)
Visiting friends	0.43 (0.01,38)	activities[3]	
and relatives			
Religious	0.33 (0.01,44)		
services			
Association	0.50 (0.01,44)		
membership			
Youngest: 66-75 yrs		Youngest: 54-74 yrs	
Association	0.52 (0.01,16)	Overall activi-	0.40 (0.05,31)
membership		ties with PAS	
Religious	0.67 (0.01,16)	Indoor activi-	0.39 (0.05,31)
services		ties with PAS	
Oldest: 82-92 yrs		Oldest: 85 yrs and over	
Listen to radio	0.45 (0.01,16)	Indoor activi-	0.44 (0.001,50)
Association	0.60 (0.01,16)	ties with PAS	
attendance		Overall activi-	0.52 (0.001,50)
		ties with PAS	
		Overall activi-	0.48 (0.001,50)
		ties with PAS	

Notes: 1 Correlations are with the ABS score unless stated to the contrary; correlation coefficients are given beside each activity score, with significance level and sample size in parentheses.
2 Indoor activities covered were: (a) handicrafts and home interests, e.g. sewing, knitting, carpentry, baking; (b) games — bingo, cards, jigsaws, dominoes, darts; (c) writing letters; (d) reading; (e) listening to radio; and (f) watching television.
3 Overall activities are indoor activities (above) and the following outdoor activities: (g) gardening, fishing or other outdoor activities; (h) attending church and other church activities; (i) visiting pub or social club; (j) attending meetings of clubs, societies, groups or other organisations; and (k) cinema, concert or other entertainment (including going out to play bingo).

Moriwaki (1974) investigated the relationship between subjective well-being and a number of other variables, notably the degree of role loss, morale, mental health and avowed happiness.

(iii) Well-being and avowed happiness

A direct comparison can be made between our own study and that of Moriwaki, in terms of avowed happiness. In both studies this measure was obtained by asking the question: 'Taking all things together, how would you say things are these days? Would you say you are very happy, pretty happy or not too happy?' Scores range from 1 for 'not too happy' to 3 for 'very happy' (Bradburn, 1969; Hall, 1976). Moriwaki found that 'the individual's self report of over-all happiness was positively related to the PAS and the ABS, although the latter was not significant, due to small sample size.' Our study confirms this pattern, with a significant positive correlation between avowed happiness and both the ABS and PAS. (Correlation coefficients were 0.59 and 0.44, respectively, both significant at the 0.001 level.)

(iv) Well-being, anxiety and physical symptoms

Moriwaki showed how the NAS is directly related to measures of mental illness, such as anxiety and worry. Although the measures used differ, our work also shows a significant positive correlation (0.40, significant at 0.001 level) between NAS and a three-item scale of psychological symptoms of anxiety suggested by Bradburn (1969, p. 108), and also between NAS and a check-list of physical symptoms of anxiety (0.46, significant at 0.001 level).

Conclusions

Our experience with the ABS with a sample of very elderly residents in old people's homes, demonstrates some of the problems of this type of technique. It is difficult and time-consuming to administer and several of its positive affect items can be seen to be outside the present experience of the elderly respondents in our sample. This may account for the somewhat higher scores on the NAS. Nevertheless, some of our findings are consistent with those of earlier work and we note that further modification of the scale, along the lines suggested by Beiser (1974) may increase its validity with this age-group. However, the problems of administering the scale must always be borne in mind and we cannot necessarily support Moriwaki's view that the ABS is the 'best predictor of psychological well-being' particularly for a sample of elderly respondents in residential care.

Notes

Chapter one: The production of welfare

1 Paul Brearley's two recent books are among the few honourable exceptions (Brearley, 1975 and 1977).

2 The distinction between 'levels of provision', 'throughout', and the 'effects of services on the attainment of their objectives' is discussed in B. Davies (1977) and is given a more focused treatment in the introduction to Part two of this book. Chapters 2 and 3 discuss the output dimensions themselves. Some earlier British literature adopts a theoretical stance which has certain key elements in common with the approach propounded in this book. (For example, see Brearley, 1977, especially chapter 3; Goldberg *et al.*, 1970, chapter 1; Fanshel, 1975; Institute of Municipal Treasurers and Accountants, 1972; and Williams, 1977.)

3 Some have argued that output or outcome should be measured at the *home* rather than the individual level (e.g., Fanshel, 1975). It may sometimes be necessary, because of the scale of the policy decision or the nature of the analysis, to work at a home level, but such output indicators can only be validly derived through the aggregation (in some sense) of output measures for individual residents. The problems of aggregation are many and are not readily overcome as is made clear by Arrow's so-called Possibility Theorem and the vast theoretical literature it spawned (Arrow, 1951; Sen, 1970 and 1977).

4 These factors of intermediate causal priority are called 'endogenous'. Factors whose causation is considered outside the theoretical argument because they are not to any great degree influenced by factors discussed in that argument are called 'exogenous'.

5 See, for example, Hall (1976), the papers presented at a seminar of the Organisation for Economic Co-operation and Development (1974), and Roos and Roos (1976).

6 The analytical approach of the Institute of Operational Research

210

adopted just such a constraint, arguing that the 'state of dependency best describes that aspect of the quality of life which is said to be responsive to the "good" done [by the health and welfare services]' (Fanshel, 1975, p. 349). This approach stands in stark contrast to the view, just a couple of years earlier, of a DHSS witness to the House of Commons Expenditure Committee (Eighth Report of the Expenditure Committee, 1971-2, response to question 13):

> In looking at the needs of the elderly there has been a tendency, certainly in the bulk of the research that has been done, to look at dependency and to measure outputs, and so on, and success in terms of how you reduce the dependency of the elderly. Certainly a number of attempts have been made to measure dependency comparatively successfully. We will go on improving this, but dependency is only one measure. We would hope to take it further . . . into the general welfare of the elderly. We want to promote something much more positive than simply reducing dependency. . . . We . . . want people to live a more constructive, socially oriented life, more integrated with the community. It is when you move into those intangibles that the measurements become so difficult.

7   It may be useful to give an example of the way in which the production relations approach focuses on important research questions. The meta-theory shows that given adequate measurement of inputs and outputs, relative and 'absolute' technical efficiency of homes is indicated by the precise size and sign of residuals from the estimated relation between inputs and outputs (the production function), whilst additional information on input prices (or at least ratios of prices) allows the computation of economic efficiency.
8   The cost and production functions are actually 'mathematical duals' (Diewert, 1974). The exact specification of one implies a unique specification for the other.
9   To the best of our knowledge there have been no production function studies of personal social services, although some 'close relatives' are discussed in the text below. A review of production function techniques and the preliminary estimation of an 'intermediate output production function' is reported in Knapp (1977a). In the health services field numerous examples abound; see Feldstein (1967) for an early attempt to estimate a production function for British hospitals, and Feldstein (1974) for a comprehensive review of subsequent developments. Verry and Davies (1975) have applied the production function model to British universities.
10   See B. Davies (1977) or Knapp (1981) for fuller discussions of the differences between final and intermediate output.

Chapter two: The psychological well-being of residents

1 This is clearly not an exhaustive list of the ratings, scales and indices that have been suggested for the measurement of psychological well-being with populations of elderly respondents. Some of the articles and books cited in this section will give the reader some idea of the range of alternatives, whilst others are referred to in the sections that follow. Very few British studies have used subjective well-being measures, the apparent exceptions being those of Abrams (1978), Bigot (1974), Fleming (1976), Knapp (1976, 1977b), Savage *et al.* (1977), Luker (1979), and the North London Polytechnic Survey Research Unit (see Appendix B to this chapter) and the Personal Social Services Research Unit, University of Kent at Canterbury.

2 *Concurrent validity* is a measure of how well a scale can describe a present criterion (as compared with *predictive validity* which refers to a future criterion). See, for example, Moser and Kalton (1971, p. 356).

3 The validity of a scale is its success 'in measuring what it sets out to measure, so that differences between individual's scores can be taken as representing the differences in the characteristic under study' (Moser and Kalton, 1971, p. 355). A scale has *face validity* if each item appears relevant to the characteristic being examined, whilst the more systematic *content validity* further requires that the items between them cover the whole range of the characteristic.

4 From the Kansas City study of Neugarten and her colleagues, correlation coefficients of 0.55 and 0.58 were found between the LSR on the one hand and the two indices, LSI-A and LSI-B, on the other (sample of 89 respondents aged fifty and over). The correlation between the two indices was 0.73. Whilst these three scores cannot be regarded as independent, their intercorrelations do provide a useful check on the concurrent validity of the indices. Similar results were later found by Wood, Wylie and Sheafor (1969) from their study of 100 'rural elderly' and by Lohmann (1977) in her study of the over-60s in Knoxville, Tennessee.

5 Pearson correlation coefficients in this case were 0.39 and 0.47 (sample of 52 respondents aged fifty and above), the LSI-B scale once again performing slightly better than LSI-A.

6 Rogers' positive regard and self-regard, and Maslow's esteem needs seem to be related to items 14 and 17, whilst the nearest to a salient item in LSI-B is the question: 'Do you ever worry about your ability to do what people expect of you — to meet demands that people make on you?' Again Maslovian actualisation of potential is well covered in LSI-A by items 2, 17 and 19 whereas nothing in LSI-B related directly to it. Initiative, as stressed by both Rogers and Maddi, is covered by items 16, and item 8 corresponds directly to Rogers' fulfilled person who is open to new experiences.

7 Wood *et al.* recommended reducing the number of items from twenty to thirteen, omitting items 5, 8, 10, 11, 13, 14 and 15, and

suggested a 2-1-0 scoring scheme, allowing for 'don't know' responses. This actually raised the correlation between LSI-A and LSR.

8 The three usable factors were mood tone (items 3, 4, 5, 6, 7, 18), zest for life (items 1, 8, 9, 10, 15, 16) and congruence between desired and achieved goals (items 12, 13, 19). The fourth factor was resolution and fortitude (items 2, 17, 20). The two remaining items (11 and 14) performed 'quite poorly in contributing to the total LSI-A score' and were thus omitted.

9 Klemmack, Carlson and Edwards (1974) took the 'best ten' items revealed by Adams' (1969) re-examination of LSI-A and compared them with a Social Isolation Index and a Willingness-to-Live Index. The LSI-A appeared to overlap with the Social Isolation Index to a considerable extent.

10 These were: acceptance-contentment (items 4, 5, 6, 9) and achievement-fulfilment (items 13, 14, 17, 18).

11 Nancy Lohmann's (1977) matrix of intercorrelations between four variants of the LSI (and, incidentally, with and between other psychological well-being measures) gives an indication of the importance of some of the refinements. The relevant sub-matrix is:

	LSI-B	LSI (Wood)	LSI (Adams)
LSI-A	0.628	0.941	0.989
LSI (Adams)	0.644	0.952	
LSI (Wood)	0.635		

12 These judges were a psychologist and a nurse in one home, and a psychologist, a superintendent, a chaplain, two social workers and three matrons in the other home. The ultimate criterion of validity was the judgment of the person with the higher inter-judge correlation. The correlation of the scale with this criterion was 0.70 overall.

13 Lohmann's (1977) study found the PGC morale scale to be highly correlated with both the LSI-A (0.76) and the LSI-B (0.74) for her sample of 259 older people from Tennessee. Morris, Wolf and Klerman (1975) compared the PGC with a number of depression scales, finding them to be fairly congruent inasmuch as a common theme appeared to run through them. However, this should not be taken as a suggestion that depression should be subsumed under a morale concept without investigation in its own right (Challis, 1978).

14 The dimensions were agitation (items 5, 8, 15, 17, 22 and 30), attitude towards own ageing (items 1, 2, 6, 9, 11) and lonely dissatisfaction (items, 3, 4, 10, 13, 18, 19).

15 The PGC morale scale does not appear to have been used in any British study. The scale is, however, currently being used as part of an outcome measurement in the Kent Community Care Project administered jointly by Kent County Council Social Services Department and the Personal Social Services Research Unit. We hope to be able to report on the usefulness of this particular measure of psychological well-being at a later date.

16 Lohmann's (1978) study of seven frequently-used life satisfaction measures found a construct, termed 'life satisfaction', shared by six of the measures, but that no single measure adequately covered the construct. A new instrument was thus suggested.

Chapter three: Other outputs

1 In this book we do not discuss the social worker's role in helping the ageing resident to face and accept death, other than in our treatment of beneficial and ameliorative environments in general, nor do we discuss the social worker's role in helping a resident's significant others to cope with bereavement, loss and grief. Helen Zach (1978) has recently presented some of the issues and problems, listing a number of relevant studies. A more lengthy consideration is given in the comprehensive and informative textbook of Atchley (1977, chapter 10).

2 Our discussion of morbidity is necessarily partial in a number of respects. We do not, for example, give any more than brief accounts of the processes of physiological and psychological ageing, nor can we even hope to scan the vast and burgeoning literature dealing with health status indicators for general populations. Our treatment of these subjects must necessarily be restricted to those aspects which impinge upon our production model for the elderly residents of old people's homes.

3 The weight of support for functional measures of physical health or morbidity is clearly indicated by, for example, the constituent indices of most 'need indicators' or by the methods used in carrying out the surveys recommended by the Chronically Sick and Disabled Persons Act. On the psychological side, Jerome Fisher has most persuasively argued for social assessment. He suggests that the concepts of social competence and effectiveness replace that of mental impairment (Fisher and Pearce, 1967; Fisher, 1973).

4 One of the best studies to be found in the international literature is that conducted by the Batelle Human Research Centre in Washington. Four output dimensions are distinguished — mental status, functional status (the activities of daily living), psychopathology, and psychological well-being. A total of 429 patients in six nursing homes were studied at two points in time, five months apart. Very few changes were found, a fact which probably mainly reflects the very short time interval that elapsed between assessments. (McCaffree and Harkins, 1976).

5 Gottesman and Bourestom (1974) report an interesting phenomenon in the opposite causal direction — residents who received visits from friends and relatives were accorded better treatment by staff.

Chapter four: Resource inputs: labour and capital

1 Boldy (1976) conducted a 'diary study' of 83 wardens of grouped dwellings (sheltered housing schemes) for the elderly, looking in particular at their role, duties and activities. The findings of Boldy and Imber allow an interesting comparison between staff roles, and to some extent resident life, to be made between sheltered housing care and the more conventional residential care.

2 For a review see Kart and Manard (1976).

3 A rather less crude scaling measure was suggested by Barrett (1976), who preferred to base his indicator on the definition, implicit in DHSS design recommendations, of a domestically-scaled home as a building which, when viewed from any approach, conveyed an impression of a cluster of small houses. Two main characteristics were therefore important: the arrangement and the dimensionality of the wall surfaces. His indicator of scale was the proportion of wall surfaces less than 560 square feet in surface area.

4 Hypothermia should not be a problem encountered by the elderly in residential care. In the community the problem has recently been shown to be more prevalent than previously imagined (Wicks, 1978, and see the brief survey in Challis, 1978).

5 Unfortunately the classification scheme is not widely available, although a specimen Census form is given in DHSS (1975). The resultant 'Fabric Index' was used in some of our earlier research and detailed in Knapp (1978b), for example. We are grateful to Valerie Imber for details of the classification.

6 See also the appendix to Davies and Knapp (1978) for a brief resumé of some of the principles of capital cost measurement.

Chapter five: Social environment

1 An alternative classification of services and interventions for the elderly, and one that draws heavily on the competence-press model of Lawton, has recently been proposed by Golant and McCaslin (1977). These two authors classify services and interventions by reference to two hierarchically ordered dimensions — competence and independence.

2 Some discussions of institutional environments maintain a distinction between regime and social control, on the one hand, and individuality, independence, and residents' rights on the other. We discuss them together here as they are very closely related, but we do maintain the distinction between *social* control and *motor* control. One of the most recent and interesting reviews of the 'relocation' literature regards the concept of control as the key element in understanding the diverse findings on the influence of relocation on the well-being of the aged (Schulz and Brenner, 1977).

3 Manard *et al.* (1977, pp. 18-20) record a number of variations in this 'type' of privacy between different types of home and between

home staff of different statuses.

4 It would be a mistake to restrict a discussion of furniture and equipment to the oft-quoted importance of reinforcing a resident's sense of individuality. Equipment can be labour-saving and can compensate for the disabilities of residents that can otherwise handicap attempts to help them to do more for themselves. There is of course a large literature on aids to nursing. What is less developed are studies of the ways in which equipment can contribute to the quality of life in homes by allowing residents to do things for themselves and by releasing staff for activities that contribute more directly to the psychological needs of residents.

Chapter six: Personal characteristics and experiences

1 Savage *et al.* (1977) review a number of studies of the personality characteristics of older people, with particular emphasis on British studies.
2 Details of these dimensions are given in Turner (1969), Appendix C.
3 We have already touched on the importance of experiences prior to admission in the prediction of well-being in our discussion of relocation in section 5.3.7 above. Similarly, our later discussion of individual characteristics at the point of entry (section 6.3) will develop some of the arguments introduced in the previous chapter.
4 Morris's study is discussed in more detail in section 6.3 below.
5 We have added the descriptions in square brackets to this quotation to clarify the nature of the study by Dr Spasoff and his colleagues.
6 The term adjustment is used here simply to mean 'adjustment to the residential home'. The term is not used in the sense commonly assumed in the American gerontological literature — that is, adjustment to ageing as some global process.

Chapter seven: Concluding discussion

1 In comparison with the approaches developed in the USA, the British literature on old people's homes seems almost obstinately atheoretical in its treatment of the role of social environment. No doubt this is partly because what major British works there have been have reflected the intellectual ambitions of British social administration and social work more than that of the basic social sciences. Although they give great insight into causal processes, little of the work combines sustained logical argument about the complex causal processes with the testing of the argument against formal evidence carefully analysed. Perhaps only specialists in well established disciplines can bring to bear the rigorous training required for this. The numbers in these disciplines are small by American standards. Perhaps, it is for this reason that we are so theoretically dependent on a literature intended to develop theory

for institutions so different from our own.
2 Examples of this are voluntary visiting to homes and schemes to adopt a resident as a 'quasi-parent'.
3 Cmnd 6149.
4 See, for instance, Andersen and Hull (1969), Davis and Russell (1972), Harris (1975), Havighurst (1974) — particularly the papers of Curran, Lave and Lave, and Prosser — Hellinger (1977), Hixson and Worthington (1977), Lave, Lave and Silverman (1973), Leveson (1968), Pauly (1974), Pauly and Drake (1970), Ro (1969), Ro and Auster (1969), Russell (1973), and Shulman and Galanter (1976).

Appendix B: The use of Bradburn's Affect Balance Scale with the elderly in residential care

1 MIND, National Association for Mental Health, London and formerly of North London Polytechnic.
2 Department of Applied Social Studies, Polytechnic of North London.
3 Median age of respondents — Moriwaki's study — 'psychiatric out-patient group' = 67.5 yrs; 'normal church group' = 69.5 yrs; the median age of our quality of life study = 81 yrs.
4 Mean score for 1975 Quality of Life Survey of Great Britain, undertaken by the SSRC Survey Unit (n = 932) (Hall, 1976).

Bibliography

Abrams, M. (1978), *Beyond Three-Score and Ten*, Age Concern, Mitcham.

Abrams, P. (1977), 'Community Care: Some Research Problems and Priorities', *Policy and Politics*, 6, pp. 126-51.

Adams, D.L. (1969), 'Analysis of a Life Satisfaction Index', *Journal of Gerontology*, 24, pp. 470-4.

Adams, D.L. (1971), 'Correlates of Satisfaction Among the Elderly', *Gerontologist*, 11, pp. 64-8.

Age Concern and National Corporation for the Care of Old People (1977), *Report of the Working Party on Voluntary Homes*, London.

Aiken, M., and Hage, J. (1966), 'Organizational Alienation: a Comparative Analysis', *American Sociological Review*, 31, pp. 497-507.

Aldrich, C.K. (1964), 'Personality Factors and Mortality in the Relocation of the Aged', *Gerontologist*, 5, p. 92.

Allardt, E. (1973), *About Dimensions of Welfare: An Exploratory Analysis of a Comparative Scandinavian Study*, Research Report No. 1, University of Helsinki.

Allen, D. (1977), 'The Residential Task — Is There One?', *Social Work Today*, 9, 11 October, pp. 20-2.

Aloia, A.J. (1973), 'Relationships Between Perceived Privacy Options, Self-Esteem, and Internal Control Among Aged People', Doctoral dissertation, California School of Professional Psychology.

Alutto, T., and Acito, F. (1973), 'Decisional Participation and Sources of Job Satisfaction', mimeograph, University of New York at Buffalo.

Anderson, N., Holmberg, R.H., Schneider, R.E., and Stone, L.B. (1969), *Policy Issues Regarding Nursing Homes: Findings from a Minnesota Study*, Institute of Interdisciplinary Studies, Minneapolis.

Andersen, R., and Hull, J. (1969), 'Hospital Utilisation and Cost Trends in Canada and the United States', *Health Services Research*, 4, pp. 198-222.

Apte, R.Z. (1968), *Halfway Houses*, Bell, London.

218

Arrow, K.J. (1951), *Social Choice and Individual Values*, Wiley, New York.

Atchley, R.C. (1977), *The Social Forces in Later Life*, Wadsworth, Belmont, California.

Atkinson, J.W. (1957), 'Motivational Determinants of Risk-Taking Behaviour', *Psychological Review*, 64, pp. 359-72.

Averill, J. (1973), 'Personal Control Over Aversive Stimuli and its Relationship to Stress', *Psychological Bulletin*, 80, pp. 286-303.

Bader, J., and Lawton, M.P. (1969), 'Wish for Privacy by Old and Young', mimeograph, Philadelphia Geriatric Center.

Baltz, T.M., and Turner, J.G. (1977), 'Development and Analysis of a Nursing Home Aide Screening Device', *Gerontologist*, 17, pp. 66-9.

Barker, R. (1968), *Ecological Psychology*, Stanford University Press.

Barrett, A. (1976), 'User Requirements in Purpose-Built Local Authority Residential Homes for Old People — the Notion of Domesticity in Design', PhD. thesis, University of Wales.

Barton, R. (1966), *Institutional Neurosis*, John Wright, Bristol.

Bates, K. (1976), 'A Study of Reactions to Admission to Homes for the Elderly', MPhil. thesis, University of Nottingham.

Battelle Health Care Study Centre (1977), 'Long Term Care Case Mix, Employee Time and Costs', mimcograph, Seattle, Washington.

Battista, J., and Almond, R. (1973), 'The Development of Meaning in Life', *Psychiatry*, 36, pp. 409-27.

Beattie, W.M., and Bullock, J. (1964), 'Evaluating Services and Personnel in Facilities for the Aged', in M. Leeds and H. Shore (eds), *Geriatric Institutional Management*, Putnam, New York.

Beiser, M. (1974), 'Components and Correlates of Mental Well-Being', *Journal of Health and Social Behaviour*, 15, pp. 320-7.

Bennett, A.E., Deane, M., Elliott, A., and Holland, W.W. (1968), 'Care of Old People in Residential Homes', *British Journal of Preventive and Social Medicine*, 22, pp. 193-8.

Bennett, R.G. (1963), 'The Meaning of Institutional Life', *Gerontologist*, 3, pp. 117-25.

Bennett, R.G. (1970), 'Social Context — a Neglected Variable in Research on Ageing', *International Journal of Ageing and Human Development*, 1, pp. 97-116.

Bennett, R.G., and Eisdorfer, C. (1975), 'The Institutional Environment and Behavior Change', in S. Sherwood (ed,), *Long Term Care*, Spectrum, New York.

Bennett, R.G., and Nahemow, L. (1965a), 'The Relations Between Social Isolation, Socialisation and Adjustment in Residents of a Home for the Aged', in M.P. Lawton (ed.), *Proceedings of Institute on Mentally Impaired Aged*, Maurice Jacob Press, Philadelphia.

Bennett, R.G., and Nahemow, L. (1965b), 'Institutional Totality and Criteria of Social Adjustment in Residential Settings for the Aged', *Journal of Social Issues*, 21, pp. 44-78.

Bennett, R.G., and Nahemow, L. (1972), 'Socialisation and Social Adjustment in Five Residential Settings for the Aged', in D.P. Kent, R. Kastenbaum, and S. Sherwood (eds), *Research Planning and*

Action for the Elderly, Behavioral Publications, New York.

Berliner, J.S. (1972), *Economy, Society and Welfare*, Praeger, New York.

Berlyne, D.E. (1960), *Conflict, Arousal and Curiosity*, McGraw-Hill, New York.

Bigot, A. (1974), 'The Relevance of American Life Satisfaction Indices for Research on British Subjects Before and After Retirement', *Age and Ageing*, 3, pp. 113-21.

Bild, B., and Havighurst, R.J. (1976), 'Senior Citizens in Great Cities: the Case of Chicago', *Gerontologist*, 16, pp. 1-88.

Billis, D. (1975), 'Managing to Care', *Social Work Today*, 6, pp. 38-43.

Binstock, R. (1966), 'Some Deficiencies of Gerontological Research in Social Welfare', *Journal of Gerontology*, 21, pp. 157-60.

Blau, P.M. (1964), *Exchange and Power in Social Life*, Wiley, New York.

Blau, P.M. (1970), 'Decentralisation in Bureaucracies', in M.N. Zald (ed.), *Power in Organisations*, Vanderbilt University Press.

Blunden, R., and Kushlick, A. (1974), 'Research and the Care of Elderly People', Research Report 110, Health Care Evaluation Research Team, Winchester.

Boldy, D. (1976), 'A Study of the Wardens of Grouped Dwellings for the Elderly', *Social and Economic Administration*, 10, pp. 59-67.

Bradburn, N.M. (1969), *The Structure of Psychological Well-Being*, Aldine, Chicago.

Bradburn, N.M., and Caplovitz, D. (1965), *Reports on Happiness: a Pilot Study of Behaviour Related to Mental Health*, Aldine, Chicago.

Brearley, C.P. (1975), *Social Work, Ageing and Society*, Routledge & Kegan Paul, London.

Brearley, C.P. (1977), *Residential Work with the Elderly*, Routledge & Kegan Paul, London.

Breytspraak, L.M., and George, L.K. (1977), 'Measurement of Self-Concept and Self-Esteem in Older People: the State of the Art', paper presented to the Gerontological Society, San Francisco.

British Association of Social Workers (1977), 'Guidelines for Social Work with the Elderly', *Social Work Today*, 8, 12 April, pp. 8-15.

Brophy, J.G., Ernst, M., and Shore, H. (1977), 'A Short-Form for Assessing Sensory Loss in the Elderly', mimeograph, North Texas State University.

Bull, C.N., and Aucoin, J.B. (1975), 'Voluntary Association Participation and Life Satisfaction: a Replication Note', *Journal of Gerontology*, 30, pp. 73-6.

Bultena, G. (1968), 'Age Grading in the Social Interaction of an Elderly Male Population', *Journal of Gerontology*, 23, pp. 539-43.

Bultena, G. (1974), 'Structural Effects on the Morale of the Aged: a Comparison of Age-segregated and Age-integrated Communities'. In G.F. Gubrium (ed.) *Late Life: Communities and Environmental Policy*, Charles C. Thomas, Springfield, Illinois.

Bultena, G., and Marshall, D.G. (1969), 'Structural Effects on the Morale of the Aged', paper read to American Sociological

Association, San Francisco.

Bultena, G., and Wood, V. (1969), 'Normative Attitudes Toward the Aged Role among Migrant and Non-Migrant Retirees', *Gerontologist*, 9, pp. 204-8.

Burgess, E.M., Cavan, R., and Havighurst, R.J. (1947), *Your Activities and Attitudes*, Science Research Associates, Chicago.

Butler, R.N., and Perlin, S. (1957), 'Depressive Reactions in the Aged: the Function of Denial, Awareness and Insight', paper presented to American Psychiatric Association, Chicago.

Calhoun, J. (1963), 'Population Density and Social Pathology', in L. Duhl (ed.), *The Urban Condition*, Basic Books, New York.

Callahan, J.J. (1979), 'The Organisation of the Long Term Care System and the Potential for a Single Agency Option', University Health Policy Consortium, Brandeis University, Waltham, Massachusetts.

Cameron, P. (1975), 'Mood as an Indicant of Happiness: Age, Sex, Social Class, and Situational Differences', *Journal of Gerontology*, 30, pp. 216-24.

Campbell, A., and Converse, P. (1970), *Monitoring the Quality of American Life*, Russell Sage Foundation, New York.

Cannell, C.F., Lawson, S.A., and Hauser, D.L. (1975), 'A Technique for Evaluating Interviewer Performance', mimeograph, Survey Research Center, University of Michigan, Ann Arbor.

Cantril, H. (1965), *The Pattern of Human Concern*, Rutgers University Press.

Carp, F.M. (1966), *A Future for the Aged*, University of Texas Press.

Carstairs, V., and Morrison, N. (1971), *The Elderly in Residential Care*, Scottish Home and Health Department, Edinburgh.

Cartwright, A., Hockey, L., and Anderson, J. (1973), *Life before Death*, Routledge & Kegan Paul, London.

Cavan, R., Burgess, E., Havighurst, R., and Goldhamer, H. (1949), *Personal Adjustment in Old Age*, Science Research Associates, Chicago.

Challis, D.J. (1978), 'The Measurement of Outcome in Social Care of the Elderly', discussion paper, Personal Social Services Research Unit, University of Kent at Canterbury.

Chang, B.L. (1977), 'The Relationship of Generalised Expectancies and Situational Control of Daily Activities to Morale of the Institutionalised Aged', paper presented to Gerontological Society Conference, San Francisco.

Cheshire County Council, Social Services Department (1976), 'Brief for the Architect of Residential Homes For Old People', mimeograph, Chester.

Cicirelli, V.G. (1977), 'Relationship of Siblings to the Elderly Person's Feelings and Concerns', *Journal of Gerontology*, 32, pp. 317-22.

Coe, R.M. (1965), 'Self-conception of Institutionalisation', in A.M. Rose and W.A. Peterson (eds), *Older People and their Social World*, F.A. Davis, Philadelphia.

Coleman, P. (1976), 'Sources of Self-esteem in the Elderly — Development of and First Results with a Measuring Instrument for

Use in a Longitudinal Study of Relocation', paper presented to British Psychological Society, York.

Copeland, J.R.M. *et al.* (1976), 'A Semi-Structured Clinical Interview for the Assessment and Diagnosis of Mental State in the Elderly: the Geriatric Mental State Scheme', *Psychological Medicine*, 6, pp. 439-49.

Crawford, M.P. (1971), 'Retirement and Disengagement', *Human Relations*, 24, pp. 255-78.

Cumming, E., and Henry, W.E. (1961), *Growing Old: The Process of Disengagement*, Basic Books, New York.

Curran, W.J. (1974), 'A National Survey and Analysis of State "Certificate-of-Need" Laws for Health Facilities', in C.C. Havighurst (ed.), *Regulating Health Facilities Construction*, American Enterprise Institute for Public Policy Research, Washington, D.C.

Curry, T.J., and Ratliff, B.W. (1973), 'The Effects of Nursing Home Size on Resident Isolation and Satisfaction', *Gerontologist*, 13, pp. 295-8.

Davies, B.P. (1968), *Social Needs and Resources in Local Services*, Michael Joseph, London.

Davies, B.P. (1975), 'Social and Economic Indicators: the Academic's Contribution', paper presented at Statistics Users Conference, London.

Davies, B.P. (1976), 'Causal Processes and Techniques in the Modelling of Policy Outcomes', in K. Young (ed.), *Essays on the Study of Urban Politics*, Macmillan, London.

Davies, B.P. (1977), 'Needs and Outputs', in H. Heisler (ed.), *Foundations of Social Administration*, Macmillan, London.

Davies, B.P. (1978), *Universality, Selectivity and Effectiveness in Social Policy*, Heinemann, London.

Davies, B.P. (1979), 'Territorial Justice and the Regions', discussion paper 134, Personal Social Services Research Unit, University of Kent at Canterbury.

Davies, B.P., and Knapp, M.R.J. (1978), 'Hotel and Dependency Costs of Residents in Old Peoples Homes', *Journal of Social Policy*, 7, pp. 1-22.

Davies, L., Hastrop, K., and Bender, A.E. (1975), 'Protein in the Diet of Old Age Pensioners Receiving Meals-on-Wheels', *Modern Geriatrics*, 5, pp. 12-20.

Davies, M. (1977), *Support Systems in Social Work*, Routledge & Kegan Paul, London.

Davies, R.M., and Duncan, I.B. (1975), 'Allocation and Planning of Local Authority Residential Accommodation for the Elderly in Reading', mimeograph, Operational Research (Health Services) Unit, University of Reading.

Davis, K., and Russell, L. (1972), 'The Substitution of Hospital Outpatient Care for Inpatient Care', *Review of Economics and Statistics*, 54 (2), pp. 109-20.

DeLong, A.J. (1967), 'An Outline of the Environmental Language of the Older Person', paper presented to American Association of Homes for the Aged.

DeLong, A.J. (1974), 'Environments for the Elderly', *Journal of Communications*, 24, pp. 101-12.

Department of Health and Social Security (1975), *The Census of Residential Accommodation 1970. Volume 1: Residential Accommodation for the Elderly and the Younger Physically Handicapped*, HMSO, London.

Department of Health and Social Security (1976a), 'Some Aspects of Residential Care', *Social Work Service*, 10, pp. 3-17.

Department of Health and Social Security (1976b), *Manpower and Training for the Social Services*, HMSO, London.

Department of Health and Social Security (1976c), *Lifestyle for the Elderly*, HMSO, London.

Department of Health and Social Security (1977), *Residential Homes for the Elderly: Arrangements for Health Care*, HMSO, London.

Department of Health and Social Security (1979), *Health and Personal Social Services Statistics for England 1978*, HMSO, London.

Diewert, W.E. (1974), 'Applications of Duality Theory', in M.D. Intrilligator and D.A. Kendrick (eds), *Frontiers of Quantitative Economics, Vol. 2*, North-Holland, Amsterdam.

Doke, L.A., and Risley, T.R. (1972), 'The Organisation of Day-Care Environments. Required Versus Optional Activities', *Journal of Applied Behavioural Analysis*, 5, pp. 405-20.

Dominic, J.R., Greenblatt, D.L., and Stotsky, B.A. (1968), 'The Adjustment of Aged Persons in Nursing Homes. The Patients' Report', *Journal of American Geriatrics Society*, 16, pp. 63-7.

Dominic, J.R., Greenblatt, D.L., and Stotsky, B.A. (1968a), 'The Adjustment of Aged Persons in Nursing Homes. The Nurses' Report', *Journal of American Geriatrics Society*, 16, pp. 436-9.

Dorset County Council, Social Services Department (1977), 'Evaluation of the First Year of a New Home for the Elderly', mimeograph.

Dowd, J.J. (1975), 'Ageing as Exchange: a Preface to Theory', *Journal of Gerontology*, 30, pp. 584-94.

Drevenstedt, J. (1975), 'Scale-Checking Styles on the Semantic Differential Scale among Older People', *Journal of Gerontology*, 30, pp. 170-3.

Duncan, T.L.C. (1971), *Measuring Housing Quality*, occasional paper 20, Centre for Urban and Regional Studies, University of Birmingham.

East Sussex County Council Social Services Department (1975), *The Elderly: Main Report of Findings*, mimeograph, Lewes.

Edwards, J., and Klemmack, D. (1973), 'Correlates of Life Satisfaction: a Re-examination', *Journal of Gerontology*, 28, pp. 497-502.

Eighth Report of the Expenditure Committee (1971-2), *Relationship of Expenditure to Needs*, HCCP 515 (1971-2), HMSO.

Elias, B.M. (1977), 'Residential Environment and Social Adjustment among Older Widows' (abstract), mimeograph, University of Guelph, Ontario, Canada.

Erikson, E.H. (1963), *Childhood and Society*, Macmillan, New York.

Exton-Smith, A.N. (1968), 'Health and Nutrition of the Elderly', *Royal Society of Health Journal*, pp. 205-8.

Exton-Smith, A.N. (1970), 'Nutrition Surveys and the Problems of Detection of Malnutrition in the Elderly', *Nutrition*, 24, pp. 218-25.

Fairhurst, E. (1978), 'Talk and the Elderly in Institutions', paper presented to annual conference of British Society of Social and Behavioural Gerontology, Edinburgh.

Fanshel, S. (1972), 'A Meaningful Measure of Health for Epidemiology', *International Journal of Epidemiology*, 1, pp. 319-37.

Fanshel, S. (1975), 'The Welfare of the Elderly: a Systems Analysis Viewpoint', *Policy Sciences*, 6, pp. 343-7.

Fawcett, G., Stonner, D., and Zepelin, H. (1976), 'Locus of Control Perceived, Constraint, and Morale Among Institutionalised Aged', paper presented at Gerontological Society Conference, New York.

Feder, J.M. (1977), *Medicare: The Politics of Federal Hospital Insurance*, D.C. Heath, Lexington, Massachusetts.

Feldstein, M.S. (1967), *Economic Analysis for Health Service Efficiency*, North-Holland, Amsterdam.

Feldstein, M.S. (1974), 'Economic Studies of Health Economics', in M. Intrilligator and D. Kendrick (eds), *Frontiers of Quantitative Economics*, Vol. 2, North-Holland, Amsterdam.

Felton, B., and Kahana, E. (1974), 'Adjustment and Situationally-Bound Locus of Control among Institutionalised Aged', *Journal of Gerontology*, 29, pp. 295-301.

Fisher, J. (1973), 'Competence, Effectiveness, Intellectual Functioning, and Ageing', *Gerontologist*, 13, pp. 62-8.

Fisher, J., and Pearce, M. (1967), 'Dimensions of Intellectual Functioning of the Aged', *Journal of Gerontology*, 22, pp. 166-73.

Fiske, D.W., and Maddi, S.R. (eds) (1961), *Functions of Varied Experience*, Dorsey Press, Homewood, Illinois.

Fleming, R.W. (1976), 'Changes in Life Satisfaction and Self-Help Activities Following the Introduction of Residents' Meetings and a Self-Help Clinic in an Old People's Home', mimeograph, London Borough of Newham.

Fried, C. (1974), *Medical Experimentation: Personal Integrity and Social Policy*, North-Holland, Amsterdam.

Fromm, E. (1947), *Man for Himself*, Holt, Reinhardt & Winston, New York.

Goffman, E. (1961), *Asylums*, Anchor Books, Doubleday, New York.

Golant, S.M., and McCaslin, R. (1977), 'A Functional Classification of Services for Older People', mimeograph, Department of Geography, University of Chicago.

Goldberg, E.M., Mortimer, A., and Williams, B.T. (1970), *Helping the Aged*, Allen & Unwin, London.

Goldsmith, S. (1971), 'Appraisal (of an Old People's Home)', *Architects Journal*, 29 September, pp. 704-13.

Gottesman, L.E. (1972), 'Nursing Home Performance as Related to Resident Traits, Ownership, Size, and Source of Payment', *American Journal of Public Health*, 64, pp. 269-76.

Gottesman, L.E., and Bourestom, N.C. (1974), 'Why Nursing Homes Do What They Do', *Gerontologist*, 14, pp. 501-5.

Gouldner, A.W. (1963), 'Cosmopolitans and Locals: Toward an Analysis of Latent Social Roles – I and II', *Administrative Science Quarterly*, pp. 281-306, and pp. 444-80.

Graney, M.J. (1973), 'The Affect Balance Scale and Old Age', *Social Abstracts*, 21.

Graney, M.J. (1974), 'The Aged and Their Environment: the Study of Intervening Variables', in J.F. Gubrium (ed.), *Late Life: Communities and Environmental Policy*, Charles C. Thomas, Springfield, Illinois.

Graney, M.J. (1975), 'Happiness and Social Participation in Ageing', *Journal of Gerontology*, 30, pp. 701-6.

Graney, M.J. (1977), 'An Exploration of Social Factors Influencing the Sex Differential in Mortality', paper presented to Gerontological Society Annual Meeting, San Francisco.

Grant, G.W.B., and Moores, B. (1977), 'Resident Characteristics and Staff Behaviour in Two Hospitals for the Mentally-Retarded', *American Journal of Mental Deficiency*, 82, pp. 259-65.

Greenfield, P. (1976), 'Medical Care in Old Peoples Homes', in Department of Health and Social Security, *A Lifestyle for the Elderly*, HMSO, London.

Greenwald, S.R., and Linn, M.W. (1970), 'What Wives Say about Nursing Homes', *Journal of American Geriatrics Society*, 18, pp. 166-71.

Greenwald, S.R., and Linn, M.W. (1971), 'Intercorrelation of Data on Nursing Homes', *Gerontologist*, 11, pp. 337-40.

Greenwood, R. (1978), 'Politics and Public Bureaucracies: a Reconsideration', *Policy and Politics*, 6, pp. 403-19.

Gresham, M.I. (1976), 'The Infantilization of the Elderly: a Developing Concept', *Nursing Forum*, 15, pp. 195-210.

Grusky, O. (1959), 'Role Conflict in Organisations', *Administrative Science Quarterly*, 3, pp. 452-72.

Gubrium, J.F. (1970), 'Environmental Effects on Morale in Old Age and the Resources of Health and Solvency', *Gerontologist*, 10, pp. 294-7.

Gubrium, J.F. (1972), 'Toward a Socio-Environmental Theory of Ageing', *Gerontologist*, 12, pp. 281-4.

Gubrium, J.F. (1974), 'On Multiple Realities in a Nursing Home', in J.F. Gubrium (ed.), *Late Life: Communities and Environmental Policy*, Charles C. Thomas, Springfield, Illinois.

Hall, J. (1976), 'Subjective Measures of Quality of Life in Britain: 1971 to 1975', *Social Trends*, 7, pp. 47-60.

Hall, J., and Ring, J. (1974), 'Indicators of Environmental Quality of Life Satisfaction: Subjective Approach', mimeograph, SSRC Survey Unit, London.

Hall, R.H. (1967), 'Some Organizational Considerations in the Professional-Organizational Relationship', *Administrative Science Quarterly*, 12, pp. 461-78.

Haringey Social Services Department (1978), 'London Borough of Haringey Old People's Homes — Identification of Resident Condition, Standards of Care, Staffing Levels and Future Policies', mimeograph.

Harris, A.I. (1968), *Social Welfare for the Aged*, HMSO, London.

Harris, D. (1977), 'Seven Models of Residential Care', *Social Work Today*, 9, 30 August, pp. 19-20.

Harris, H. (1977), 'Workhouse? Hotel? It's All Just the Bleedin' Same', *Social Work Today*, 9, 11 November, pp. 13-15.

Harris, H., Lipman, A., and Slater, R. (1977), 'Architectural Design: the Spatial Location and Interactions of Old People', *Gerontology*, 23, pp. 390-400.

Harris, J.M., Veit, S.W., Allen, G.J., and Chinsky, J.M. (1974), 'Aide-Resident Ratio and Ward Population Density as Mediators of Social Inter-Action', *American Journal of Mental Deficiency*, 79, pp. 320-6.

Harris, S.E. (1975), *The Economics of Health Care: Finance and Delivery*, McCulchan, California.

Hathaway, S., and McKinley, D. (1951), *The Minnesota Multiphasic Personality Inventory*, Psychological Corporation, New York.

Havighurst, C.C. (1974), *Regulating Health Facilities Construction*, American Enterprise Institute for Public Policy Research, Washington, D.C.

Havighurst, R.J. (1968), Personality and Patterns of Ageing', *Gerontologist*, 8, pp. 20-3.

Havighurst, R.J., and Albrecht, R. (1953), *Older People*, Longmans, New York.

Havighurst, R.J., Munnichs, J.M.A., Neugarten, B.L. and Thomae, H. (1969), *Adjustment to Retirement: A Cross-National Study*, Van Gorcum, Amsterdam.

Heal, K., Sinclair, I.A.G., and Troop, J. (1973), 'The Development of a Social Climate Questionnaire for Use in Approved Schools and Community Homes', *British Journal of Sociology*, 24, pp. 223-35.

Hellinger, F.J. (1977), 'Substitutability among Different Types of Care Under Medicare', *Health Services Research*, 12 (1), pp. 11-18.

Helson, H. (1964), *Adaptation Level Theory*, Harper & Row, New York.

Henry, J. (1957), 'Types of Institutional Structure', in M. Greenblatt (ed.), *The Patient and the Mental Hospital*, Free Press, Glencoe, Illinois.

Hirsch, F. (1977), *Social Limits to Growth*, Routledge & Kegan Paul, London.

Hitch, D., and Simpson, A. (1972), 'An Attempt to Assess a New Design in Residential Homes for the Elderly', *British Journal of Social Work*, 2, pp. 481-501.

Hixson, J.S., and Worthington, P.N. (1977), 'An Administered Price System for Hospitals', *Social Science and Medicine*, 11, pp. 801-7.

Hobman, D. (1978), 'Standards of Care in the Private Sector', *Social*

Work Today, 9, 16 May, p. 22.

Holdsworth, M.D. (1978), 'Catering and Nutrition in Residential Homes for the Elderly', paper presented at annual conference of British Society of Social and Behavioural Gerontology, Edinburgh.

Holland, T. (1973), 'Organizational Structure and Institutional Care', *Journal of Health and Social Behaviour*, 14, pp. 241-51.

Hopkins, T. (1979a), 'Child Care at a Profit', *New Society*, 38 (863), 19 April, pp. 135-6.

Hopkins, T. (1979b), private correspondence.

Imber, V. (1977), *A Classification of Staff in Homes for the Elderly* (Statistical and Research Report 18, DHSS), HMSO, London.

Institute of Municipal Treasurers and Accountants (1972), *Output Measurement: Personal Social Services*, IMTA, London.

Isaacs, B., Livingstone, M., and Neville, Y. (1972), *Survival of the Unfittest*, Routledge & Kegan Paul, London.

Ittleston, W.H., Proshansky, H.M., and Rivlin, L.G. (1970), 'Bedroom Size and Social Interaction on the Psychiatric Ward', *Environment and Behaviour*, 2, pp. 255-70.

Jackson, D.W. (1974), 'Relationship of Residence, Education, and Socialisation to Cognitive Tasks in Normal People of Advanced Old Age', *Psychological Reports*, 35, pp. 423-6.

Jackson, J.M. (1964), 'Toward the Comparative Study of Mental Hospitals: Characteristics of the Treatment Environment', in A.F. Wessen (ed.), *The Psychiatric Hospital as a Social System*, Charles C. Thomas, Springfield, Illinois.

Jackson, J.S., Herzog, A.R., Monteiro, R.C., and Chatters, L. (1977), 'Background Factors and Subjective Well-Being in Blacks', mimeograph, University of Michigan.

Jenkins, J., Felce, D., Lunt, B., and Powell, L. (1976), 'Research in Residential Environments of the Elderly: an Applied Behavioural Approach', research report 122, Health Care Evaluation Research Team, Winchester.

Jenkins, J., Felce, D., Lunt, B., and Powell, L. (1977), 'Increasing Engagement in Activity of Residents in Old People's Homes by Providing Recreational Materials', *Behaviour Research and Therapy*, 15, pp. 429-34.

Jones, D.C. (1975), 'Spatial Proximity, Interpersonal Conflict, and Friendship Formation in the Intermediate-Care Facility', *Gerontologist*, 15, pp. 150-4.

Kahana, E. (1974), 'Matching Environments to Needs of the Aged: a Conceptual Scheme', in J.F. Gubrium (ed.), *Late Life: Communities and Environmental Policy*, Charles C. Thomas, Springfield, Illinois.

Kahana, E. and Coe, R.M. (1969), 'Dimensions of Conformity: a Multi-Disciplinary View', *Journal of Gerontology*, 24, pp. 76-81.

Kahana, E., and Kahana, B. (1970), 'Changes in Mental States of Elderly Patients in Age Integrated and Age Segregated Hospital Milieu', *Journal of Abnormal Psychology*, 75, pp. 177-81.

Kalish, R.A. (1976), 'Death and Dying in a Social Context', in R. Binstock and E. Shanas (eds), *Handbook of Ageing and Social*

Sciences, Van Nostrand Reinhold, New York.

Karcher, C.J., and Linden, L.L. (1974), 'Family Rejection of the Aged and Nursing Home Utilization', *International Journal of Ageing and Human Development*, 5, pp. 231-44.

Kart, C.S., and Manard, B.B. (1976), 'Quality of Care in Old Age Institutions', *Gerontologist*, 16, pp. 250-6.

Kasarda, J. (1974), 'The Structural Implications of Social System Size: a Three Level Analysis', *American Sociological Review*, 39, pp. 19-28.

Kast, F.R., and Rosenzweig, J.E. (1973), *Contingency Views of Organisation and Management*, Social Research Associates.

Katz, D., and Kahn, R.L. (1966), *The Social Psychology of Organisations*, Wiley, New York.

Kellam, S.G., Shmelzer, J., and Berman, A. (1966), 'Variations in the Atmospheres of Psychiatric Wards', *Archives of General Psychiatry*, 14, pp. 561-70.

King, R.D., and Raynes, N.V. (1968), 'An Operational Measure of Inmate Management in Residential Institutions', *Social Science and Medicine*, 2, pp. 41-53.

King, R.D., Raynes, N.V., and Tizard, J. (1971), *Patterns of Residential Care*, Routledge & Kegan Paul, London.

Kleemeier, R.W. (1961), 'The Use and Meaning of Time in Special Settings', in R.W. Kleemeier (ed.), *Aging and Leisure*, Oxford University Press, New York.

Klemmack, D.L., Carlson, J.R., and Edwards, J.N. (1974), 'Measures of Well-Being: an Empirical and Critical Assessment', *Journal of Health and Social Behaviour*, 15, pp. 267-74.

Knapp, M.R.J. (1976), 'Predicting the Dimensions of Life Satisfaction', *Journal of Gerontology*, 31, pp. 595-604.

Knapp, M.R.J. (1977a), 'An Empirical Production Function for Old People's Homes: a Survey of Alternative Functional Forms and Some Preliminary Estimates', discussion paper 70, Personal Social Service Research Unit, University of Kent at Canterbury.

Knapp, M.R.J. (1977b), 'The Activity Theory of Ageing: an Examination in the English Context', *Gerontologist*, 17, pp. 553-9.

Knapp, M.R.J. (1977c), 'The Design of Residential Homes for the Elderly: an Examination of Variations with Census Data', *Socio-Economic Planning Sciences*, 11, pp. 205-12.

Knapp, M.R.J. (1978a), 'Cost Functions for Care Services for the Elderly', *Gerontologist*, 18, pp. 30-6.

Knapp, M.R.J. (1978b), 'Economies of Scale in Residential Care', *International Journal of Social Economics*, 5, pp. 81-92.

Knapp, M.R.J. (1979), 'On the Determination of the Manpower Requirements of Old People's Homes', *Social Policy and Administration*, 13 (3), pp. 219-36.

Knapp, M.R.J. (1981), *The Economics of Social Care*, Macmillan, London (forthcoming).

Kosberg, J.I. (1971), 'The Relationship between Organisational Characteristics and Treatment Resources in Nursing Homes', PhD.

thesis, University of Chicago.

Kosberg, J.I. (1973), 'Difference in Proprietary Institutions Caring for Affluent and Nonaffluent Elderly', *Gerontologist*, 13, pp. 299-304.

Kosberg, J.I. (1974), 'Making Institutions Accountable: Research and Policy Issues', *Gerontologist*, 14, pp. 510-16.

Kosberg, J.I., Cohen, S.Z., and Mendlovitz, A. (1972), 'Comparison of Supervisors' Attitudes in a Home for the Aged', *Gerontologist*, 12, pp. 241-5.

Kushlick, A. (1967), 'A Method of Evaluating the Effectiveness of a Community Health Service', *Social and Economic Administration*, 1 (4), pp. 29-48.

Kushlick, A. (1974), 'Improving Services for the Mentally Handicapped', research report 114, Health Care Evaluation Research Team, Winchester.

Kushlick, A., and Blunden, R. (1974), 'Proposals for Setting Up and Evaluation of an Experimental Service for the Elderly', research report 107, Health Care Evaluation Research Team, Winchester.

Kutner, B. (1969), 'The Calculus of Services for the Aged', *Canadian Medical Association Journal*, 98, pp. 775-80.

Langner, T.S. (1962), 'A Twenty-Two Item Screening Score of Psychiatric Symptoms Indicating Impairment', *Journal of Health and Human Behaviour*, 3, pp. 269-76.

Larson, R. (1978), 'Thirty Years of Research on the Subjective Well-Being of Older Americans', *Journal of Gerontology*, 33, pp. 109-25.

Lave, J.R., and Lave, L.B. (1974), 'The Supply and Allocation of Medical Resources: Alternative Control Mechanisms', in C.C. Havighurst (ed.), *Regulating Health Facilities Construction*, American Enterprise Institute for Public Policy Research, Washington, D.C.

Lave, J.R., Lave, L.B., and Silverman, L.P. (1973), 'A Proposal for Incentive Reimbursement for Hospitals', *Medical Care*, 11 (2), pp. 79-90.

Lawton, M.P. (1970a), 'Institutions for the Aged: Theory, Content, and Methods for Research', *Gerontologist*, 10, pp. 305-12.

Lawton, M.P. (1970b), 'Planning Environments for the Elderly', *Journal of American Institute of Planners*, 36, pp. 124-9.

Lawton, M.P. (1970c), 'Assessment, Integration and Environments for Older People', *Gerontologist*, 10, pp. 38-46.

Lawton, M.P. (1972a), 'The Dimensions of Morale', in D.P. Kent *et al.* (eds), *Research Planning and Action for the Elderly*, Behavioural Publications, New York.

Lawton, M.P. (1972b), 'Assessing the Competence of Older People', in D.P. Kent *et al.* (eds), *Research Planning and Action for the Elderly*, Behavioural Publications, New York.

Lawton, M.P. (1975a), 'The PGC Morale Scale: a Revision', *Journal of Gerontology*, 30, pp. 85-9.

Lawton, M.P. (1975b), *Planning and Managing Housing for the Elderly*, Wiley, New York.

Lawton, M.P. (1976), 'Morale: What are we Measuring?', mimeograph,

Philadelphia Geriatric Center.

Lawton, M.P., Brody, E.M., and Turner-Massey, P. (1978), 'Short - Range Effects of Community Housing', *Gerontologist*, 18, pp. 133-7.

Lawton, M.P., and Cohen, J. (1974), 'The Generality of Housing Impact on the Well-Being of Older People', *Journal of Gerontology*, 29, pp. 194-204.

Lawton, M.P., Liebowitz, B., and Charon, H. (1970), 'Physical Structure and the Behaviour of Senile Patients Following Ward Remodelling', *International Journal of Ageing and Human Development*, 1.

Lawton, M.P., and Nahemow, L. (1973), 'Ecology and the Aging Process', in C. Eisdorfer and M.P. Lawton (eds), *The Psychology of Adult Development and Ageing*, American Psychological Association, Washington.

Lawton, M.P., Nahemow, L., and Teaff, J. (1975), 'Housing Characteristics and the Well-Being of Elderly Tenants in Federally Assisted Housing', *Journal of Gerontology*, 30, pp. 601-7.

Lawton, M.P., Patnaik, B., and Kleban, M.H. (1976), 'The Ecology of Adaptation to a New Environment', *International Journal of Ageing and Human Development*, 7, pp. 15-26.

Lawton, M.P., and Simon, B. (1968), 'The Ecology of Social Relationships in Housing for the Elderly', *Gerontologist*, 8, pp. 108-15.

Lawton, M.P., and Yaffe, S. (1970), 'Mortality, Morbidity and Voluntary Changes of Residence by Older People', *Journal of American Geriatrics Society*, 18, pp. 823-31.

Leveson, I. (1968), 'Medical Care Cost Incentives: Some Questions and Approaches for Research', *Inquiry*, 5 (4), pp. 3-13.

Levey, S., Ruchlin, H.J., Stotsky, B.A., Kinloch, D.R., and Oppenheim, W. (1973), 'An Appraisal of Nursing Home Care', *Journal of Gerontology*, 28, pp. 222-8.

Lewin, K. (1935), *A Dynamic Theory of Personality*, McGraw-Hill, New York.

Lewin, K. (1946), 'Behaviour and Development as a Function of the Total Situation', in L. Carmichael (ed.), *Manual of Child Psychology*, Wiley, New York.

Lewin, K. (1952), 'Group Decision and Social Change', in G. Swanson, T. Newcomb, and E. Hartley (eds), *Readings in Social Psychology*, Holt, Reinhardt & Winston, New York.

Lieberman, M.A. (1961), 'Relationship of Mortality Rates to Entrance to a Home for the Aged', *Geriatrics*, 16, pp. 515-19.

Lieberman, M.A. (1965), 'Psychological Correlates of Impending Death: Some Preliminary Observations', *Journal of Gerontology*, 20, pp. 181-90.

Lieberman, M.A. (1969), 'Institutionalisation of the Aged: Effects on Behaviour', *Journal of Gerontology*, 24, pp. 330-40.

Lieberman, M.A. (1974), 'Relocation Research and Social Policy', *Gerontologist*, 14, pp. 494-501.

Lieberman, M.A., Brock, V., and Tobin, S.S. (1968), 'Psychological

Effects of Institutionalisation', *Journal of Gerontology*, 23, pp. 343-53.

Liebowitz, B. (1974), 'Impact of Intra-Institutional Relocation', *Gerontologist*, 14, pp. 293-5.

Linn, M.W. (1974), 'Predicting Quality of Patient Care in Nursing Homes', *Gerontologist*, 14, pp. 225-7.

Linn, M.W., and Gurel, L. (1972), 'Family Attitudes in Nursing Home Placement', *Gerontologist*, 12, pp. 220-4.

Lipman, A.R. (1967), 'Chairs as Territory', *New Society*, 9, pp. 564-6.

Lipman, A.R. (1968), 'Some Problems of Direct Observation in Architectural Social Research', *Architects Journal*, 147, pp. 1349-56.

Lipman, A.R., and Slater, R. (1975), 'Architectural Design Implications of Residential Homes for Old People', SSRC final report, London.

Lipman, A.R., and Slater, R. (1977a), 'Homes for Old People: Towards a Positive Environment', *Gerontologist*, 17, pp. 146-56.

Lipman, A.R., and Slater, R. (1977b), 'Status and Spatial Appropriation in Eight Homes for Old People', *Gerontologist*, 17, pp. 250-5.

Lohmann, N. (1977), 'Correlations of Life Satisfaction, Morale, and Adjustment Measures', *Journal of Gerontology*, 32, pp. 73-5.

Lohmann, N. (1978), 'A Construct Validation of Seven Measures of Life Satisfaction Adjustment and Morale', mimeograph, West Virginia University.

Lopata, H.Z. (1973), *Widowhood in an American City*, Schenkman, Cambridge, Massachusetts.

Lowenthal, M.F., and Haven, C. (1968), 'Interaction and Adaptation: Intimacy as a Critical Variable', *American Sociological Bulletin*, 33, pp. 20-30.

Luker, K.A. (1979), 'Measuring Life Satisfaction in an Elderly Female Population', *Journal of Advanced Nursing*, 4, pp. 503-11.

Lunt, B., Felce, D., Jenkins, J., and Powell, L. (1977), 'Organising Recreational Activity Sessions in a Home for the Elderly Mentally Infirm: the Effect of Different Levels of Staff Input on Resident Participation', research report 130, Health Care Evaluation Research Team, Winchester.

Lupton, T. (1971), *Management and the Social Sciences*, 2nd edn, Penguin, London.

Maas, H.S., and Kuypers, J.A. (1974), *From Thirty to Seventy*. Josey-Bass, San Francisco.

McCaffree, K.M. (1977), 'Returns to Equity Capital in Nursing Homes', discussion paper no. 7, Centre for Health Services Research, University of Washington, Seattle.

McCaffree, K.M., and Harkins, E.B. (1976), 'Evaluation of the Outcomes of Nursing Home Care', Executive Summary, Battelle Centre, Washington.

McCaffree, K.M., Muller, L., Ramathan, K.V., Maher, M., and Miller, L.C. (1975), *Profit and Growth: Allowances for Owner/Operator Contributions in a Cost Related Prospective Payment for Services System for Nursing Home Care*, American Health Care Association,

Washington, D.C.

McCaffree, K.M., Winn, S., Bennett, C.A., Morrow, G., and Crowley, D. (1977), 'Cost Data Reporting System for Nursing Home Care: final report', US Department of Commerce, Springfield, Virginia.

McClannahan, L.E. (1973a), 'Design of Living Environments for Nursing Home Residents', PhD. thesis, University of Kansas.

McClannahan, L.E. (1973b), 'Therapeutic and Prosthetic Living Environments for Nursing Home Residents', *Gerontologist*, 13, pp. 424-9.

McClannahan, L.E., and Risley, T.R. (1974), 'Design of Living Environments for Nursing Home Residents. Recruiting Attendance at Activities', *Gerontologist*, 14, pp. 236-40.

McClannahan, L., and Risley, T. (1975), 'Design of Living Environments for Nursing-Home Residents: Increasing Participation in Recreation Analysis', *Journal of Applied Behavioral Analysis*, 8, pp. 261-8.

McClelland, D.C. (1951), *Personality*, William Sloane Associates, New York.

McClelland, D.C., Atkinson, J.W., Clark, R.A., and Lowell, E.L. (1953), *The Achievement Motive*, Appleton-Century-Crofts, New York.

MacDonald, M.L., and Butler, A.K. (1974), 'Reversal of Helplessness: Producing Walking Behaviour in Nursing Home Wheelchair Residents Using Behavioural Modification Procedures', *Journal of Gerontology*, 29, pp. 97-101.

McKennell, A. (1974), 'Monitoring the Quality of American Life', in B. Strumpel (ed.), *Cognition and Affect in Judgements of Subjective Well-Being*, ISR, University of Michigan.

McQuillam, F.L.M. (1974), *Fundamentals of Nursing Home Administration*, W.B. Saunders, Pennsylvania.

Maddi, S.R. (1961), 'Affective Tone During Environmental Regularity and Change', *Journal of Abnormal and Social Psychology*, 62, pp. 338-45.

Maddi, S.R., and Andrews, S.L. (1966), 'The Need for Variety in Fantasy and Self-Description', *Journal of Personality*, 34, pp. 610-25.

Manard, B.B., Woehle, R.E., and Heilman, J.M. (1977), *Better Homes for the Old*, Lexington Books, Lexington, Massachusetts.

Mangold, R.F. (1977), 'The Effects of an Adult Education Programme on the Life Situation of Nursing Care Patients', mimeograph, Grand Rapids Public Schools.

Mangum, W.P. (1971), 'Adjustments in Special Residential Settings for the Aged: an Enquiry Based on the Kleemeier Conceptualisation', doctoral dissertation, University of South Carolina.

Markson, E.W., and Cumming, J.H. (1974), 'Social Consequences of Physical Impairments in an Ageing Population', *Gerontologist*, 9, pp. 39-46.

Martin, D. (1955), 'Institutionalisation', *Lancet*, 269, pp. 1188-90.

Martin, D.N., and Peckford, R.W. (1977), 'Hearing Impairment in Homes for the Elderly', mimeograph, North Yorkshire County

Council Social Services Department.

Maslow, A.H. (ed.) (1959), *New Knowledge in Human Values*, Harper & Row, New York.

Maslow, A.H. (1970), *Motivation and Personality*, 2nd edn, Harper & Row, New York.

Mathieu, R.P. (1971), *Hospital and Nursing Home Management*, W.B. Saunders, Pennsylvania.

Maxwell, R.J., Bader, J., and Watson, W. (1972), 'Territory and Self in a Geriatric Setting', *Gerontologist*, 12, pp. 413-17.

Meacher, M. (1972), *Taken for a Ride*, Longman, London.

Mendelson, M. (1974), *Tender Loving Greed*, Knopf, New York.

Messer, M. (1967), 'The Possibility of an Age-Concentrated Environment Becoming a Normative System', *Gerontologist*, 7, 247-50.

Milgram, S. (1965), 'Some Conditions of Obedience and Disobedience to Authority', *Human Relations*, 18, pp. 57-76.

Miller, D.B., and Barry, J.T. (1976), 'The Relationship of Off Premises Activities to the Quality of Life of Nursing Home Patients', *Gerontologist*, 16, pp. 61-4.

Minge, M.R., and Bowman, T. (1969), 'Attendants' Views of Causes of Short-Term Employment at an Institution for the Mentally Retarded', *Mental Retardation*, 7, pp. 28-30.

Mischel, W. (1973), 'Toward a Cognitive Social Learning Reconceptualization of Personality', *Psychological Review*, 80, pp. 252-83.

Molberg, E., and Brothen, T. (1977), 'Factors Affecting Nursing Homes Nursing Assistants' Intentions to Seek New Employment', mimeograph, University of Minnesota.

Montgomery, J.E. (1965), 'Living Arrangements and Housing of the Rural Aged in a Central Pennsylvania Community', Public Health Service, Washington.

Mooney, G.H. (1978), 'Planning for Balance of Care of the Elderly', *Scottish Journal of Political Economy*, 25, pp. 149-64.

Moos, R.H. (1972), 'Assessment of the Psychological Environments of Community-Orientated Psychiatric Treatment Programmes', *Journal of Abnormal Psychology*, 79, pp. 9-18.

Moos, R.H. (1974a), *Evaluating Treatment Environments: A Social Ecological Approach*, Wiley, New York.

Moos, R.H. (1974b), *Community Orientated Programmes Environment Scales Manual*, Consulting Psychological Press, Palo Alto.

Moos, R. (1975), 'Evaluating and Changing Community Settings', paper presented to American Psychological Association, Chicago.

Moos, R.H., Gauvain, M., Lemke, S., Max, W., and Mehren, B. (1979), 'Assessing the Social Environments of Sheltered Care Settings', *Gerontologist*, 19, pp. 74-82.

Moos, R.H., and Houts, P. (1970), 'Differential Effects of the Social Atmospheres of Psychiatric Wards', *Human Relations*, 23, pp. 47-70.

Moriwaki, S.Y. (1974), 'The Affect Balance Scale: a Validity Study with Aged Samples', *Journal of Gerontology*, 29, pp. 73-8.

Morris, J.N. (1974), 'Changes in Morale Experienced by Applicants to a Long-Term Care Facility as they Progress Along the Institutional Path', PhD. thesis, Brandeis University.

Morris, J.N. (1975), 'Changes in Morale Experienced by Elderly Institutional Applicants Along the Institutional Path', *Gerontologist*, 15, pp. 345-9.

Morris, J.N., and Sherwood, S. (1975), 'A Retesting and Modification of the PGC Morale Scale', *Journal of Gerontology*, 30, pp. 77-84.

Morris, J.N., Wolf, R.S., and Klerman, L.V. (1975), 'Common Themes Among Morale and Depression Scales', *Journal of Gerontology*, 30, pp. 209-15.

Morris, P. (1969), *Put Away*, Routledge & Kegan Paul, London.

Moser, C.A., and Kalton, G. (1971), *Survey Methods in Social Investigation*, Heinemann, London.

Murray, H.A. (1938), *Explorations in Personality*, Oxford University Press, New York.

Nahemow, L., and Bennett, R. (1968), 'Attitude Change with Institutionisation', unpublished report (cited in Bennett, 1970).

National Corporation for the Care of Old People (1976), *Day Care for the Elderly: The Role of Residential Homes*, Homes Advice Broadsheet no. 2, NCCOP, London.

Neill, J.E., McGuinness, B., and Warburton, R.W. (1976), 'Views of Social Workers in Homes for Children, Homes for the Elderly, Hostels and Day Centres in One Division of Hampshire County Council', mimeograph, National Institute for Social Work, London.

Neugarten, B.L. (1964), 'A Developmental View of Adult Personality', in J.E. Birren (ed.), *Relations of Development and Ageing*, Charles C. Thomas, Springfield, Illinois.

Neugarten, B.L. (1968), *Middle Age and Ageing*, University of Chicago Press.

Neugarten, B.L., Berkovitz, H., and associates (1964), *Personality in Middle and Late Life*, Atherton Press, New York.

Neugarten, B.L., Havighurst, R.J., and Tobin, S.S. (1961), 'The Measurement of Life Satisfaction', *Journal of Gerontology*, 16, pp. 134-43.

Noelker, L.S., and Harel, Z. (1977), 'Predictors of Well-Being and Survival Among Institutionalised Aged', paper presented to Gerontological Society Annual Meeting, San Francisco.

Oberleder, M. (1962), 'An Attitude Scale to Determine Adjustment in Institutions for the Aged', *Journal of Chronic Diseases*, 15, pp. 915-23.

O'Donnell, J.M., Collins, J.L., and Schuler, S. (1978), 'Psychological Perceptions of the Nursing Home: a Comparative Analysis of Staff, Resident, and Cross-Gerontological Perspectives', *Gerontologist*, 18, pp. 267-71.

Olsen, R. (1978), 'The Needs of the Elderly', *Social Work Today*, 9, 21 February, p. 17.

Organisation for Economic Cooperation and Development (1974), *Subjective Elements of Well-Being*, OECD, Paris.

Osmond, H. (1957), 'Function as a Basis of Psychiatric Ward Design', *Mental Hospitals*, 8, pp. 23-9.

Pace, C., and Stern, G. (1958), 'An Approach to the Measurement of Psychological Characteristics of College Environments', *Journal of Educational Psychology*, 49, pp. 269-77.

Palfrey, C. (1976), 'Three Models of Residential Homes for the Elderly', mimeograph, Gwent County Council Social Services Department, Cwmbran.

Palmore, E. (ed.) (1974), *Normal Ageing*, vol 2, Duke University Press.

Palmore, E., and Kivett, V. (1977), 'Change in Life Satisfaction: a Longitudinal Study of Persons Aged 46-70', *Journal of Gerontology*, 32, pp. 311-16.

Palmore, E., and Luikart, C. (1972), 'Health and Social Factors Related to Life Satisfaction', *Journal of Health and Social Behaviour*, 13, pp. 68-80.

Parkes, C.M. (1972a), *Bereavement*, International Universities Press, New York.

Parkes, C.M. (1972b), 'Components of the Reaction to Loss of a Limb, Spouse or Home', *Journal of Psychosomatic Research*, 16.

Pastalan, L.A. (1968), 'Privacy as an Expression of Human Territoriality', paper presented to Symposium on Spatial Behavior, University of Michigan.

Patterson, E.A. (1977), 'Care-Work: the Social Organisation of Old People's Homes', PhD. thesis, University of Aberdeen.

Paulig, K., and McGee, J. (1977), 'Situational Variation and Sex Differentiation in Group Interaction Patterns of the Elderly', paper presented to Gerontological Society Conference, San Francisco.

Paulson, S.R. (1974), 'Causal Analysis of Inter-Organisational Relations: an Axiomatic Theory Revisited', *Administrative Science Quarterly*, 19, pp. 319-37.

Pauly, M.V. (1974), 'The Behaviour of Non-Profit Monopolies: Alternative Models of the Hospital', in C.C. Havighurst (ed.), *Regulating Health Facilities Construction*, American Enterprises Institute for Public Policy Research, Washington, D.C.

Pauly, M.V., and Drake, D.F. (1970), 'The Effect of Third-Party Methods of Reimbursement on Hospital Performance', in H.E. Klarman (ed.), *Empirical Studies in Health Economics*, Johns Hopkins Press, Baltimore.

Payne, C. (1977), 'Caring for the Care-Givers', *Social Work Today*, 8, 18 January, 14, pp. 14-15.

Payne, C. (1978), 'What Kind of Care?', *Social Work Today*, 9, 25 July, p. 25.

Peace, S.M., Hall, J.F., and Hamblin, G.R. (1979), *The Quality of Life of the Elderly in Residential Care*, Survey Research Unit Research Report 1, North London Polytechnic.

Peck, R.C. (1955), 'Psychological Developments in the Second Half of Life', in J.E. Anderson (ed.), *Psychological Aspects of Ageing*, American Psychological Association.

Perrow, C. (1972), *Complex Organizations*, Scott Freeman, Glenview,

Illinois.

Personal Social Services Council (1975), *Living and Working in Residential Homes*, PSSC, London.

Personal Social Services Council (1977), *Residential Care Reviewed*, PSSC, London.

Piaget, J., and Inhelder, B. (1970), *The Psychology of the Child*, Basic Books, New York.

Pierce, R.C., and Clark, M.M. (1973), 'Measurement of Morale in the Elderly', *International Journal of Ageing and Human Development*, 4, pp. 83-101.

Pincus, A. (1968), 'The Definition and Measurement of the Institutional Environment in Homes for the Aged', *Gerontologist*, 8, pp. 207-10.

Pincus, A. (1968a), 'Toward a Conceptual Framework for Studying Institutional Environments in Homes for the Aged', Doctoral dissertation, University of Wisconsin.

Pincus, A., and Wood, V. (1970), 'Methodological Issues in Measuring the Environment in Institutions for the Aged and its Impact on Residents', *International Journal of Ageing and Human Development*, 1, pp. 117-26.

Pitt, B. (1974), *Psychogeriatrics*, Churchill Livingstone, Edinburgh.

Plank, D. (1977), 'Caring for the Elderly: Report of a Study of Various Means of Caring for Dependent Elderly People in Eight London Boroughs', Greater London Council Research memorandum.

Plank, D. (1978), 'The Policy Context', paper presented at SSRC-sponsored conference, Canterbury.

Pope, P.J. (1977), 'Emergency Admissions into Old People's Homes', mimeograph, Mid-Glamorgan Social Services Department, Cardiff.

Pope, P.J. (1978), 'Admissions to Residential Homes for the Elderly', *Social Work Today*, 9, 18 July, pp. 12-16.

Powell, L., Felce, D., Jenkins, J., and Lunt, B. (1977), 'Increasing Engagement in a Home for the Elderly by Providing an Indoor Gardening Activity', research report 128, Health Care Evaluation Research Team, Winchester.

Prosser, D.M. (1978), 'Finding a Fair Example of Working: Reply to Payne', *Social Work Today*, 9, 8 August, p. 11.

Prosser, R.A. (1974), 'Certificates of Need for Health Care Facilities: a Dissenting View', in C.C. Havighurst (ed.), *Regulating Health Facilities Construction*, American Enterprise Institute for Public Policy Research, Washington, D.C.

Pugh, D.S., Hickson, D.J., Hinings, C.R., and Turner, C. (1968), 'Dimensions of Organization Structure', *Administrative Science Quarterly*, 13, pp. 65-105.

Pyrek, J.D., and Snyder, L.H. (1977), 'The Human Development Inventory: a Measurement Instrument With Programmatic Application', mimeograph, Ebenezer Society, Minneapolis.

Raynes, N.V., Pratt, M.W., and Roses, S. (1979), *Organisational Structure and the Care of the Mentally Retarded*, Croom Helm, London.

Reichard, S., Livson, F., and Petersen, P.G. (1962), *Ageing and Personality*, Wiley, New York.
Reiter, J., and Nuehring, E. (1968), 'The Effects of Four Environmental Dimensions on the Adjustment of Ambulatory Residents of Nursing Homes: a Methodological Approach', mimeograph, University of Wisconsin.
Ro, K.-K. (1969), 'Incremental Pricing Would Increase Efficiency in Hospitals', *Inquiry*, 6 (1), pp. 28-36.
Ro, K.-K., and Auster, R. (1969), 'An Output Approach to Incentive Reimbursement', *Health Services Research*, 4 (3), pp. 177-87.
Robb, B. (1967), *Sans Everything – A Case to Answer*, Nelson, London.
Rodstein, M., Savitsky, E., and Starkman, R. (1976), 'Initial Adjustment to a Long-Term Care Institution: Medical and Behavioral Aspects', *Journal of American Geriatrics Society*, 24, pp. 65-71.
Rogers, C.R. (1959), 'A Theory of Therapy Personality and Interpersonal Relationships', in S. Koch (ed.), *Psychology*, vol. 3, McGraw-Hill, New York.
Rogers, C.R. (1961), *On Becoming a Person*, Houghton Miffin, Boston.
Romaniuk, M., Hoyer, F.W., and Romaniuk, J.G. (1977), 'Helpless Self-Attitudes of the Elderly: the Effect of Patronizing Statements', mimeograph, Hutchings Psychiatric Center, New York.
Roos, J.P., and Roos, B. (1976), 'Welfare Research and the Development of a Multi-Dimensional Concept of Welfare', in Eurosocial report no. 11, *Use of Social Research in the Preparation, Implementation, and Evaluation of Social Welfare Programmes*, Vienna.
Rose, A. (1965), 'Group Consciousness Among the Ageing', in A. Rose and W.A. Peterson (eds), *Older People and their Social World*, Davis, Philadelphia.
Rosencranz, H.A. (1974), 'Sociology of ageing', in W.C. Bier (ed.), *Ageing: Its Challenge to the Individual and to Society*, Fordham University Press.
Rosow, I. (1963), 'Adjustment of the Normal Aged', in R.H. Williams, C. Tibbitts, and W. Donahue (eds), *Processes of Ageing*, vol. 2, Atherton Press, New York.
Rosow, I. (1967), *Social Integration of the Aged*, Free Press, New York.
Rubenstein, J., and Rubenstein, B. (1972), 'Effect of Young Persons on Nursing Home Patients', *Geriatrics*, 27, p. 124 and p. 130.
Russell, L. (1973), 'The Impact of Extended-Care Facility Benefit on Hospital Use and Reimbursements Under Medicare', *Journal of Human Resources*, 8 (1), pp. 57-72.
Savage, R.D., Gaber, L.B., Britton, P.G., Bolton, N., and Cooper, A. (1977), *Personality and Adjustment in the Aged*, Academic Press, London.
Schmidt, M.G. (1975), 'Interviewing the "Old Old" ', *Gerontologist*, 15, pp. 544-7.
Schoenberg, B.C., Carr, A.C., Peretz, D., and Kutscher, A.H. (1972),

Psychological Aspects of Terminal Care, Columbia University Press.

Schooler, K.K. (1970a), 'Residential Physical Environment and Health of the Aged', mimeograph, Brandeis University.

Schooler, K.K. (1970b), 'Effect of Environment on Morale', *Gerontologist*, 10, pp. 194-7.

Schooler, K.K. (1974), 'Response of the Elderly to Environment: a Stress-Theoretical Perspective', paper presented to Gerontological Society Conference, Manhatten, Kansas.

Schulz, R. (1976), 'Effect of Control and Predictability on the Physical and Psychological Well-Being of the Institutional Aged', *Journal of Personality and Social Psychology*, 33, pp. 563-73.

Schulz, R., and Alderman, D. (1973), 'Effect of Residential Change on the Temporal Distance of Death of Terminal Cancer Patients', *Omega: Journal of Death and Dying*, 4, pp. 157-62.

Schulz, R., and Brenner, G. (1977), 'Relocation of the Aged: a Review and Theoretical Analysis', *Journal of Gerontology*, 32, pp. 323-33.

Schwartz, A.N. (1975), 'An Observation on Self-Esteem as the Linchpin of Quality of Life for the Aged. An Essay', *Gerontologist*, 15, pp. 470-2.

Schwartz, A.N., and Proppe, H. (1969), 'Perception of Privacy Among Institutionalised Aged', *Proceedings of 77th Annual Convention*, American Psychological Association.

Schwartz, A.N., and Proppe, H. (1970), 'Toward Person/Environment Transactional Research in Ageing', *Gerontologist*, 10, pp. 228-32.

Scottish Education Department, Social Work Services Group (1976), *Residential Census and Unit Return Forms, 1976-77, (and notes for guidance)*, Edinburgh.

Seelbach, W.C., and Sauer, W.J. (1977), 'Filial Responsibility Expectations and Morale Among Aged Parents', *Gerontologist*, 17, pp. 492-9.

Seligman, M.E. (1975), *Helplessness*, Freeman, San Francisco.

Sen, A.K. (1970), *Collective Choice and Social Welfare*, Oliver & Boyd, London.

Sen, A.K. (1977), 'Social Choice Theory: a Re-examination', *Econometrica*, 45 (1), pp. 53-89.

Shanas, E. (1961), 'Family Relationships of Older People', Health Information Foundation, research series 20, University of Chicago.

Shanas, E., Townsend, P., Wedderburn, D., Friis, H., Milhøj, P., and Stehouwer, J. (1968), *Older People in Three Industrial Societies*, Atherton Press, New York.

Sherman, E., and Newman, E.S. (1977), 'The Meaning of Cherished Personal Possessions for the Elderly', *International Journal of Ageing and Human Development*, 8, pp. 181-92.

Sherwood, S. (1972), 'Social Gerontology and Research Strategies', in D.P. Kent *et al.* (eds), *Research Planning and Action for the Elderly*, Behavioural Publications, New York.

Sherwood, S., Morris, J.N., and Barnhart, E. (1975), 'Developing a System for Assigning Individuals into an Appropriate Residential Setting', *Journal of Gerontology*, 30, pp. 331-42.

Sherwood, S., and Nadelson, T. (1972), 'Alternate Predictions Concerning Despair in Old Age', in D.P. Kent *et al.* (eds), *Research Planning and Action for the Elderly*, Behavioral Publications, New York.

Shulman, D., and Galanter, R. (1976), 'Reorganising the Nursing Home Industry: a Proposal', *Milbank Memorial Fund Quarterly*, 54, pp. 129-43.

Silverstone, B., and Wynter, L. (1975), 'The Effects of Introducing a Heterosexual Living Space', *Gerontologist*, 15, pp. 83-7.

Sinclair, I. (1971), *Hostels for Probationers*, HMSO, London.

Skoglund, J. (1978), 'A Comparative Factor Analysis of Attitudes Toward Societal Relations of the Elderly', *International Journal of Ageing and Human Development*, 8, pp. 277-91.

Slater, R. (1968), 'The Adjustment of Residents in Old People's Homes: Consideration of Important Factors', *British Journal of Geriatric Practice*, 5, pp. 299-302.

Slater, R., and Lipman, A.R. (1977), 'Staff Assessments of Confusion and the Situation of Confused Residents in Homes for Old People', *Gerontologist*, 17, pp. 523-30.

Smith, J.J., and Lipman, A.R. (1972), 'Staff Assessment of "Confusion" and the Situation of Confused Residents in Homes for Old People', mimeograph.

Snyder, L.H., Rupprecht, P., Pyrek, J., Brekhus, S., and Moss, T. (1978), 'Wandering', *Gerontologist*, 18, pp. 272-80.

Somers, H.M., and Somers, A.R. (1967), *Medicare and the Hospitals*, Brookings Institute, Washington, D.C.

Sommer, R., and Osmond, H. (1960), 'Symptoms of Institutional Care', *Social Problems*, 3, pp. 244-53.

Spasoff, R.A., Kraus, A.S., Beattie, E.J., Holden, D.E.W., Lawson, J.S., Rosenburg, M., and Woodcock, G.M. (1978), 'A Longtitudinal Study of Elderly Residents of Long-Stay Institutions', *Gerontologist*, 18, pp. 281-92.

Srole, L. (1956), 'Social Integration and Certain Corollaries', *American Sociological Review*, 21, pp. 709-16.

Stanton, A.H., and Schwartz, M.S. (1954), *The Mental Hospital*, Basic Books, New York.

Stanton, B.R. (1971), *Meals for the Elderly*, King Edward's Hospital Fund, London.

Stathopoulos, P. (1977), 'Gerontologists and Advocacy', mimeograph, Brandeis University.

Stern, G. (1970), *People in Context*, Wiley, New York.

Stern, G., Stein, M., and Bloom, B. (1956), *Methods in Personality Assessment*, Free Press, New York.

Stevenson, O. *et al.* (1978), 'Social Work Research Project: Final Report', mimeograph.

Stotsky, B.A. (1967), 'A Controlled Study of Factors in the Successful Adjustment of Mental Patients to Nursing Homes', *American Journal of Psychiatry*, 123, pp. 1243-51.

Streib, G.F. (1971), 'New Roles and Activities for Retirement', in

Bibliography

G.L. Maddox (ed.), *The Future of Ageing and the Aged*, SNPA Foundation, Atlanta.

Sumner, G., and Smith, R. (1969), *Planning Local Authority Services for the Elderly*, Allen & Unwin, London.

Teaff, J.D., Lawton, M.P., Nahemow, L., and Carlson, D. (1978), 'Impact of Age Integration on the Well-Being of Elderly Tenants in Public Housing', *Journal of Gerontology*, 33, pp. 126-33.

Thomas, N., Gough, J., and Spencely, H. (1979), *An Evaluation of the Group Unit Design for Old People's Homes*, DHSS, London.

Thormalen, P.W. (1965), *A Study of on-the-ward Training of Trainable Mentally Retarded Children in a State Institution*, Sacramento, California, Department of Mental Hygiene.

Thurnher, M. (1974), 'Goals, Values and Life Evaluations at the Pre-Retirement Stage', *Journal of Gerontology*, 29, pp. 85-96.

Titmuss, R. (1972), *The Gift Relationship*, Allen & Unwin, London.

Tizard, B., Cooperman, O., Joseph, A., and Tizard, J. (1972), 'Environmental Effects on Language Development: a Study of Young Children in Long-Stay Residential Nurseries', *Child Development*, 43, pp. 337-58.

Tizard, J. (1964), *Community Services for the Mentally Handicapped*, Oxford University Press.

Tizard, J., Sinclair, I., and Clarke, R.V.G. (1975), *Varieties of Residential Experience*, Routledge & Kegan Paul, London.

Tobin, S.S., and Lieberman, M.A. (1976), *Last Home for the Aged*, Jossey-Bass, San Francisco.

Townsend, J., and Kimbell, A. (1975), 'Caring Regimes in Elderly Persons' Homes', *Health and Social Services Journal*, 11 October, p. 2286.

Townsend, J., Kimbell, A., and Bird, M. (1974), 'A Study of Various Aspects of Regime and Activities in Elderly Persons' Homes and Their Effect Upon the Residents', mimeograph, Cheshire County Council Social Services Department.

Townsend, P. (1962), *The Last Refuge*, Routledge & Kegan Paul, London.

Tunstall, J. (1966), *Old and Alone*, Routledge & Kegan Paul, London.

Turner, B.F. (1969), 'Psychological Predictors of Adaptation to the Stress of Institutionalisation in the Aged', unpublished Doctoral thesis, University of Chicago.

Turner, B.F., Tobin, S.S., and Lieberman, M.A. (1972), 'Personality Traits as Predictors of Institutional Adaptation Among the Aged', *Journal of Gerontology*, 27, pp. 61-8.

Utting, B. (1977), 'Residential Care — the End or the Beginning', *Social Work Today*, 19, 11 October, pp. 14-17.

Verry, D.W., and Davies, B.P. (1975), *University Costs and Outputs*, Elsevier, Amsterdam.

Wager, R. (1972), *Care of the Elderly*, Institute of Municipal Treasurers and Accountants, London.

Walton, R. (1978), 'The Survival Syndrome', *Social Work Today*, 9, 11 April, p. 20.

Bibliography

Ward, L. (1977), 'Social Work By Social Workers', *Social Work Today*, 8, 18 January, pp. 1-2.
Weinstock, C.S. (1974), 'Successful Ageing: a Psychological Viewpoint', in W.C. Bier (ed.), *Ageing: Its Challenge to the Individual and to Society*, Fordham University Press.
Weiss, L.J. (1977), 'Intimacy: an Intervening Factor in Adaptation', paper presented to Gerontological Society Conference, San Francisco.
White, R.W. (1959), 'Motivation Reconsidered: the Concept of Competence', *Psychological Review*, 66, pp. 297-333.
Wicks, M. (1978), *Old and Cold: Hypothermia and Social Policy*, Heinemann, London.
Wilkinson, R.K. (1973), 'House Prices and the Measurement of Externalities', *Economic Journal*, 83, pp. 72-86.
Williams, A. (1977), 'Measuring the Quality of Life of the Elderly', in L. Wingo and A. Evans (eds), *Public Economics and the Quality of Life*, Johns Hopkins University Press.
Williams, A., and Anderson, R. (1975), *Efficiency in the Social Services*, Basil Blackwell, Oxford, and Martin Robertson, London.
Williams, G. (Chairman) (1967), *Caring for People. Report of a Committee of Enquiry set up by the National Council of Social Services*, Allen & Unwin, London.
Wilson, J. (1977), 'Dear Howard Harris', *Social Work Today*, 9, 29 November, p. 9.
Wilson, J.Q. (1974), 'The Politics of American Business Regulation', in J. McKie (ed.), *Social Responsibility and the Business Predicament*, Brookings Institute, Washington, D.C.
Wilson, N. (1967), 'Correlates of Avowed Happiness', *Psychological Bulletin*, 67, pp. 294-306.
Wilson, S.H. (1978), 'Nursing Home Patients' Rights: Are They Enforceable?', *Gerontologist*, 18 (3), pp. 255-61.
Wing, J.K., and Brown, G.W. (1970), *Institutionalism and Schizophrenia*, Cambridge University Press.
Wiseman, M., and Silverman, G. (1974), 'Evaluating Social Services: Did the General Accounting Office Help?', *Social Service Review*, 48, pp. 315-26.
Wittels, I., and Botwinick, J. (1974), 'Survival in Relocation', *Journal of Gerontology*, 29, pp. 440-3.
Wolk, S., and Kurtz, J. (1975), 'Positive Adjustment and Involvement During Ageing and Expectancy for Internal Control', *Journal of Consulting and Clinical Psychology*, 43, pp. 173-8.
Wolk, S., and Telleen, S. (1976), 'Psychological and Social Correlates of Life Satisfaction as a Function of Residential Constraint', *Journal of Gerontology*, 31, pp. 89-98.
Wood, V., Wylie, M., and Sheafor, B. (1969), 'An Analysis of a Short Self-Report Measure of Life Satisfaction: Correlation with Rater Judgements', *Journal of Gerontology*, 24, pp. 465-9.
Wright, K.G. (1974), 'Alternative Measures of Output of Social Programmes: the Elderly', in A.J. Culyer (ed.), *Economic Policies*

and Social Goals, Martin Robertson, London.

Wright, K.G. (1978), 'Output Measurement in Practice', in A.J. Culyer and K.G. Wright (eds), *Economic Aspects of Health Services*, Martin Robertson, London.

Wylie, M.L. (1970), 'Life Satisfaction as a Program Impact Criterion', *Journal of Gerontology*, 25, pp. 36-40.

Yawney, B.A., and Slover, D.L. (1973), 'Relocation of the Elderly', *Social Work*, 18, pp. 86-95.

Zach, H. (1978), 'Death and Dying – Loss and Mourning', *Social Work Today*, 9, 13 June, pp. 11-12.

Zimbardo, P., Haney, C., and Banks, W.C. (1975), 'A Prandellian Prison', in E. Krupat (ed.), *Psychology is Social*, Scott, Foresman, Glenview, Illinois.

Index

Abrams, M., 212, 218
Abrams, P., 7, 218
accommodation to social environment, 125, 127, 129
accountability, 10, 133, 176; political accountability, 84
Acito, F., 80, 218
activation, 37, 46, 50, 116
activity, 26-9, 30, 31, 35, 42, 44, 60, 68, 75, 77, 78, 81, 82, 92, 96, 98, 100-1, 103, 104, 110, 111, 113, 119, 126, 133, 137, 138, 141, 142, 154, 157, 158, 159, 167, 183, 196, 201, 207-9, 216; see also engaged activity
Activity Theory of Ageing, 30, 40, 138, 168, 207
Adams, D. L., 44, 213, 218
adaptation, 126, 131, 141, 148; psychological and behavioural adaptation, 33
adaptation level, 127, 128, 180
adaptive behaviour, 127, 180
adaptive demands of the environment, 148
adaptive responses, 144, 155
adjustment, 25, 33, 68, 125-6, 131, 134, 140-1, 148, 149, 151, 153, 154, 155-61, 181, 184, 216; see also development task adjustment
admission to the home, 61-3, 80, 111, 137, 144-5, 148, 149-61, 170, 184; admission practices, 156; emergency admissions, 150
affect, 25, 39, 41, 45-8, 50, 51-2, 53, 68, 97, 118, 119, 127, 128, 131, 138, 143, 145, 168, 171, 204-9; affective responses, 127;

see also happiness; life satisfaction; morale; psychological well-being
Affect Balance Scale, 26, 40, 45-8, 51, 52, 168, 171, 204-9
Age Concern, 4, 218
ageing, 58-9, 171, 207, 214; socio-environmental theory of ageing, 131; typologies of ageing, 30-1, 168
agitation, 51, 171, 213
Aiken, M., 80, 81, 218
aims, see objectives
Albrecht, R., 40, 226
Alderman, D., 56, 238
Aldrich, C. K., 156, 218
Allardt, E., 12, 218
Allen, D., 4, 218
Allen, G. J., 76, 226
Almond, R., 33, 219
Aloia, A. J., 137, 218
altruism, 6-7
Alutto, T., 80, 218
Andersen, R., 217, 218
Anderson, J., 62, 221
Anderdon, N., 76, 90, 91, 218
Anderson, R. 17, 241
Andrews, S. L., 232
anomie, 39; Srole's Anomie Scale, 51
anxiety, 39, 46, 50, 51, 59, 63, 95, 148, 152, 156, 209
approach motive, 27, 37
Apte, R. Z., 110, 218
architects, 91, 92, 96, 100, 102
architectural characteristics, see design of home
Arrow, K. J., 210, 219
assimilation of social environment,

243

125, 127, 128
Aston Group, 79, 85, 175-6
Atchley, R. C., 55-6, 63, 134, 214, 219
Atkinson, J. W., 28, 37, 219, 232
attitude, *see* resident attitudes; staff attitudes
Attitude Inventory, 52
Aucoin, J. B., 155, 220
Auster, R., 217, 237
autonomy, 35, 134, 135, 143, 156, 167, 176, 183
Averill, J., 133, 219
avoidance motive, 27, 37

Bader, J., 96, 135, 219, 233
Balance of Care Model, 17-18
Baltz, T. M., 87, 177, 219
Banks, W. C., 88, 242
Barker, R., 109, 219
Barnhart, E., 128, 238
Barrett, A., 89, 92-103, 113, 182, 215, 219
Barry, J. T., 138, 233
Barton, R., 100, 159, 219
Bates, K., 159, 219
bathrooms and toilets, 73-4, 89, 93, 94, 99-100, 102, 103, 136, 182
Battelle Health Care Study Centre, 73, 74-5, 175, 214, 219
Battista, J., 33, 219
Beattie, E. J., 149, 153, 157-9, 239
Beattie, W. M., 91, 219
Bebbington, A. C., viii
bedrooms, 89, 93, 94, 95-7, 99, 102, 103, 116, 136, 145, 167, 182; distribution within home, 89; number of residents per bedroom, 77; residents' preferences, 96; sharing, 7
Beiser, M., 47-8, 205, 209, 219
Bender, A. E., 107, 222
benefits to residents not contributing directly to psychological well-being, 55-61, 169; *see also* outputs; significant others
Bennett, A. E., 135, 219
Bennett, C. A., 73-5, 175, 232
Bennett, R. G., 55, 109, 111-13, 114, 141, 142, 143, 149, 151, 157, 178-9, 219, 234
bereavement, 55, 63, 154, 156, 214
Berkovitz, H., 234
Berliner, J. S., 17, 220
Berlyne, D. E., 128, 220

Berman, A., 110, 228
Bevan, A., 90, 167
Bigot, A., 44, 212, 220
Bild, B., 47, 220
Billiis, D., 10, 220
Binstock, R., 17, 38
Bird, M., 240
Blau, P. M., 81, 131, 220
block treatment, 93, 99, 110, 112
Bloom, B., 109, 120, 239
Blunden, R., 26, 28, 57, 138, 220, 229
Boldy, D., 213, 220
Bolton, N., 212, 216, 237
boredom, 34, 205
Botwinick, J., 56, 241
Bourestom, N. C., 214, 225
Bowman, T., 83, 233
Bradburn, N. M., 39, 45-8, 52, 204-9
Brearley, C. P., 36, 38, 87, 150, 210, 220
Brekhus, S., 59, 135, 143, 239
Brenner, G., 56, 144, 152-3, 156, 183, 215, 237
Breytspraak, L. M., 39, 220
British Association of Social Workers, 85, 150, 156, 220
Britton, P. G., 212, 216, 237
Brody, E. M., 92, 230
Brophy, J. G., 58-9, 220
Brothen, T., 76, 83, 233
Brown, G. W., 110, 241
building design, *see* design of home; design recommendations
Bull, C. N., 155, 220
Bullock, J., 91, 219
Bultena, G., 45, 141-2, 143, 183, 220-1
bureaucracy, Weber's theory of, 79
bureaucratic ideologies, 83, 84
Burgess, E. M., 39, 40, 52, 221
Butler, A. K., 57, 232
Butler, R. N., 154, 221

Calhoun, J., 128, 221
Callahan, J. J., 221
Cameron, P., 39, 221
Campbell, A., 52, 221
Cannell, C. F., 204, 221
Cantril, H., 52-3, 221
capital, 7, 18, 69, 75, 88-106, 172-85, 197; capital expenditure, 104, 106, 188, 192, 193; rate of return, 190, 191, 192, 195, 196
Caplovitz, D., 39, 45-8, 220

Carlson, D., 142, 240
Carlson, J. R., 213, 228
Carp, F. M., 56, 144, 221
Carr, A. C., 143, 237
Carstairs, V., 72, 89, 90, 221
Cartwright, A., 62, 221
Cavan, R., 39, 40, 52, 140, 221
census of residential accommodation,
    70, 89-91, 95-100, 104-6, 182
centralisation, 79, 80-1, 84, 175-6
Challis, D. J., viii, 58, 59, 60, 171,
    213, 215, 221
Chang, B. L., 134, 221
charges, 189-90, 194, 198-9
Charon, H., 96, 230
Chatters, L., 52, 227
Cheshire County Council, Social
    Services Department, 28, 60,
    88, 111, 113, 221
children, care of, 80, 111, 178, 192
Chinsky, J. M., 76, 226
choice, 38, 99, 100, 114, 115, 119,
    136, 143
Cicirelli, V. G., 63, 221
citizens' outputs, 169-70
Clark, M. M., 39, 51, 236
Clark, R. A., 37, 232
Clarke, R. V. G., 80, 182, 240
cleanliness, 16, 61, 171, 182
coding behaviour, 109, 125, 146
Coe, R. M., 112, 221, 227
Cohen, J., 57, 230
Cohen, S. Z., 87, 229
Coleman, P., 39, 149, 221-2
Collins, J. L., 122, 234
communication, 71, 80, 81-2, 92,
    110, 115, 116, 136, 137, 138-41,
    176, 183; see also interaction
Community Oriented Programmes
    Environment Scale (COPES),
    121-4
community services, 4, 18
competence, 35, 40, 61, 98, 99, 109,
    120-32, 137, 140, 143, 144, 146,
    159-60, 180, 214, 215
compliance, 125
conformity, 112, 151, 157
confused residents, 3, 4, 59, 60, 88,
    98, 129, 141, 143, 145
confusion, 59-60, 68, 76, 113, 134,
    184, 205
congregation, 108, 111, 114-20, 141-3,
    179; see also social distance,
    spatial proximity
congruence, 119; environmental

congruence, 14, 25, 27-8, 29-38,
    60, 109, 115, 118, 120, 121, 125,
    128, 137, 147, 148, 168, 179-80,
    181, 199; goal congruence, 41,
    42, 44, 171, 202, 213
consequences of care, see outputs
consumables, 7, 69, 106-7, 182
Contingency Theory, 83-4, 85, 176
continuity, 168; of environment,
    104, 118, 141, 143-6, 149, 183;
    of relationships, 83; of self, 39,
    119, 183; see also relocation
control, 55, 56, 67, 68, 84, 120;
    of capital, 193; motor control,
    98, 119, 134-5, 183, 215; psycho-
    motor control, 135, 182; psycho-
    pharmacological control, 135,
    182; social control, 114, 133,
    138, 139, 215; see also institutional
    control
controllability and predictability
    of relocation, 144, 156
Converse, P., 52, 221
Cooper, A., 212, 216, 237
Cooperman, O., 76, 80, 240
Copeland, J. R. M., 59, 222
corridors, 88, 94, 95, 98, 102, 103
cost, 16, 73, 74, 90, 106, 169, 177,
    189-90, 191, 192, 195, 196, 197,
    198, 215; cost-effectiveness,
    4, 199; function, 15, 197, 198,
    211; minimisation, 193; replace-
    ment cost depreciation, 197, 198
Crawford, M. P., 28, 222
Crowley, D., 73-5, 175, 232
culture, 83, 187; subculture of ageing,
    141-3
Cumming, E., 30, 39, 40, 56, 222
Cumming, J. H., 232
Curran, W. J., 217, 222
Curry, T. J., 16, 45, 76, 91, 92, 175
    222

Davies, B. P., 11, 12, 15, 90, 168,
    185, 194, 197, 210, 211, 215,
    222, 240
Davies, L., 107, 222
Davies, M., 14, 222
Davies, R. M., 62, 222
Davis, K., 217, 222
day-care services, 3, 61, 104, 138;
    as determinant of staffing levels,
    73-4, 175
Deane, M., 135, 219
death, 35, 42, 55-7, 61, 63, 75, 87,

Index

134, 142, 149, 153, 154, 214;
social death, 55, 56, 87; *see also*
bereavement; mortality
De Long, A. J., 109, 125, 127, 222-3
demand, 95, 104, 174, 189, 190,
192-3; demands of political
accountability, 84; *see also* need
demographic trends, effects on policy,
192-3
Department of Health and Social
Security, 5, 9, 70, 71, 72, 85-6,
89-105, 138, 145, 182, 189, 211,
215, 223; Social Work Service,
9, 133
dependency, 4, 17, 57, 68, 71, 73-5,
78, 93, 100, 102, 113, 119, 129,
133, 134, 135, 138, 145, 150,
158, 159, 174-5, 190
depersonalisation, 93, 112, 113, 117,
118, 145, 175, 183
depression, 39, 59, 63, 134, 152,
154, 156, 205, 213
design of home, 13, 16, 60, 76,
88-106, 115, 116, 135, 136,
172, 175, 177, 182. design recommendations, 89, 90, 92, 95, 97,
99, 102, 105, 194; as determinant
of staffing levels, 71, 73-4, 75;
micro-design, 102-3, 122
developmental stages, 36, 52
developmental task, 30, 31, 36, 46,
47, 52
developmental task adjustment, 47-8,
50, 154
deviance, 112, 142
diet, 6, 10, 61, 63, 93, 103, 106-7,
171, 173, 182, 199
Diewart, W. E., 211, 223
dignity, 26, 38
dining rooms, 89, 93, 94, 99, 100,
182; as determinant of staffing
levels, 73-4
disability, *see* dependency; residents'
characteristics
discharging, 75, 80, 158
disengagement, 28, 30, 125, 142,
158-9
Disengagement Theory, 28, 30, 40,
138, 168
documentation, 84
Doke, L. A., 27, 100, 223
domains of living, 52
domestic v. institutional design, 90-1,
92-3, 94, 95, 98, 99, 101, 103,
178, 182, 215

domiciliary services, 3, 61, 192
Dominic, J. R., 151, 223
doors, 94, 96, 102, 103, 129, 182
Dorset County Council, Social Services
Department, 134, 145, 223
Dowd, J. J., 31, 131, 223
Drake, D. F., 217, 235
Drevenstedt, J., 48, 223
Duncan, I. B., 62, 222
Duncan, T. L. C., 105, 223

East Sussex County Council, Social
Services Department, 139, 223
economics, 7, 17, 18, 62, 67, 70,
104, 106, 165, 172, 187, 198
economies of scale, 12, 167, 191
Edwards, J. N., 45, 213, 223, 228
effectiveness, 18, 62, 69, 74, 81, 83,
137, 192, 199; *see also* cost, cost-
effectiveness; outputs
efficiency, 10, 74, 133, 185, 195,
197-8, 211
ego-differentiation, 36
ego-integration, 31, 35-6, 41, 46,
49-50
ego-preoccupation, 36
ego-transcendence, 36, 41
Eighth Report of the Expenditure
Committee, 211, 223
Eisdorfer, C., 112, 142, 219
Elias, B. M., 140, 223
Elliott, A., 135, 219
employment function, 73; *see also*
staff
endogeneity, 8, 14, 67, 210
engaged activity, 25, 26-9, 168, 171
engagement, 25, 31, 72, 137, 138
Engagement Theory, *see* Disengagement Theory
entrance and exit points, 93-4
environmental docility hypothesis,
120, 124, 125-7, 141, 180
environmental press, 56, 59, 109, 114,
120-32, 146, 179, 180, 183, 215; alpha
press, 126, 130; beta press, 126
equilibrium between environmental
press and individual competence,
127
Erikson, E. H., 31, 34-6, 39, 41, 123,
154, 224
Ernst, M., 58-9, 220
exchange theory, 109, 131, 132; *see
also* transactional models
exogeneity, 8, 14, 67, 210
expectations, 6, 14, 55, 134, 144, 159

experiences of residents prior to
  admission, 7, 14, 18, 68, 149-52,
  157, 161, 181, 184, 216
Exton-Smith, A. N., 107, 224
'extra care' units, 3

fabric index for old people's homes,
  74, 105, 215
Fairhurst, E., 139, 140, 183, 224
Fanshel, S., 17-18, 58, 210, 211, 224
Fawcett, G., 134, 224
Feder, J. M., 224
Felce, D., 26, 72, 137-8, 227, 231,
  236
Feldstein, M. S., 211, 224
Felton, B., 134, 224
final output, see output
financial accounts, 194-5, 196
financial exploitation of residents,
  193-6, 199
fire, 61, 101, 194
fire precautions, 94, 95, 101-2, 169-70,
  194
fire regulations, 94, 190
Fisher, J., 214, 224
Fiske, D. W., 34, 37, 128, 224
fit, see congruence
Fleming, R. W., 212, 224
flexibility of care, 81, 91, 98, 174, 183
food, see diet
formalisation, 79-80, 81, 84, 91, 110,
  112, 176, 182
frailty, see dependency; residents'
  characteristics
Fried, C., 156, 224
friendship, 92, 94-5, 138, 140-1, 143,
  150, 157; see also interaction;
  social niches
Friis, H., 63, 238
Fromm, E., 34, 36, 123, 224
furniture, 89, 97, 182; residents' own
  furniture, 107; see also personal
  possessions of residents

Gaber, L. B., 212, 216, 237
Galanter, R., 197, 217, 239
Gauvain, M., 122, 233
George, L. K., 39, 220
gerontology, 11, 16, 17, 18, 38,
  45, 55, 57, 96, 107, 129
goals, 33, 121, 154, 171, 202; goals
  of care, see objectives
Goffman, E., 76, 80, 108, 109, 110-14,
  115, 133, 141, 146, 148, 178,
  224

Golant, S. M., 61, 126, 134, 215,
  224
Goldberg, E. M., 50, 120, 224
Goldhamer, H., 40, 52, 221
Goldsmith, S., 91, 96, 99, 100, 224
Gottesman, L. E., 91, 214, 224
Gough, J., 91, 106, 240
Gouldner, A. W., 6, 225
Graney, M. J., 47, 56, 130, 142,
  143, 204, 207-8, 225
Grant, G. W. B., 76, 225
Greenblatt, D. L., 151, 223
Greenfield, P., 71, 225
Greenwald, S. R., 16, 63, 92, 225
Greenwood, R., 83-4, 225
Gresham, M. L., 134, 225
group unit design, 91, 93, 106, 182
Grusky, O., 81, 225
Gubrium, J. F., 87, 118, 126, 131,
  141, 142, 183, 225
Gurel, L., 62, 231

Hage, J., 80, 81, 218
Hall, J. F., 26, 48, 52, 60, 204-9,
  210, 217, 225, 235
Hall, R. H., 80, 226
Hamblin, G., 26, 48, 204-9, 235
Haney, C., 88, 242
happiness, 36, 39, 46, 53, 171, 205,
  207, 209
Harel, Z., 56, 234
Haringey London Borough, Social
  Services Department, 100, 226
Harkins, E. B., 16, 50, 214, 231
Harris, A. I., 89, 226
Harris, D., 86, 132, 226
Harris, H., 89, 132, 137, 226
Harris, J. M., 76, 226
Harris, S. E., 217, 226
Hastrop, K., 107, 222
Hathaway, S., 39, 226
Hauser, D. L., 204, 211
Haven, C., 141, 231
Havighurst, C. C., 217, 226
Havighurst, R. J., 31, 38-9, 40-5,
  47, 50, 52, 201-3, 212, 220, 221,
  226, 234
head of home, see staff, supervisory
Heal, K., 111, 226
health, 57-60, 62, 74, 125, 136, 131,
  141, 152, 154-5, 159, 184, 204,
  214; biological health, 57; func-
  tion health, 57, 58, 59, 126,
  152, 171, 214; self-rated health,
  39, 57, 58, 140, 141, 154-5, 158,

171; social health, *see* functional
health; *see also* competence,
dependency; residents' character-
istics
health authorities, 4, 71
health care, 18, 71, 74, 80, 81, 153,
157, 198, 211
hedonism, 46
Heilman, J. M., 56, 72, 215, 217,
232
Hellinger, F. J., 217, 226
Helson, H., 127, 226
Henry, J., 82, 226
Henry, W. E., 30, 39, 40, 222
Herzog, A. R., 52, 227
Hickson, D. J., 85, 236
Hinings, C. R., 85, 236
Hirsch, F., 6-7, 226
'hit and run' workers, 82, 173
Hitch, D., 92, 226
Hixson, J. S., 217, 226
Hobman, D., 90, 226-7
Hockey, L., 62, 221
Holden, D. E. W., 149, 153, 157-9,
239
Holdsworth, M. D., 107, 227
Holland, T., 80, 227
Holland, W. W., 135, 219
Holmberg, R. H., 76, 90, 91, 218
homes: age, 96, 97; general resources,
101; original function, 73, 90,
96, 97, 99, 100, 104, 143, 182;
state of repair, 103
Homes for the Aged Descriptive
Questionnaire, 109, 115-18, 130,
179
homogeneity, 110, 113-18, 130,
141-3, 183
Hopkins, T., 192, 227
hospitals, *see* health care
housing departments, 4
Houts, P., 120, 233
Hoyer, F. W., 86, 139-40, 237
Hull, J., 217, 218
humanist psychologists, 33-8
hypothermia, 107, 215

identity, 35, 94, 137, 160
illness, 42; *see also* health
Imber, V., 70, 78, 173, 182, 215, 227
impulse control, 119
incentive reimbursement, 197-200
independence, 26, 38, 61, 93, 95,
98, 99, 100, 121, 122, 133-4, 137,
142, 167, 178, 183, 215

individuality, 38, 78, 81, 82, 83, 87,
110, 112, 119, 133-4, 183, 215,
216
'infantilisation' of residents, 134
Inhelder, B., 127, 236
inputs, 5, 7-9, 13, 16, 18, 24, 54, 57,
61, 63-4, 67-161, 166, 172-85,
194, 199, 211; quasi-inputs and
non-resource inputs, 7-9, 18, 29,
50, 57, 67-8, 77, 106-7, 108-61,
168, 170, 172-85, 194; resource
inputs, 3, 4, 6, 7-9, 10-11, 13, 16,
18, 37, 67-8, 69-107, 116-17, 119,
124, 128, 135, 161, 166, 170,
172-85; *see also* capital; consumables; diet; manpower; social
environment; staff
input-output function, *see* production
function
Institute of Municipal Treasurers and
Accountants (IMTA), 10, 210, 227
institutional control, 108, 114-20, 121,
179, 183
institutionalisation, 68, 71, 128-9,
148, 152, 154-61, 167; stages of,
160, 179; *see also* domestic v.
institutional design
'institutional neurosis', 100, 159
integrity, 123
intellect, 59, 80, 138
interaction, 6, 26-9, 94-5, 96, 100,
110, 113, 114, 115, 123, 129,
131, 137 138-41, 142, 148, 150,
151-2, 183, 201; resident-
community interaction, 93-4,
138-41, 151, 160; resident-resident
interaction, 94-5, 97-8, 126, 137,
138-41, 159; resident-staff interaction, 76, 78, 83, 86-7, 96, 97-8,
99, 102, 113, 121, 122, 138-41,
174, 176; *see also* communication;
friendship; social distance
internal scale of homes, 94-5, 182
intimacy, 35, 135, 136, 183
intra-psychic symptoms, 39
Isaacs, B., 62, 227
isolation, 16, 35, 59, 62, 91, 92, 96,
115, 117, 141, 143, 151, 152,
213; Adult Isolation Index, 151-2;
Pre-Entry Isolation Index, 151-2
Ittleston, W. H., 96, 136, 227

Jackson, D. W., 157, 227
Jackson, J. M., 117, 227
Jackson, J. S., 52, 227

Jenkins, J., 26, 72, 137-8, 227, 231, 236
joint financing, 72, 173
joint supply, 187
Jones, D. C., 227
Joseph, A., 76, 80, 240

Kahana, B., 142, 227
Kahana, E., 30, 108, 109, 112, 115, 118-20, 128, 130, 133, 134-5, 142, 146 179, 224, 227
Kahn, R. L., 17, 228
Kalish, R. A., 63, 227-8
Kalton, G., 212, 234
Karcher, C. J., 62, 228
Kart, C. S., 17, 86, 92, 105, 214, 228
Kasarda, J., 91, 228
Kast, F. R., 83, 228
Katz, D., 17, 228
Kellam, S. G., 110, 228
Kimbell, A., 28, 60, 111, 113, 178, 240
King, R. D., 76, 80, 82, 86, 111, 112-14, 133, 178-9
Kinloch, D. R., 17, 90, 91, 230
Kivett, V., 53, 235
Kleban, M. H., 126, 230
Kleemeier, R. W., 108, 109, 114-20, 126, 133, 146, 150, 179, 228
Klemmack, D. L., 45, 213, 228
Klerman, L. V., 39, 213, 234
Knapp, M. R. J., 12, 13, 15, 28, 30, 44, 45, 71, 73-4, 89-91, 95-100, 105, 138, 174, 177, 182, 197, 211, 212, 215, 222, 228
Kosberg, J. E., 38, 87, 101, 228-9
Kraus, A. S., 149, 153, 157-9, 239
Kurtz, J., 154, 241
Kushlick, A., 10, 26, 28, 57, 79, 82, 138, 171, 183, 220, 229
Kutner, B., 40, 159, 229
Kutscher, A. H., 143, 237
Kuypers, J. A., 149, 150, 231

labour, see manpower; staff
land costs, 197, 198
Langner, T. S., 39, 229
Larson, R., 38, 44, 57, 229
laundry, 74
Lave, J. R., 217, 229
Lave, L. B., 217, 229
Lawson, J. S., 149, 153, 157-9, 239
Lawson, S. A., 204, 221
Lawton, M. P., 16, 17, 38-9, 40, 48-51, 52, 56, 57, 92, 94, 95, 96, 101,

102-3, 109, 115, 119, 120, 124-30, 137, 141, 142, 146, 180, 181, 183, 215, 219, 229-30, 240
Lemke, S., 122, 233
Leveson, I., 217, 230
Levey, S., 17, 90, 91, 230
Lewin, K., 108-9, 115, 131, 230
Lieberman, M. A., 31, 56, 139, 144, 145, 146, 147-9, 150, 152, 154, 156, 171, 181, 184, 230-1, 240
Liebowitz, B., 56, 96, 231
life satisfaction, 11, 16, 25, 30, 31, 36, 38-45, 47, 48, 50-3, 55, 119, 126, 127, 134, 141, 142, 159-60, 168, 171, 204, 214
Life Satisfaction Index, 16, 38-9, 40, 42-5, 50, 52-3, 145, 168, 171, 212, 213
Life Satisfaction Ladder, 52-3
Life Satisfaction Rating Scale, 38-9, 40-2, 50, 52, 168, 171, 201-3, 212, 213
lift, 89, 102, 182
Linden, L. L., 62, 228
Linn, M. W., 16, 62, 63, 76, 91, 92, 101, 175, 225, 231
Lipman, A. R., 59-60, 76, 89, 91, 93, 97-8, 99, 100, 102, 103, 113, 126, 137 141, 143, 154, 179, 181, 226, 231, 239
'Living Environments' approach, 100
Livingstone, M., 62, 227
Livson, F., 237
Lohmann, N., 39, 40, 212, 213, 214, 231
loneliness, 39, 42, 51, 123, 139, 154, 171, 205, 213
longitudinal studies, 53
Lopata, H. Z., 63, 231
Lowell, E. L., 37, 232
Lowenthal, M. F., 141
Luikart, C., 53, 57, 235
Luker, K. A., 212, 231
Lunt, B., 26, 72, 137-8, 227, 231, 236
Lupton, T., 83, 231

Maas, H. S., 149, 150, 231
McCaffree, K. M., 16, 50, 73-5, 106, 175, 214, 231-2
McCaslin, R., 61, 126, 134, 215, 224
McClannahan, L. E., 26, 72, 100, 103, 138, 142, 232
McClelland, D. C., 28, 34, 37, 130, 180, 232

Index

MacDonald, M. L., 57, 232
McGee, J., 131, 235
McGuiness, B., 76, 99, 101, 175, 234
McKennell, A., 60, 232
McKinley, D., 39, 226
McQuillam, F. L. M., 232
Maddi, S. R., 27, 34, 37, 42, 128, 180, 212, 224, 232
Maher, M., 106, 231
management, 8
Manard, B. B., 17, 56. 72, 86, 92, 105, 215, 217, 228, 232
Mangold, R. F., 44, 232
Mangum, W. P., 118, 125-6, 232
manpower input, 8, 18, 69-88, 106, 172-85; see also staff
Markson, E. W., 56, 232
Marshall, D. G., 141, 220-1
Martin, D., 148, 232
Martin, D. N., 59, 232
Maslow, A. H., 11-12, 31, 34, 41, 61, 123, 212, 233
Mathieu, R. P., 233
Max, W., 122, 233
Maxwell, R. J., 135, 233
Meacher, M., 51, 60, 143, 157, 233
Mehren, B., 122, 233
Mendelson, M., 233
Mendlovitz, A., 87, 229
mental health, see residents' characteristics
mentally handicapped and ill, 27, 29, 46, 138, 167, 175, 177, 209
Messer, M., 142, 233
meta-theory, 14-15, 187
Milgram, S., 88, 233
Milhøj, P., 63, 238
milieu, see social environment
Miller, D. B., 138, 233
Miller, L. C., 106, 231
Minge, M. R., 83, 233
Ministry of Health, 90, 92, 94
Mischel, W., 88, 233
Molberg, E., 76, 83, 233
Monteiro, R. C., 52, 227
Montgomery, J. E., 150, 233
mood, 39, 41, 44, 154, 171, 203, 213
Mooney, G. H., 17-18, 233
Moores, B., 76, 225
Moos, R. H., 32, 33, 109, 115, 120-4, 129, 130, 133, 137, 146, 179-80, 233
morale, 25, 38-40, 47, 48-51, 52-3, 55, 61, 63, 91-2, 103, 104, 106,

119, 127, 128, 134, 138, 141, 142, 143, 154, 168, 171, 208, 209; morale scales, 47; see also Philadelphia Geriatric Center Morale Scale
morbidity, 23, 57-60, 144, 148, 149, 154-5, 156, 169, 171, 214
Moriwaki, S. Y., 46-7, 204, 206, 207, 209, 217, 233
Morris, J. N., 39, 50, 51, 128, 149, 153-5, 181, 184, 213, 216, 234, 238
Morris, P., 76, 234
Morrison, N., 72, 89, 90, 221
Morrow, G., 73-5, 175, 232
mortality, 23, 55-7, 63, 134, 142, 144, 155, 156, 169, 171
Mortimer, A., 50, 224
Moser, C. A., 212, 234
Moss, T., 59, 135, 143, 239
motivation, 28, 82
motivational tendencies, 120
motor control, see control
Muller, L., 106, 231
multiple realities, 118
Munnichs, J. M. A., 45, 52, 226
Murray, H. A., 108-9, 115, 120, 121, 123, 124, 126, 130, 133, 137, 141, 179 183, 234

Nadelson, T., 35-6, 154, 239
Nahemow, L., 16, 92, 111, 112, 124-30, 142, 143, 149, 151, 157, 180, 219, 230, 234, 240
National Association of Social Workers (USA), 160
National Corporation for the Care of Old People (NCCOP), 138, 218, 234
needs, 7, 23, 26, 27, 32, 34, 36, 38, 60-1, 84, 109, 115, 118, 120, 123, 128, 130, 146, 147, 149, 150, 153, 158, 169, 179, 190, 193, 194, 199, 211, 212, 214, 216; need gratification, 119; need-press model, 109, 115, 120-32, 137, 141, 146, 179-80; need-press model equilibrium, 127, 180, 199, 215; psychosocial needs, 135, 177; viscerogenic needs, 120; see also personality
Neill, J. E., 76, 99, 101, 175, 234
Neugarten, B. L., 29, 31-2, 38-9, 40-5, 47, 50, 52, 145, 201-3, 212, 216, 234

250

Neville, Y., 62, 227
Newman, E. S., 107, 145, 238
Noelker, L. S., 56, 234
normative argument, 178
normative information, 111, 112, 126, 130
norms, 68, 109, 142, 143, 151, 154, 157, 190
Nuehring, E., 118, 237
nursing care, 70, 71; v. social care, 70
nursing homes, 3, 16, 62, 70, 72, 74, 86, 87, 90, 111, 119, 122, 157, 167, 191, 195
nursing qualifications, 71-2, 74, 85-6, 117, 172-3, 177, 216
nurture, 61, 103, 107, 171, 182, 193, 199; see also cleanliness; diet; warmth
nutrition, see diet

Oberleder, M., 154, 160, 234
objectives of care, 4, 9-12, 14, 26, 55, 57, 93, 110, 166, 194, 196; see also philosophy of care
occupational pensions, 190
O'Donnell, J. M., 122, 234
Olsen, R., 88, 234
Oppenheim, W., 17, 90, 91, 230
Organisation for Economic Cooperation and Development, 52, 210, 234
organisational characteristics of homes, 79-85, 119, 121, 122, 175, 182
organisational characteristics of local authorities, 79-85, 176
orientation of care, 80-1, 113
orientation period, 157
Osmond, II., 95, 148, 235, 239
outputs, 5-7, 9-12, 15, 16, 17, 18, 23, 24,-64, 68, 72, 73, 77, 78-9, 86, 87, 88, 113, 114, 147, 154, 165-72, 177, 180, 185, 194, 196, 197, 199, 210, 211; intermediate outputs, 7, 16, 17, 54, 91, 169, 180, 210, 211; see also benefits to residents not contributing directly to psychological well-being; citizens' outputs; psychological well-being; significant others
ownership of homes, 3-4, 17, 72-3, 90, 182, 188, 191-2, 193, 196; housing associations, 191; inter-sectoral coordination, 188-93; see also private old people's homes, voluntary old people's homes

Pace, C., 109, 120, 235
Palfrey, C., 132, 235
Palmore, E., 53, 57, 235
Parkes, C. M., 156, 235
participation, 30, 100, 116, 121, 122, 137-8, 151-2, 157, 183
Pastalan, L. A., 135-7, 183, 235
Patnaik, B., 126, 230
patronising statements, 134, 139-40, 183
Patterson, E. A., 78, 87, 235
Paulig, K., 235
Paulson, S. R., 80, 235
Pauly, M. V., 217, 235
Payne, C., 86, 132, 235
Peace, S. M., 26, 48, 204-9, 235
Pearce, M., 214, 224
Peck, R. C., 36, 39, 41, 235
Peckford, R. W., 59, 232
perceptions: residents', 130, 156, 180; significant others', 6; staff, 81, 117, 130, 180, 182
Peretz, D., 143, 237
Perlin, S., 154, 221
Perrow, C., 81-2, 235
personal possessions of residents, 107, 111, 112, 119, 145, 183
personal social services, 10, 23, 106, 128, 132, 150, 215; inter-sectoral coordination, 118-93; substitution between, 4, 10, 173, 174; see also community services; day services; domiciliary services; private old people's homes; voluntary provision
Personal Social Services Council, 4, 9-10, 86-7, 128, 133, 136, 137, 150, 166, 182, 183, 236
Personal Social Services Research Unit, vii-viii, 212, 213
personality: interaction with environment, 33, 60; residents', 8, 14, 25, 27, 29-38, 50, 59, 68, 108-9, 119, 120, 124, 126, 147-9, 181, 184, 216; staff, 79, 87-8, 176, 177, 182, 183; theory, 11-12, 25, 29, 30-1, 33-8, 40-2, 49-50, 52, 113, 123-4, 147-9, 166, 168, 180
Peterson, P. G., 237
Philadelphia Geriatric Center (PGC) morale scale, 38, 40, 48-51, 52, 57, 119, 153, 168, 171, 213
philosophy of care, 9-10, 112, 113. 166

Index

physical capacity, *see* dependency; residents' characteristics
physically handicapped, 27, 29, 95, 143, 167
physiotherapy, 72, 172, 183
Piaget, J., 127, 236
Pierce, R. C., 39, 51, 236
Pincus, A., 108, 109, 115-20, 130, 133, 146, 179, 236
Pitt, B., 59, 236
Plank, D., 5, 130, 140, 236
planning, *see* policy
policy 6, 18-19, 56, 61, 67-8, 188-200
policy-makers, 8, 80, 85, 176
Pope, P. J., 150-1, 156-7, 236
positive regard, 34-6, 41, 123, 212
positive self-regard, 34, 41, 46, 123, 212
Powell, L., 26, 72, 137-8, 227, 231, 236
power model of ageing, *see* transactional model
Pratt, M. W., 76, 79-85, 113, 121-2, 175, 236
preparation for admission, 150, 151, 152-6, 184
prices, 185, 193, 211
privacy, 38, 96, 103, 110, 112, 114-15, 116, 118, 119, 122, 135-7, 138-41, 156, 159, 167, 183, 199, 215
private old people's homes, 19, 72-3, 74, 90, 167, 188-93, 193-200; communication, 191-2; inspection, 194, 199; registration, 193-200
privatisation of welfare, 188-200
production function, 15, 17, 73, 104, 197, 198, 211
production relations, *see* production function; production of welfare approach
production of welfare approach, 5, 7, 8, 12-5, 16, 18-9, 25, 29, 54, 57, 58, 67, 75, 77, 78, 89, 96, 107, 118, 124, 130, 132, 152, 158, 160-1, 165, 172-85, 195, 198; application, 165-85; empirical investigation, 185-8; and policy, 188-200; schematic representation, 186
productivity, 185; marginal, 79, 104, 172
profit, 90, 192-3, 196, 197-8; non-profit homes, 119
programme of care, 81, 86, 133, 167; clarity, 121
Proppe, H., 136-7, 238

252

Proshansky, H. M., 96, 136, 227
Prosser, D. M., 217, 236
Prosser, R. A., 132, 236
prostheses, 10, 57, 71, 95, 101, 103, 129, 134, 137, 138, 182
provisions, *see* consumables; diet
psychological well-being: residents', 10, 12, 23, 25-53, 55, 57, 60, 61, 64, 92, 108, 153-4, 169, 171, 178, 187, 199, 206-9, 212, 213, 214; significant others', 61-3; *see also* affect; happiness; life satisfaction; morale; well-being
psychophysiological symptoms, 39, 171, 214
psychosocial milieu, 115
'psychosocial staffing', 72, 86
Public Assistance Institutions, 90
Pugh, D. S., 85, 236
Pyrek, J. D., 58, 59, 135, 143, 236, 239

quality of care, 16-17, 25, 54, 62, 63, 76, 77-9, 81, 82-3, 85-8, 90, 91, 92, 96, 101, 105, 113-14, 168, 170, 173, 174, 176; control of, 196-7, 199; *see also* staff quality
quality of life, 4, 5-7, 8, 10, 11, 12-13, 17, 25, 26, 33, 47, 54, 62, 76, 77, 85, 87, 88, 90, 95, 101, 110, 138, 141, 166, 168, 170, 173, 174, 177, 178, 180-1, 193, 195, 204, 216
Quality of Life Survey, 206-7, 217
queueing, 93, 99

Ramathan K. V., 106, 231
Ratcliff, B. W., 16, 45, 76, 91, 92, 175, 222
Raynes, N. V., 76, 79-85, 111, 112-14, 121-2, 133, 175-6, 178-9, 228, 236
reciprocity, 126
'reciprocity multiplier', 6
recreation, 52, 63, 167; *see also* activities
regime, 71, 78, 79, 80-1, 84, 87, 96, 110, 112, 113, 114, 115, 116, 117, 118, 133-4, 139, 183, 215
registration of homes, 193-200
Reichard, S., 31, 237
Reiter, J., 118, 237
relationships, *see* friendships,

interaction
relative deprivation, 154
relatives, *see* significant others
reliability, 7, 26, 32, 42, 48, 50, 52,
    53, 57, 119, 130, 151, 157, 166,
    168-9, 170, 187-8
religion, 52, 208; church, 104
relocation, 31, 56, 126, 142, 143-6,
    148, 149-53, 156, 215, 216
Resident Management Practices Scale,
    80, 86, 111, 178
residents' attitudes, 14, 39, 42, 86,
    134, 140, 150, 152-3, 171, 181,
    184, 213
residents' characteristics, 6, 18, 29,
    31, 32, 57, 68, 73, 74-5, 114,
    119, 124, 137, 174, 180-1, 184,
    185; age, 30-1, 71, 113, 114, 115,
    122, 127, 130, 141-3, 192, 204,
    208; capacity for self care, 57,
    58, 60, 68, 71, 75, 134, 149,
    154-5, 160, 166, 174, 204; com-
    pensation for disability, 61; con-
    tinence, 75, 143; as determinent of
    staff numbers, 71; ethnicity, 114,
    141-3; health status, *see* health;
    level of functioning, 114, 141-3;
    marital status, 96, 148, 155, 158,
    159, 160; mental status, 47, 59-60,
    62, 74-5, 171, 181, 184, 204,
    214; permanency, 114, 141-3;
    see also short-stay residents; at
    point of entry, 124, 149, 152-5,
    157, 161, 170, 181, 216; religion,
    114, 141-3; sex, 56, 114, 130,
    141-3, 192; *see also* dependency;
    personality; residents' rights
residents' rights, 38, 134, 156, 193,
    195, 215
resolution and fortitude, 41, 44,
    201-2, 213
resources, *see* inputs
respect, 38
retirement, 44, 142, 154
rigidity v. creativity, 59, 112, 133,
    174, 183
Ring, J., 60, 225
risk, 61, 84, 128, 133, 169-70, 183
Risley, T. R., 26, 27, 72, 100, 223,
    232
Rivlin, L. G., 96, 136, 227
Ro, K. -K., 217, 237
Robb, B., 90, 237
Rodstein, M., 157, 237
Rogers, C. R., 31, 34, 36, 41-2, 46,
    47, 123, 212, 237

role, 29-30, 33, 47, 82, 109, 114,
    126, 127, 129, 131, 142, 159,
    174
role perceptions of staff, 8, 13, 215
Romaniuk, J. G., 86, 139-40, 183,
    237
Romaniuk, M., 86, 139-40, 237
room reserved for residents' private
    use, 73-4
Roos, B., 210, 237
Roos, J. P., 210, 237
Rose, A., 142, 237
Rosenburg, M., 149, 153, 157-9, 239
Rosencranz, H. A., 29, 237
Rosenzweig, J. E., 83, 228
Roses, S., 76, 79-85, 113, 121-2, 175,
    236
Rosow, I., 39, 47, 125, 141, 237
routine, 112, 113, 118, 133, 183
routinisation, 125
Rubenstein, B., 142, 237
Rubenstein, J., 142, 237
Ruchlin, H. J., 17, 90, 91, 230
Rupprecht, P., 59, 135, 143, 239
Russell, L., 217, 237

salary, 7, 170, 190, 197
sanctions, 111, 133
satisfaction, 48, 49, 91, 118, 150,
    153, 155, 156, 159, 213; long term
    satisfaction, 47-8, 171
Sauer, W. J., 63, 238
Savage, R. D., 31, 44, 212, 216, 237
Savitsky, E., 157, 237
Schmelzer, J., 110, 228
Schmidt, M. G., 45, 237
Schneider, R. E., 76, 90, 91, 218
Schoenberg, B. C., 143, 237
Schooler, K. K., 39, 51, 92, 103, 104,
    105, 128, 177, 238
Schuler, S., 122, 234
Schulz, R., 56, 134, 144, 152-3, 156,
    183, 215, 238
Schwartz, A. N., 136-7, 238
Schwartz, M. S., 81, 239
Scottish Education Department,
    Social Work Services Group,
    89, 238
seats, 94, 95
secondment, 69
security, 94, 156
Seelbach, W. C., 63, 238
segregation, 108, 113, 114-20, 141-3,
    154, 179, 183
self-actualisation, 31-2, 34, 41, 49,
    100, 127, 212

self-concept, 39, 40, 41-2, 102, 171, 202-3
self-control, 26
self-determination, 134
self-esteem, 26, 39, 131, 212
self-image, *see* self-concept
self-regard, 34-6, 50, 137; *see also* positive self-regard
Seligman, M. E., 134, 238
Sen, A. K., 210, 238
sensory acuity, 58-9, 60, 68, 125, 171, 184, 204
Shanas, E., 63, 150, 238
Sheafor, B., 44, 212, 241
Sheltered Care Environment Scale (SCES), 121-4
Sherman, E., 107, 145, 238
Sherwood, S., 35-6, 38, 50, 51, 128, 154, 234, 238-9
shop, 101, 167
Shore, H., 58-9, 220
short-stay residents, 4, 111, 143, 150, 170
Shulman, D., 197, 217, 239
significant others, 3, 6, 7, 42, 52, 54, 61-3, 71, 72, 75, 92, 104, 141, 150, 151, 158-9, 168, 169-71, 208, 214; outputs enjoyed by, 61-3; *also see* perceptions, psychological well-being
Silverman, L. P., 17, 217, 229, 241
Silverstone, B., 142-3, 239
Simon, B., 124, 125, 230
Simpson, A., 92, 226
Sinclair, I. A. G., 32-3, 76, 80, 111, 182, 226, 239, 240
siting of home, 83, 104
sitting rooms, 89, 93, 94, 97-9, 143, 182; as determinent of staffing levels, 73-4
size of home, 12-13, 16, 17, 71, 73-4, 83, 90-2, 94, 96, 97, 167, 178, 182
size of living unit, 80, 90-2, 93, 178
Skoglund, J., 239
Slater, R., 59-60, 76, 89, 91, 93, 97-8, 99, 100, 102, 103, 113, 137, 140, 143, 179, 181, 226, 231, 239
Slover, D. L., 31, 155-61, 184, 241
Smith, J. J., 126, 141, 154, 239
Smith, R., 89, 168, 240
Snyder, L. H., 58, 59, 135, 143, 236, 239
social distance, 113, 114, 117, 137, 141, 179, 183; *see also* congregation; spatial proximity
social ecology model, 109, 115, 120-30, 247
social environment, 7, 18, 25, 29-33, 42, 57, 60, 68, 69, 72, 76, 78-9, 83, 86, 87-8, 90, 91, 106, 108-46, 153, 154, 157, 177, 179-80, 181, 183, 185, 199, 216
social indicators, 52, 206
'Social Indicators Movement', 11
social integration, 6, 17, 23, 61, 141, 142, 151, 157, 183
socialisation, 112, 151, 152, 157
social milieu, *see* social environment
social niches, 29, 92
social services departments, 4, 5, 6, 10, 84, 174, 194
social welfare paradigm, 9-12, 16, 18, 33-4, 35, 53, 61, 63-4, 67-8, 84, 155, 166
social work, 5, 72, 84, 145, 150, 166, 213, 214, 216
Somers, A. R., 239
Somers, H. M., 239
Sommer, R., 148, 239
Spasoff, R. A., 149, 153, 157-9, 216, 239
spatial proximity, 94, 97, 100, 102, 114, 131, 137, 143, 182
specialisation, 80, 82, 85, 176
Spencely, H., 91, 106, 240
spontaneity, 121, 122
Srole, L., 39, 47, 51, 239
stability, 125
staff, 7, 16, 150, 151, 182-3; accommodation, 101-2; attitudes, 7-8, 18, 68, 86, 87-8, 90, 96, 124, 172, 176, 177, 182; care, 7, 70, 71, 73, 76, 78, 81, 82-3, 88, 92, 96-7, 101, 174, 197; care tasks, 71, 77-8; characteristics, 79, 85-8, 182; domestic, 70, 71, 73, 76, 78, 96-7, 117, 175, 197; domestic tasks, 71, 77-8; hours, 4, 69, 76, 81, 90, 175, 182; morale, 81, 83, 92, 101, 176; night, 73, 96, 101-2, 190; norms, 190; numbers, 69, 72-6, 90, 96, 97, 133, 135, 182; office and secretarial, 70, 73; qualifications, 5, 85-8, 133, 176, 182; quality 69, 77-9, 82, 92, 172, 175-7, 182; recruitment, 101; roles, 80; stress, 86; supervisory, 9, 70, 73, 76, 78, 80-1, 82, 92, 96, 101-2, 173; super-

visory tasks, 71; support, 86,
176; training, 9, 69, 85-8, 176,
177, 182, 199; turnover, 76, 83,
101, 176, 182; types, 9, 70-2,
172-4, 182, 215-16
staff-resident ratios, 71, 72-6, 77,
97, 114, 174, 182, 189
standardisation, 84
standards of care, *see* quality of care
Stanton, A. H., 81, 239
Stanton, B. R., 107, 239
Starkman, R., 157, 237
Stathopoulos, P., 72, 239
statistical techniques, 13, 15, 39,
47, 49, 117, 123, 128, 148, 168,
177
status quo, satisfaction with, 39, 40,
51, 119; *see also* Disengagement
Theory
Stehouwer, J., 63, 238
Stein, M., 109, 120, 239
Stern, M., 109, 120, 121, 123, 141,
235, 239
Stevenson, O., 62, 239
stigma, 139
stimulation, 110, 115, 119, 128,
137-8, 167, 183
stimuli, 27-8, 37, 109, 120, 127,
129, 141, 155, 180
Stone, L. B., 76, 90, 91, 218
Stonner, D., 134, 224
Stotsky, B. A., 17, 90, 91, 151, 223,
230, 239
Streib, G. F., 134, 239
stress, 126, 128, 131, 141, *see also*
staff stress
'structure', 119
successful care, *see* outputs
Sumner, G., 89, 168, 240
supply of residential home places,
190, 191, 192
'supra-personal environment', 115,
118, 125, 141-3, 184; *see also*
homogeneity, residents' characteristics
survival, 134, 144; *see also* adjustment;
death; mortality
systems analysis, 14-15, 17-18

talk, 76, 80, 81-2, 97, 137, 139-40,
175, 183; *see also* interaction
task performance, 126; *see also*
developmental task adjustment
Teaff, J. D., 16, 92, 142, 230, 240
Telleen, S., 30, 45, 134, 154, 241

temporary residents, *see* short-stay
residents
tension creation and reduction, 118,
128, 180
therapeutic community, 3, 10
therapists: occupational, 74; physical,
74; speech, 74
therapy, 63, 100
Thomae, H., 45, 52, 226
Thomas, N., 91, 106, 240
Thormalen, P. W., 76, 240
Thurnher, M., 46, 240
time-sampling, 26-7
Titmuss, R., 6, 240
Tizard, B., 76, 80, 240
Tizard, J., 76, 80, 82, 86, 112-14,
182, 228, 240
Tobin, S. S., 31, 38-9, 40-5, 50, 52,
139, 144, 145, 147-9, 150, 152,
181, 184, 201-13, 212, 234, 240
totality, 10, 76, 89, 108, 109, 110-15,
120, 141, 146, 159, 178-9, 182;
Index of Totality, 111; *see also*
social environment
Townsend, J., 28, 60, 111, 113, 240
Townsend, P., 17, 63, 77, 88-9, 90,
91, 103, 148, 178, 182, 238,
240
transactional model of ageing, 126,
128, 130-2, 280
transfer function, *see* production
function
transport, 104
Troop, J., 111, 226
Tunstall, J., 51, 240
Turner, B. F., 31, 147-9, 154, 160,
181, 184, 216, 240
Turner, C., 85, 236
Turner, J. G., 87, 177, 219
Turner-Massey, P., 92, 230

uncertainty, 34
uniformity, 99
Utting, B., 133, 183, 240

validity, 7, 18, 26, 37-8, 39, 40-2,
44, 47, 50, 51, 52, 58, 77, 85,
117, 118, 129, 153, 168-9, 170,
179, 187-8, 206, 209, 210, 212,
213
Veit, S. W., 76, 226
Verry, D. W., 211
visitors, 100, 101, 116, 136, 138,
140-1, 151, 159, 183, 208, 214,
217

voluntary old people's homes, 72-3, 90, 167, 188-93, 193-200; inspection, 194, 199; registration, 193-200
voluntary organisations, 192, 207
voluntary provision, 4, 19
volunteers, 72, 74, 141, 217

Wager, R., 12, 90, 106, 139, 240
Walton, R., 78, 240
wandering, 119, 134-5
Warburton, R. W., 76, 99, 101, 175, 234
Ward, L., 85, 241
Ward Armosphere Scale (WAS), 121
warmth, 61, 103, 171, 182, 199; see also hypothermia
Watson, W., 135, 233
Weber, M., 79
Wedderburn, D., 63, 238
Weinstock, C. S., 131, 241
Weiss, L. J., 137, 241
welfare, see well-being
well-being, 6, 7, 10, 17, 28, 54, 68, 78, 88, 106, 109, 114, 119, 124 134, 137, 141, 142, 144, 145, 148, 149, 150, 151, 152, 157, 160, 168, 170, 173, 177, 180, 181, 196, 207-9; on admission to home, 153-4; see also psychological well-being
White, R. W., 128, 241
Wicks, M., 215, 241

Wilkinson, R. K., 105, 241
Williams, A., 17, 210, 241
Williams, B. T., 50, 244
Williams, G., 72, 89, 90, 241
Wilson, J., 143, 241
Wilson, J. Q., 200, 241
Wilson, N., 39, 241
Wilson, S. H., 241
Wing, J. K., 110, 241
Winn, S., 73-5, 175, 232
Wiseman, M., 17, 241
Wittels, I., 56
Woehle, R. E., 56, 72, 215, 217, 232
Wolf, R. S., 39, 213, 234
Wolk, S., 30, 45, 134, 154, 241
Wood, V., 44, 115, 117, 130, 142, 212, 213, 221, 236, 241
Woodcock, G. M., 149, 153, 157-9, 239
Worthingon, P. N., 217, 226
Wright, K. G., 17, 50, 58, 171, 241-2
Wylie, M. L., 38, 44, 55, 212, 241, 242
Wynter, L., 142-3, 239

Yaffe, S., 56, 230
Yawney, B. A., 31, 155-61, 184, 241

Zach, H., 63, 214, 242
Zepelin, H., 134, 234
zest (v. apathy), 41-2, 44, 48-50, 171, 201, 213
Zimbardo, P., 88, 242

Routledge Social Science Series

Routledge & Kegan Paul   London, Henley and Boston

39 Store Street,
London WC1E 7DD
Broadway House,
Newtown Road,
Henley-on-Thames,
Oxon RG9 1EN
9 Park Street,
Boston, Mass. 02108

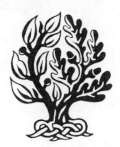

Contents

International Library of Sociology 2
General Sociology 2
Foreign Classics of Sociology 2
Social Structure 3
Sociology and Politics 3
Criminology 4
Social Psychology 4
Sociology of the Family 5
Social Services 5
Sociology of Education 5
Sociology of Culture 6
Sociology of Religion 6
Sociology of Art and Literature 6
Sociology of Knowledge 6
Urban Sociology 7
Rural Sociology 7
Sociology of Industry and
Distribution 7
Anthropology 8
Sociology and Philosophy 8

International Library of
Anthropology 9
International Library of Phenomen-
ology and Moral Sciences 9
International Library of Social
Policy 9
International Library of Welfare and
Philosophy 10
Library of Social Work 10
Primary Socialization, Language and
Education 12
Reports of the Institute of
Community Studies 12
Reports of the Institute for Social
Studies in Medical Care 13
Medicine, Illness and Society 13
Monographs in Social Theory 13
Routledge Social Science Journals 13
Social and Psychological Aspects of
Medical Practice 14

*Authors wishing to submit manuscripts for any series
in this catalogue should send them to the Social Science Editor,
Routledge & Kegan Paul Ltd, 39 Store Street,
London WC1E 7DD.*

● *Books so marked are available in paperback.*
○ *Books so marked are available in paperback only.*
*All books are in metric Demy 8vo format (216 × 138mm approx.)
unless otherwise stated.*

International Library of Sociology
General Editor   John Rex

GENERAL SOCIOLOGY

Barnsley, J. H. The Social Reality of Ethics. *464 pp.*
Brown, Robert. Explanation in Social Science. *208 pp.*
● Rules and Laws in Sociology. *192 pp.*
Bruford, W. H. Chekhov and His Russia. *A Sociological Study. 244 pp.*
Burton, F. and **Carlen, P.** Official Discourse. *On Discourse Analysis, Government Publications, Ideology. About 140 pp.*
Cain, Maureen E. Society and the Policeman's Role. *326 pp.*
● **Fletcher, Colin.** Beneath the Surface. *An Account of Three Styles of Sociological Research. 221 pp.*
Gibson, Quentin. The Logic of Social Enquiry. *240 pp.*
Glassner, B. Essential Interactionism. *208 pp.*
Glucksmann, M. Structuralist Analysis in Contemporary Social Thought. *212 pp.*
Gurvitch, Georges. Sociology of Law. *Foreword by Roscoe Pound. 264 pp.*
Hinkle, R. Founding Theory of American Sociology 1881–1913. *About 350 pp.*
Homans, George C. Sentiments and Activities. *336 pp.*
Johnson, Harry M. Sociology: *A Systematic Introduction. Foreword by Robert K. Merton. 710 pp.*
● **Keat, Russell** and **Urry, John.** Social Theory as Science. *278 pp.*
Mannheim, Karl. Essays on Sociology and Social Psychology. *Edited by Paul Keckskemeti. With Editorial Note by Adolph Lowe. 344 pp.*
Martindale, Don. The Nature and Types of Sociological Theory. *292 pp.*
● **Maus, Heinz.** A Short History of Sociology. *234 pp.*
Myrdal, Gunnar. Value in Social Theory: *A Collection of Essays on Methodology. Edited by Paul Streeten. 332 pp.*
Ogburn, William F. and **Nimkoff, Meyer F.** A Handbook of Sociology. *Preface by Karl Mannheim. 656 pp. 46 figures. 35 tables.*
Parsons, Talcott and **Smelser, Neil J.** Economy and Society: *A Study in the Integration of Economic and Social Theory. 362 pp.*
Payne, G., Dingwall, R., Payne, J. and **Carter, M.** Sociology and Social Research. *About 250 pp.*
Podgórecki, A. Practical Social Sciences. *About 200 pp.*
Podgórecki, A. and **Łos, M.** Multidimensional Sociology. *268 pp.*
Raffel, S. Matters of Fact. *A Sociological Inquiry. 152 pp.*
● **Rex, John.** Key Problems of Sociological Theory. *220 pp.*
  Sociology and the Demystification of the Modern World. *282 pp.*
● **Rex, John.** (Ed.) Approaches to Sociology. *Contributions by Peter Abell, Frank Bechhofer, Basil Bernstein, Ronald Fletcher, David Frisby, Miriam Glucksmann, Peter Lassman, Herminio Martins, John Rex, Roland Robertson, John Westergaard and Jock Young. 302 pp.*
Rigby, A. Alternative Realities. *352 pp.*
Roche, M. Phenomenology, Language and the Social Sciences. *374 pp.*
Sahay, A. Sociological Analysis. *220 pp.*
Strasser, Hermann. The Normative Structure of Sociology. *Conservative and Emancipatory Themes in Social Thought. About 340 pp.*
Strong, P. Ceremonial Order of the Clinic. *267 pp.*
Urry, John. Reference Groups and the Theory of Revolution. *244 pp.*
Weinberg, E. Development of Sociology in the Soviet Union. *173 pp.*

FOREIGN CLASSICS OF SOCIOLOGY

● **Gerth, H. H.** and **Mills, C. Wright.** From Max Weber: *Essays in Sociology. 502 pp.*

● **Tönnies, Ferdinand.** Community and Association *(Gemeinschaft und Gesellschaft).\Translated and Supplemented by Charles P. Loomis. Foreword by Pitirim A. Sorokin. 334 pp.*

SOCIAL STRUCTURE

Andreski, Stanislav. Military Organization and Society. *Foreword by Professor A. R. Radcliffe-Brown. 226 pp. 1 folder.*

Broom, L., Lancaster Jones, F., McDonnell, P. and **Williams, T.** The Inheritance of Inequality. *About 180 pp.*

Carlton, Eric. Ideology and Social Order. *Foreword by Professor Philip Abrahams. About 320 pp.*

Clegg, S. and **Dunkerley, D.** Organization, Class and Control. *614 pp.*

Coontz, Sydney H. Population Theories and the Economic Interpretation. *202 pp.*

Coser, Lewis. The Functions of Social Conflict. *204 pp.*

Crook, I. and **D.** The First Years of the Yangyi Commune. *304 pp., illustrated.*

Dickie-Clark, H. F. Marginal Situation: *A Sociological Study of a Coloured Group. 240 pp. 11 tables.*

Giner, S. and **Archer, M. S.** (Eds) Contemporary Europe: *Social Structures and Cultural Patterns, 336 pp.*

● **Glaser, Barney** and **Strauss, Anselm L.** Status Passage: *A Formal Theory. 212 pp.*

Glass, D. V. (Ed.) Social Mobility in Britain. *Contributions by J. Berent, T. Bottomore, R. C. Chambers, J. Floud, D. V. Glass, J. R. Hall, H. T. Himmelweit, R. K. Kelsall, F. M. Martin, C. A. Moser, R. Mukherjee and W. Ziegel. 420 pp.*

Kelsall, R. K. Higher Civil Servants in Britain: *From 1870 to the Present Day. 268 pp. 31 tables.*

● **Lawton, Denis.** Social Class, Language and Education. *192 pp.*

McLeish, John. The Theory of Social Change: *Four Views Considered. 128 pp.*

● **Marsh, David C.** The Changing Social Structure of England and Wales, 1871–1961. *Revised edition. 288 pp.*

Menzies, Ken. Talcott Parsons and the Social Image of Man. *About 208 pp.*

● **Mouzelis, Nicos.** Organization and Bureaucracy. *An Analysis of Modern Theories. 240 pp.*

● **Ossowski, Stanislaw.** Class Structure in the Social Consciousness. *210 pp.*

● **Podgórecki, Adam.** Law and Society. *302 pp.*

Renner, Karl. Institutions of Private Law and Their Social Functions. *Edited, with an Introduction and Notes, by O. Kahn-Freud. Translated by Agnes Schwarzschild. 316 pp.*

Rex, J. and **Tomlinson, S.** Colonial Immigrants in a British City. *A Class Analysis. 368 pp.*

Smooha, S. Israel: Pluralism and Conflict. *472 pp.*

Wesolowski, W. Class, Strata and Power. *Trans. and with Introduction by G. Kolankiewicz. 160 pp.*

Zureik, E. Palestinians in Israel. *A Study in Internal Colonialism. 264 pp.*

SOCIOLOGY AND POLITICS

Acton, T. A. Gypsy Politics and Social Change. *316 pp.*

Burton, F. Politics of Legitimacy. *Struggles in a Belfast Community. 250 pp.*

Crook, I. and **D.** Revolution in a Chinese Village. *Ten Mile Inn. 216 pp., illustrated.*

Etzioni-Halevy, E. Political Manipulation and Administrative Power. *A Comparative Study. About 200 pp.*

Fielding, N. The National Front. *About 250 pp.*

● **Hechter, Michael.** Internal Colonialism. *The Celtic Fringe in British National Development, 1536–1966. 380 pp.*

Kornhauser, William. The Politics of Mass Society. *272 pp. 20 tables.*

Korpi, W. The Working Class in Welfare Capitalism. *Work, Unions and Politics in Sweden. 472 pp.*

Kroes, R. Soldiers and Students. *A Study of Right- and Left-wing Students. 174 pp.*

Martin, Roderick. Sociology of Power. *About 272 pp.*

Merquior, J. G. Rousseau and Weber. *A Study in the Theory of Legitimacy. About 288 pp.*

Myrdal, Gunnar. The Political Element in the Development of Economic Theory. *Translated from the German by Paul Streeten. 282 pp.*

Varma, B. N. The Sociology and Politics of Development. *A Theoretical Study. 236 pp.*

Wong, S.-L. Sociology and Socialism in Contemporary China. *160 pp.*

Wootton, Graham. Workers, Unions and the State. *188 pp.*

CRIMINOLOGY

Ancel, Marc. Social Defence: *A Modern Approach to Criminal Problems. Foreword by Leon Radzinowicz. 240 pp.*

Athens, L. Violent Criminal Acts and Actors. *104 pp.*

Cain, Maureen E. Society and the Policeman's Role. *326 pp.*

Cloward, Richard A. and **Ohlin, Lloyd E.** Delinquency and Opportunity: *A Theory of Delinquent Gangs. 248 pp.*

Downes, David M. The Delinquent Solution. *A Study in Subcultural Theory. 296 pp.*

Friedlander, Kate. The Psycho-Analytical Approach to Juvenile Delinquency: *Theory, Case Studies, Treatment. 320 pp.*

Gleuck, Sheldon and **Eleanor.** Family Environment and Delinquency. *With the statistical assistance of Rose W. Kneznek. 340 pp.*

Lopez-Rey, Manuel. Crime. *An Analytical Appraisal. 288 pp.*

Mannheim, Hermann. Comparative Criminology: *A Text Book. Two volumes. 442 pp. and 380 pp.*

Morris, Terence. The Criminal Area: *A Study in Social Ecology. Foreword by Hermann Mannheim. 232 pp. 25 tables. 4 maps.*

Rock, Paul. Making People Pay. *338 pp.*

● **Taylor, Ian, Walton, Paul** and **Young, Jock.** The New Criminology. *For a Social Theory of Deviance. 325 pp.*

● **Taylor, Ian, Walton, Paul** and **Young, Jock.** (Eds) Critical Criminology. *268 pp.*

SOCIAL PSYCHOLOGY

Bagley, Christopher. The Social Psychology of the Epileptic Child. *320 pp.*

Brittan, Arthur. Meanings and Situations. *224 pp.*

Carroll, J. Break-Out from the Crystal Palace. *200 pp.*

● **Fleming, C. M.** Adolescence: Its Social Psychology. *With an Introduction to recent findings from the fields of Anthropology, Physiology, Medicine, Psychometrics and Sociometry. 288 pp.*

● The Social Psychology of Education: *An Introduction and Guide to Its Study. 136 pp.*

Linton, Ralph. The Cultural Background of Personality. *132 pp.*

● **Mayo, Elton.** The Social Problems of an Industrial Civilization. *With an Appendix on the Political Problem. 180 pp.*

Ottaway, A. K. C. Learning Through Group Experience. *176 pp.*

Plummer, Ken. Sexual Stigma. *An Interactionist Account. 254 pp.*

● **Rose, Arnold M.** (Ed.) Human Behaviour and Social Processes: *an Interactionist Approach. Contributions by Arnold M. Rose, Ralph H. Turner, Anselm Strauss, Everett C. Hughes, E. Franklin Frazier, Howard S. Becker et al. 696 pp.*

Smelser, Neil J. Theory of Collective Behaviour. *448 pp.*

Stephenson, Geoffrey M. The Development of Conscience. *128 pp.*

Young, Kimball. Handbook of Social Psychology. *658 pp. 16 figures. 10 tables.*

SOCIOLOGY OF THE FAMILY

Bell, Colin R. Middle Class Families: *Social and Geographical Mobility. 224 pp.*
Burton, Lindy. Vulnerable Children. *272 pp.*
Gavron, Hannah. The Captive Wife: *Conflicts of Household Mothers. 190 pp.*
George, Victor and **Wilding, Paul.** Motherless Families. *248 pp.*
Klein, Josephine. Samples from English Cultures.
    1. Three Preliminary Studies and Aspects of Adult Life in England. *447 pp.*
    2. Child-Rearing Practices and Index. *247 pp.*
Klein, Viola. The Feminine Character. *History of an Ideology. 244 pp.*
McWhinnie, Alexina M. Adopted Children. *How They Grow Up. 304 pp.*
● **Morgan, D. H. J.** Social Theory and the Family. *About 320 pp.*
● **Myrdal, Alva** and **Klein, Viola.** Women's Two Roles: *Home and Work. 238 pp.*
    27 tables.
Parsons, Talcott and **Bales, Robert F.** Family: Socialization and Interaction Process.
    In collaboration with James Olds, Morris Zelditch and Philip E. Slater. 456 pp.
    50 figures and tables.

SOCIAL SERVICES

Bastide, Roger. The Sociology of Mental Disorder. *Translated from the French by*
    Jean McNeil. 260 pp.
Carlebach, Julius. Caring For Children in Trouble. *266 pp.*
George, Victor. Foster Care. *Theory and Practice. 234 pp.*
    Social Security: *Beveridge and After. 258 pp.*
George, V. and **Wilding, P.** Motherless Families. *248 pp.*
● **Goetschius, George W.** Working with Community Groups. *256 pp.*
Goetschius, George W. and **Tash, Joan.** Working with Unattached Youth. *416 pp.*
Heywood, Jean S. Children in Care. *The Development of the Service for the Deprived*
    Child. Third revised edition. 284 pp.
King, Roy D., Ranes, Norma V. and **Tizard, Jack.** Patterns of Residential Care.
    356 pp.
Leigh, John. Young People and Leisure. *256 pp.*
● **Mays, John.** (Ed.) Penelope Hall's Social Services of England and Wales.
    368 pp.
Morris, Mary. Voluntary Work and the Welfare State. *300 pp.*
Nokes, P. L. The Professional Task in Welfare Practice. *152 pp.*
Timms, Noel. Psychiatric Social Work in Great Britain (1939–1962). *280 pp.*
●   Social Casework: *Principles and Practice. 256 pp.*

SOCIOLOGY OF EDUCATION

Banks, Olive. Parity and Prestige in English Secondary Education: a Study in
    Educational Sociology. *272 pp.*
● **Blyth, W. A. L.** English Primary Education. *A Sociological Description.*
    2. Background. *168 pp.*
Collier, K. G. The Social Purposes of Education: *Personal and Social Values in*
    Education. 268 pp.
Evans, K. M. Sociometry and Education. *158 pp.*
● **Ford, Julienne.** Social Class and the Comprehensive School. *192 pp.*
Foster, P. J. Education and Social Change in Ghana. *336 pp. 3 maps.*
Fraser, W. R. Education and Society in Modern France. *150 pp.*
Grace, Gerald R. Role Conflict and the Teacher. *150 pp.*
Hans, Nicholas. New Trends in Education in the Eighteenth Century. *278 pp.*
    19 tables.
●   Comparative Education: *A Study of Educational Factors and Traditions. 360 pp.*
● **Hargreaves, David.** Interpersonal Relations and Education. *432 pp.*
●   Social Relations in a Secondary School. *240 pp.*
    School Organization and Pupil Involvement. *A Study of Secondary Schools.*

● **Mannheim, Karl** and **Stewart, W. A. C.** An Introduction to the Sociology of Education. *206 pp.*
● **Musgrove, F.** Youth and the Social Order. *176 pp.*
● **Ottaway, A. K. C.** Education and Society: An Introduction to the Sociology of Education. *With an Introduction by W. O. Lester Smith. 212 pp.*
   Peers, Robert. Adult Education: *A Comparative Study. Revised edition. 398 pp.*
   Stratta, Erica. The Education of Borstal Boys. *A Study of their Educational Experiences prior to, and during, Borstal Training. 256 pp.*
● **Taylor, P. H., Reid, W. A.** and **Holley, B. J.** The English Sixth Form. *A Case Study in Curriculum Research. 198 pp.*

SOCIOLOGY OF CULTURE

   Eppel, E. M. and **M.** Adolescents and Morality: *A Study of some Moral Values and Dilemmas of Working Adolescents in the Context of a changing Climate of Opinion. Foreword by W. J. H. Sprott. 268 pp. 39 tables.*
● **Fromm, Erich.** The Fear of Freedom. *286 pp.*
●   The Sane Society. *400 pp.*
   Johnson, L. The Cultural Critics. *From Matthew Arnold to Raymond Williams. 233 pp.*
   Mannheim, Karl. Essays on the Sociology of Culture. *Edited by Ernst Mannheim in co-operation with Paul Kecskemeti. Editorial Note by Adolph Lowe. 280 pp.*
   Merquior, J. G. The Veil and the Mask. *Essays on Culture and Ideology. Foreword by Ernest Gellner. 140 pp.*
   Zijderfeld, A. C. On Clichés. *The Supersedure of Meaning by Function in Modernity. 150 pp.*

SOCIOLOGY OF RELIGION

   Argyle, Michael and **Beit-Hallahmi, Benjamin.** The Social Psychology of Religion. *256 pp.*
   Glasner, Peter E. The Sociology of Secularisation. *A Critique of a Concept. 146 pp.*
   Hall, J. R. The Ways Out. *Utopian Communal Groups in an Age of Babylon. 280 pp.*
   Ranson, S., Hinings, B. and **Bryman, A.** Clergy, Ministers and Priests. *216 pp.*
   Stark, Werner. The Sociology of Religion. *A Study of Christendom.*
      Volume II. *Sectarian Religion. 368 pp.*
      Volume III. *The Universal Church. 464 pp.*
      Volume IV. *Types of Religious Man. 352 pp.*
      Volume V. *Types of Religious Culture. 464 pp.*
   Turner, B. S. Weber and Islam. *216 pp.*
   Watt, W. Montgomery. Islam and the Integration of Society. *320 pp.*

SOCIOLOGY OF ART AND LITERATURE

   Jarvie, Ian C. Towards a Sociology of the Cinema. *A Comparative Essay on the Structure and Functioning of a Major Entertainment Industry. 405 pp.*
   Rust, Frances S. Dance in Society. *An Analysis of the Relationships between the Social Dance and Society in England from the Middle Ages to the Present Day. 256 pp. 8 pp. of plates.*
   Schücking, L. L. The Sociology of Literary Taste. *112 pp.*
   Wolff, Janet. Hermeneutic Philosophy and the Sociology of Art. *150 pp.*

SOCIOLOGY OF KNOWLEDGE

   Diesing, P. Patterns of Discovery in the Social Sciences. *262 pp.*

- **Douglas, J. D.** (Ed.) Understanding Everyday Life. *370 pp.*
- **Hamilton, P.** Knowledge and Social Structure. *174 pp.*

Jarvie, I. C. Concepts and Society. *232 pp.*

Mannheim, Karl. Essays on the Sociology of Knowledge. *Edited by Paul Kecskemeti. Editorial Note by Adolph Lowe. 353 pp.*

Remmling, Gunter W. The Sociology of Karl Mannheim. *With a Bibliographical Guide to the Sociology of Knowledge, Ideological Analysis, and Social Planning. 255 pp.*

Remmling, Gunter W. (Ed.) Towards the Sociology of Knowledge. *Origin and Development of a Sociological Thought Style. 463 pp.*

Scheler, M. Problems of a Sociology of Knowledge. *Trans. by M. S. Frings. Edited and with an Introduction by K. Stikkers. 232 pp.*

URBAN SOCIOLOGY

Aldridge, M. The British New Towns. *A Programme Without a Policy. 232 pp.*

Ashworth, William. The Genesis of Modern British Town Planning: *A Study in Economic and Social History of the Nineteenth and Twentieth Centuries. 288 pp.*

Brittan, A. The Privatised World. *196 pp.*

Cullingworth, J. B. Housing Needs and Planning Policy: *A Restatement of the Problems of Housing Need and 'Overspill' in England and Wales. 232 pp. 44 tables. 8 maps.*

Dickinson, Robert E. City and Region: *A Geographical Interpretation. 608 pp. 125 figures.*

   The West European City: *A Geographical Interpretation. 600 pp. 129 maps. 29 plates.*

Humphreys, Alexander J. New Dubliners: *Urbanization and the Irish Family. Foreword by George C. Homans. 304 pp.*

Jackson, Brian. Working Class Community: *Some General Notions raised by a Series of Studies in Northern England. 192 pp.*

- **Mann, P. H.** An Approach to Urban Sociology. *240 pp.*

Mellor, J. R. Urban Sociology in an Urbanized Society. *326 pp.*

Morris, R. N. and **Mogey, J.** The Sociology of Housing. *Studies at Berinsfield. 232 pp. 4 pp. plates.*

Mullan, R. Stevenage Ltd. *About 250 pp.*

Rex, J. and **Tomlinson, S.** Colonial Immigrants in a British City. *A Class Analysis. 368 pp.*

Rosser, C. and **Harris, C.** The Family and Social Change. *A Study of Family and Kinship in a South Wales Town. 352 pp. 8 maps.*

- **Stacey, Margaret, Batsone, Eric, Bell, Colin** and **Thurcott, Anne.** Power, Persistence and Change. *A Second Study of Banbury. 196 pp.*

RURAL SOCIOLOGY

Mayer, Adrian C. Peasants in the Pacific. *A Study of Fiji Indian Rural Society. 248 pp. 20 plates.*

Williams, W. M. The Sociology of an English Village: *Gosforth. 272 pp. 12 figures. 13 tables.*

SOCIOLOGY OF INDUSTRY AND DISTRIBUTION

Dunkerley, David. The Foreman. *Aspects of Task and Structure. 192 pp.*

Eldridge, J. E. T. Industrial Disputes. *Essays in the Sociology of Industrial Relations. 288 pp.*

Hollowell, Peter G. The Lorry Driver. *272 pp.*

- **Oxaal, I., Barnett, T.** and **Booth, D.** (Eds) Beyond the Sociology of Development.

Economy and Society in Latin America and Africa. 295 pp.

Smelser, Neil J. Social Change in the Industrial Revolution: *An Application of Theory to the Lancashire Cotton Industry, 1770–1840. 468 pp. 12 figures. 14 tables.*

Watson, T. J. The Personnel Managers. *A Study in the Sociology of Work and Employment, 262 pp.*

ANTHROPOLOGY

Brandel-Syrier, Mia. Reeftown Elite. *A Study of Social Mobility in a Modern African Community on the Reef. 376 pp.*

Dickie-Clark, H. F. The Marginal Situation. *A Sociological Study of a Coloured Group. 236 pp.*

Dube, S. C. Indian Village. *Foreword by Morris Edward Opler. 276 pp. 4 plates.*
India's Changing Villages: *Human Factors in Community Development. 260 pp. 8 plates. 1 map.*

Fei, H.-T. Peasant Life in China. *A Field Study of Country Life in the Yangtze Valley. With a foreword by Bronislaw Malinowski. 328 pp. 16 pp. plates.*

Firth, Raymond. Malay Fishermen. *Their Peasant Economy. 420 pp. 17 pp. plates.*

Gulliver, P. H. Social Control in an African Society: a Study of the Arusha, Agricultural Masai of Northern Tanganyika. *320 pp. 8 plates. 10 figures.*
Family Herds. *288 pp.*

Jarvie, Ian C. The Revolution in Anthropology. *268 pp.*

Little, Kenneth L. Mende of Sierra Leone. *308 pp. and folder.*
Negroes in Britain. *With a New Introduction and Contemporary Study by Leonard Bloom. 320 pp.*

Tambs-Lyche, H. London Patidars. *About 180 pp.*

Madan, G. R. Western Sociologists on Indian Society. *Marx, Spencer, Weber, Durkheim, Pareto. 384 pp.*

Mayer, A. C. Peasants in the Pacific. *A Study of Fiji Indian Rural Society. 248 pp.*

Meer, Fatima. Race and Suicide in South Africa. *325 pp.*

Smith, Raymond T. The Negro Family in British Guiana: *Family Structure and Social Status in the Villages. With a Foreword by Meyer Fortes. 314 pp. 8 plates. 1 figure. 4 maps.*

SOCIOLOGY AND PHILOSOPHY

Adriaansens, H. Talcott Parsons and the Conceptual Dilemma. *About 224 pp.*

Barnsley, John H. The Social Reality of Ethics. *A Comparative Analysis of Moral Codes. 448 pp.*

Diesing, Paul. Patterns of Discovery in the Social Sciences. *362 pp.*

● **Douglas, Jack D.** (Ed.) Understanding Everyday Life. *Toward the Reconstruction of Sociological Knowledge. Contributions by Alan F. Blum, Aaron W. Cicourel, Norman K. Denzin, Jack D. Douglas, John Heeren, Peter McHugh, Peter K. Manning, Melvin Power, Matthew Speier, Roy Turner, D. Lawrence Wieder, Thomas P. Wilson and Don H. Zimmerman. 370 pp.*

Gorman, Robert A. The Dual Vision. *Alfred Schutz and the Myth of Phenomenological Social Science. 240 pp.*

Jarvie, Ian C. Concepts and Society. *216 pp.*

Kilminster, R. Praxis and Method. *A Sociological Dialogue with Lukács, Gramsci and the Early Frankfurt School. 334 pp.*

● **Pelz, Werner.** The Scope of Understanding in Sociology. *Towards a More Radical Reorientation in the Social Humanistic Sciences. 283 pp.*

Roche, Maurice. Phenomenology, Language and the Social Sciences. *371 pp.*

Sahay, Arun. Sociological Analysis. *212 pp.*

● **Slater, P.** Origin and Significance of the Frankfurt School. *A Marxist Perspective. 185 pp.*

Spurling, L. Phenomenology and the Social World. *The Philosophy of Merleau-Ponty and its Relation to the Social Sciences. 222 pp.*

Wilson, H. T. The American Ideology. *Science, Technology and Organization as Modes of Rationality. 368 pp.*

International Library of Anthropology
General Editor   Adam Kuper

● Ahmed, A. S. Millennium and Charisma Among Pathans. *A Critical Essay in Social Anthropology. 192 pp.*

Pukhtun Economy and Society. *Traditional Structure and Economic Development. About 360 pp.*

Barth, F. Selected Essays. *Volume I. About 250 pp.* Selected Essays. *Volume II. About 250 pp.*

Brown, Paula. The Chimbu. *A Study of Change in the New Guinea Highlands. 151 pp.*

Foner, N. Jamaica Farewell. *200 pp.*

Gudeman, Stephen. Relationships, Residence and the Individual. *A Rural Panamanian Community. 288 pp. 11 plates, 5 figures, 2 maps, 10 tables.*

The Demise of a Rural Economy. *From Subsistence to Capitalism in a Latin American Village. 160 pp.*

Hamnett, Ian. Chieftainship and Legitimacy. *An Anthropological Study of Executive Law in Lesotho. 163 pp.*

Hanson, F. Allan. Meaning in Culture. *127 pp.*

Hazan, H. The Limbo People. *A Study of the Constitution of the Time Universe Among the Aged. About 192 pp.*

Humphreys, S. C. Anthropology and the Greeks. *288 pp.*

Karp, I. Fields of Change Among the Iteso of Kenya. *140 pp.*

Lloyd, P. C. Power and Independence. *Urban Africans' Perception of Social Inequality. 264 pp.*

Parry, J. P. Caste and Kinship in Kangra. *352 pp. Illustrated.*

Pettigrew, Joyce. Robber Noblemen. *A Study of the Political System of the Sikh Jats. 284 pp.*

Street, Brian V. The Savage in Literature. *Representations of 'Primitive' Society in English Fiction, 1858–1920. 207 pp.*

Van Den Berghe, Pierre L. Power and Privilege at an African University. *278 pp.*

International Library of Phenomenology and Moral Sciences
General Editor   John O'Neill

Apel, K.-O. Towards a Transformation of Philosophy. *308 pp.*

Bologh, R. W. Dialectical Phenomenology. *Marx's Method. 287 pp.*

Fekete, J. The Critical Twilight. *Explorations in the Ideology of Anglo-American Literary Theory from Eliot to McLuhan. 300 pp.*

Medina, A. Reflection, Time and the Novel. *Towards a Communicative Theory of Literature. 143 pp.*

International Library of Social Policy
General Editor   Kathleen Jones

Bayley, M. Mental Handicap and Community Care. *426 pp.*

Bottoms, A. E. and McClean, J. D. Defendants in the Criminal Process. *284 pp.*

Bradshaw, J. The Family Fund. *An Initiative in Social Policy. About 224 pp.*

Butler, J. R. Family Doctors and Public Policy. *208 pp.*

Davies, Martin. Prisoners of Society. *Attitudes and Aftercare. 204 pp.*

Gittus, Elizabeth. Flats, Families and the Under-Fives. *285 pp.*

Holman, Robert. Trading in Children. *A Study of Private Fostering. 355 pp.*

Jeffs, A. Young People and the Youth Service. *160 pp.*

Jones, Howard and Cornes, Paul. Open Prisons. *288 pp.*

Jones, Kathleen. History of the Mental Health Service. *428 pp.*

Jones, Kathleen with **Brown, John, Cunningham, W. J., Roberts, Julian** and **Williams, Peter.** Opening the Door. *A Study of New Policies for the Mentally Handicapped. 278 pp.*

Karn, Valerie. Retiring to the Seaside. *400 pp. 2 maps. Numerous tables.*

King, R. D. and **Elliot, K. W.** Albany: Birth of a Prison—End of an Era. *394 pp.*

Thomas, J. E. The English Prison Officer since 1850: *A Study in Conflict. 258 pp.*

Walton, R. G. Women in Social Work. *303 pp.*

● **Woodward, J.** To Do the Sick No Harm. *A Study of the British Voluntary Hospital System to 1875. 234 pp.*

International Library of Welfare and Philosophy
General Editors   Noel Timms and David Watson

● **McDermott, F. E.** (Ed.) Self-Determination in Social Work. *A Collection of Essays on Self-determination and Related Concepts by Philosophers and Social Work Theorists. Contributors: F. P. Biestek, S. Bernstein, A. Keith-Lucas, D. Sayer, H. H. Perelman, C. Whittington, R. F. Stalley, F. E. McDermott, I. Berlin, H. J. McCloskey, H. L. A. Hart, J. Wilson, A. I. Melden, S. I. Benn. 254 pp.*

● **Plant, Raymond.** Community and Ideology. *104 pp.*

Ragg, Nicholas M. People Not Cases. *A Philosophical Approach to Social Work. 168 pp.*

● **Timms, Noel** and **Watson, David.** (Eds) Talking About Welfare. *Readings in Philosophy and Social Policy. Contributors: T. H. Marshall, R. B. Brandt, G. H. von Wright, K. Nielsen, M. Cranston, R. M. Titmuss, R. S. Downie, E. Telfer, D. Donnison, J. Benson, P. Leonard, A. Keith-Lucas, D. Walsh, I. T. Ramsey. 320 pp.*

● Philosophy in Social Work. *250 pp.*

● **Weale, A.** Equality and Social Policy. *164 pp.*

Library of Social Work
General Editor   Noel Timms

● **Baldock, Peter.** Community Work and Social Work. *140 pp.*

○ **Beedell, Christopher.** Residential Life with Children. *210 pp. Crown 8vo.*

● **Berry, Juliet.** Daily Experience in Residential Life. *A Study of Children and their Care-givers. 202 pp.*

○ Social Work with Children. *190 pp. Crown 8vo.*

● **Brearley, C. Paul.** Residential Work with the Elderly. *116 pp.*

● Social Work, Ageing and Society. *126 pp.*

● **Cheetham, Juliet.** Social Work with Immigrants. *240 pp. Crown 8vo.*

● **Cross, Crispin P.** (Ed.) Interviewing and Communication in Social Work. *Contributions by C. P. Cross, D. Laurenson, B. Strutt, S. Raven. 192 pp. Crown 8vo.*

- ● **Curnock, Kathleen** and **Hardiker, Pauline.** Towards Practice Theory. *Skills and Methods in Social Assessments. 208 pp.*
- ● **Davies, Bernard.** The Use of Groups in Social Work Practice. *158 pp.*
- ● **Davies, Martin.** Support Systems in Social Work. *144 pp.*
- **Ellis, June.** (Ed.) West African Families in Britain. *A Meeting of Two Cultures. Contributions by Pat Stapleton, Vivien Biggs. 150 pp. 1 Map.*
- ● **Hart, John.** Social Work and Sexual Conduct. *230 pp.*
- ● **Hutten, Joan M.** Short-Term Contracts in Social Work. *Contributions by Stella M. Hall, Elsie Osborne, Mannie Sher, Eva Sternberg, Elizabeth Tuters. 134 pp.*
- **Jackson, Michael P.** and **Valencia, B. Michael.** Financial Aid Through Social Work. *140 pp.*
- ● **Jones, Howard.** The Residential Community. *A Setting for Social Work. 150 pp.*
- ● (Ed.) Towards a New Social Work. *Contributions by Howard Jones, D. A. Fowler, J. R. Cypher, R. G. Walton, Geoffrey Mungham, Philip Priestley, Ian Shaw, M. Bartley, R. Deacon, Irwin Epstein, Geoffrey Pearson. 184 pp.*
- **Jones, Ray** and **Pritchard, Colin.** (Eds) Social Work With Adolescents. *Contributions by Ray Jones, Colin Pritchard, Jack Dunham, Florence Rossetti, Andrew Kerslake, John Burns, William Gregory, Graham Templeman, Kenneth E. Reid, Audrey Taylor. About 170 pp.*
- ○ **Jordon, William.** The Social Worker in Family Situations. *160 pp. Crown 8vo.*
- ● **Laycock, A. L.** Adolescents and Social Work. *128 pp. Crown 8vo.*
- ● **Lees, Ray.** Politics and Social Work. *128 pp. Crown 8vo.*
- ● Research Strategies for Social Welfare. *112 pp. Tables.*
- ○ **McCullough, M. K.** and **Ely, Peter J.** Social Work with Groups. *127 pp. Crown 8vo.*
- ● **Moffett, Jonathan.** Concepts in Casework Treatment. *128 pp. Crown 8vo.*
- **Parsloe, Phyllida.** Juvenile Justice in Britain and the United States. *The Balance of Needs and Rights. 336 pp.*
- ● **Plant, Raymond.** Social and Moral Theory in Casework. *112 pp. Crown 8vo.*
- **Priestley, Philip, Fears, Denise** and **Fuller, Roger.** Justice for Juveniles. *The 1969 Children and Young Persons Act: A Case for Reform? 128 pp.*
- ● **Pritchard, Colin** and **Taylor, Richard.** Social Work: Reform or Revolution? *170 pp.*
- ○ **Pugh, Elisabeth.** Social Work in Child Care. *128 pp. Crown 8vo.*
- ● **Robinson, Margaret.** Schools and Social Work. *282 pp.*
- ○ **Ruddock, Ralph.** Roles and Relationships. *128 pp. Crown 8vo.*
- ● **Sainsbury, Eric.** Social Diagnosis in Casework. *118 pp. Crown 8vo.*
- ● Social Work with Families. *Perceptions of Social Casework among Clients of a Family Service. 188 pp.*
- **Seed, Philip.** The Expansion of Social Work in Britain. *128 pp. Crown 8vo.*
- ● **Shaw, John.** The Self in Social Work. *124 pp.*
- **Smale, Gerald G.** Prophecy, Behaviour and Change. *An Examination of Self-fulfilling Prophecies in Helping Relationships. 116 pp. Crown 8vo.*
- **Smith, Gilbert.** Social Need. *Policy, Practice and Research. 155 pp.*
- ● Social Work and the Sociology of Organisations. *124 pp. Revised edition.*
- ● **Sutton, Carole.** Psychology for Social Workers and Counsellors. *An Introduction. 248 pp.*
- ● **Timms, Noel.** Language of Social Casework. *122 pp. Crown 8vo.*
- ● Recording in Social Work. *124 pp. Crown 8vo.*
- ● **Todd, F. Joan.** Social Work with the Mentally Subnormal. *96 pp. Crown 8vo.*
- ● **Walrond-Skinner, Sue.** Family Therapy. *The Treatment of Natural Systems. 172 pp.*
- ● **Warham, Joyce.** An Introduction to Administration for Social Workers. *Revised edition. 112 pp.*
- ● An Open Case. *The Organisational Context of Social Work. 172 pp.*
- ○ **Wittenberg, Isca Salzberger.** Psycho-Analytic Insight and Relationships. *A Kleinian Approach. 196 pp. Crown 8vo.*

Primary Socialization, Language and Education

General Editor   Basil Bernstein

Adlam, Diana S., *with the assistance of Geoffrey Turner and Lesley Lineker*. Code in Context. *272 pp.*

Bernstein, Basil. Class, Codes and Control. *3 volumes.*
- 1. *Theoretical Studies Towards a Sociology of Language. 254 pp.*
  2. *Applied Studies Towards a Sociology of Language. 377 pp.*
- 3. *Towards a Theory of Educational Transmission. 167 pp.*

Brandis, W. and **Bernstein, B.** Selection and Control. *176 pp.*

Brandis, Walter and **Henderson, Dorothy.** Social Class, Language and Communication. *288 pp.*

Cook-Gumperz, Jenny. Social Control and Socialization. *A Study of Class Differences in the Language of Maternal Control. 290 pp.*

- **Gahagan, D. M.** and **G. A.** Talk Reform. *Exploration in Language for Infant School Children. 160 pp.*

Hawkins, P. R. Social Class, the Nominal Group and Verbal Strategies. *About 220 pp.*

Robinson, W. P. and **Rackstraw, Susan D. A.** A Question of Answers. *2 volumes. 192 pp. and 180 pp.*

Turner, Geoffrey J. and **Mohan, Bernard A.** A Linguistic Description and Computer Programme for Children's Speech. *208 pp.*

Reports of the Institute of Community Studies

Baker, J. The Neighbourhood Advice Centre. A Community Project in Camden. *320 pp.*

- **Cartwright, Ann.** Patients and their Doctors. *A Study of General Practice. 304 pp.*

Dench, Geoff. Maltese in London. *A Case-study in the Erosion of Ethnic Consciousness. 302 pp.*

Jackson, Brian and **Marsden, Dennis.** Education and the Working Class: *Some General Themes Raised by a Study of 88 Working-class Children in a Northern Industrial City. 268 pp. 2 folders.*

Marris, Peter. The Experience of Higher Education. *232 pp. 27 tables.*
- Loss and Change. *192 pp.*

Marris, Peter and **Rein, Martin.** Dilemmas of Social Reform. *Poverty and Community Action in the United States. 256 pp.*

Marris, Peter and **Somerset, Anthony.** African Businessmen. *A Study of Entrepreneurship and Development in Kenya. 256 pp.*

Mills, Richard. Young Outsiders: *a Study in Alternative Communities. 216 pp.*

Runciman, W. G. Relative Deprivation and Social Justice. *A Study of Attitudes to Social Inequality in Twentieth-Century England. 352 pp.*

Willmott, Peter. Adolescent Boys in East London. *230 pp.*

Willmott, Peter and **Young, Michael.** Family and Class in a London Suburb. *202 pp. 47 tables.*

Young, Michael and **McGeeney, Patrick.** Learning Begins at Home. *A Study of a Junior School and its Parents. 128 pp.*

Young, Michael and **Willmott, Peter.** Family and Kinship in East London. *Foreword by Richard M. Titmuss. 252 pp. 39 tables.*
- The Symmetrical Family. *410 pp.*

Reports of the Institute for Social Studies in Medical Care

Cartwright, Ann, Hockey, Lisbeth and Anderson, John J. Life Before Death. *310 pp.*
Dunnell, Karen and Cartwright, Ann. Medicine Takers, Prescribers and Hoarders. *190 pp.*
Farrell, C. My Mother Said. . . *A Study of the Way Young People Learned About Sex and Birth Control. 288 pp.*

Medicine, Illness and Society
General Editor W. M. Williams

Hall, David J. Social Relations & Innovation. *Changing the State of Play in Hospitals. 232 pp.*
Hall, David J. and Stacey, M. (Eds) Beyond Separation. *234 pp.*
Robinson, David. The Process of Becoming Ill. *142 pp.*
Stacey, Margaret *et al.* Hospitals, Children and Their Families. *The Report of a Pilot Study. 202 pp.*
Stimson, G. V. and Webb, B. Going to See the Doctor. *The Consultation Process in General Practice. 155 pp.*

Monographs in Social Theory
General Editor Arthur Brittan

● Barnes, B. Scientific Knowledge and Sociological Theory. *192 pp.*
Bauman, Zygmunt. Culture as Praxis. *204 pp.*
● Dixon, Keith. Sociological Theory. *Pretence and Possibility. 142 pp.*
  The Sociology of Belief. *Fallacy and Foundation. About 160 pp.*
Goff, T. W. Marx and Mead. *Contributions to a Sociology of Knowledge. 176 pp.*
Meltzer, B. N., Petras, J. W. and Reynolds, L. T. Symbolic Interactionism. *Genesis, Varieties and Criticisms. 144 pp.*
● Smith, Anthony D. The Concept of Social Change. *A Critique of the Functionalist Theory of Social Change. 208 pp.*

Routledge Social Science Journals

The British Journal of Sociology. *Editor – Angus Stewart; Associate Editor – Leslie Sklair. Vol. 1, No. 1 – March 1950 and Quarterly. Roy. 8vo. All back issues available. An international journal publishing original papers in the field of sociology and related areas.*
Community Work. *Edited by David Jones and Marjorie Mayo. 1973. Published annually.*
Economy and Society. *Vol. 1, No. 1. February 1972 and Quarterly. Metric Roy. 8vo. A journal for all social scientists covering sociology, philosophy, anthropology, economics and history. All back numbers available.*

Ethnic and Racial Studies. *Editor – John Stone. Vol. 1 – 1978. Published quarterly.*
Religion. Journal of Religion and Religions. *Chairman of Editorial Board, Ninian Smart. Vol. 1, No. 1, Spring 1971. A journal with an inter-disciplinary approach to the study of the phenomena of religion. All back numbers available.*
Sociology of Health and Illness. *A Journal of Medical Sociology. Editor – Alan Davies; Associate Editor – Ray Jobling. Vol. 1, Spring 1979. Published 3 times per annum.*
Year Book of Social Policy in Britain. *Edited by Kathleen Jones. 1971. Published annually.*

Social and Psychological Aspects of Medical Practice
Editor   Trevor Silverstone

Lader, Malcolm. Psychophysiology of Mental Illness. *280 pp.*
● **Silverstone, Trevor** and **Turner, Paul.** Drug Treatment in Psychiatry. *Revised edition. 256 pp.*
Whiteley, J. S. and **Gordon, J.** Group Approaches in Psychiatry. *240 pp.*